Transparent Communication of Health Risks

Rocio Garcia-Retamero · Mirta Galesic
Editors

Transparent Communication of Health Risks

Overcoming Cultural Differences

Springer

Editors
Rocio Garcia-Retamero
Departamento de Psicología Experimental
Facultad de Psicología
University of Granada
Granada, Spain
and
Center for Adaptive Behavior and Cognition
Max Planck Institute for Human Development
Berlin, Germany

Mirta Galesic
Center for Adaptive Behavior and Cognition
Max Planck Institute for Human Development
Berlin, Germany

ISBN 978-1-4614-4357-5 ISBN 978-1-4614-4358-2 (eBook)
DOI 10.1007/978-1-4614-4358-2
Springer New York Heidelberg Dordrecht London

Library of Congress Control Number: 2012952273

Printed on acid-free paper

Springer is part of Springer Science+Business Media (www.springer.com)

To our families

Foreword

The value placed on informed medical decisions, and even on individual autonomy in medical choices, has changed dramatically from our past history. In the 1500s, physicians were fined for telling patients the names of medicines; a 1938 U.S. Federal Register notice recommended that drug labels be written "only in such medical terms as are not likely to be understood by the ordinary individual." Today, however, the value of individual autonomy and effective patient communication is widely recognized.

Of course, to be informed, patients must understand the risks and benefits of their health options, whether for treatment or for screening, including the numeric likelihoods of both risks and benefits. As a result, numeric information increasingly is provided to the public and patients in efforts to produce better health outcomes (e.g., How much will I decrease my risk of heart disease if I exercise and diet?; What are my chances of getting cancer?) and reduce provider liability. Implicitly, it is assumed that the information is understood and used and that it leads to more informed medical decisions.

According to economic theory, consumers require this information to compare alternatives for markets to function efficiently. Accessible information about the risks and benefits of health options presumably accomplishes this by making qualities of health care (otherwise unobservable to the individual) more transparent. As a result, everyone involved in a transaction – policy makers, healthcare providers, and patients – has access to essential information and can use this information in making choices. Providing more information and more access to information about choice options is intended to empower patients and other decision makers and to motivate efficient markets.

Thus, the increasing emphasis of public policy in health domains has been to provide information and choice in order to tap into the power of informed consumers and improve health outcomes and the efficacy of health care. However, not everyone has the ability to use complex and often numeric health information. This innumeracy (and sometimes graph illiteracy) has a profound impact on patients' and others' ability to understand and use information about the risks and benefits of treatment options. It is naïve, for example, to think it sufficient to simply tell patients that 10%

of people experience a side effect. In many cases, the patients will not be able to understand that information or incorporate it into their decision making. Comprehension, a basic building block of good decision making, is difficult with numeric information. The unfortunate result is that this combination of policy shifts with skill differences may exacerbate health disparities as those with more skills take advantage of the information-rich environment while those with fewer skills fall further behind. Just because information is provided does not mean that this information is comprehensible or useable.

In decision making, people who are more numerate understand numbers better than the less numerate. But numeracy goes beyond comprehension to influence what information is processed and how it is processed and used. For example, numeracy is associated with susceptibility to how people frame information. Imagine, for example, that two patients are told about the side effects of a medication. Emily hears that 12% of patients will suffer a drug side effect whereas John is told that 88% of patients won't develop the side effect. Less numerate individuals (but not the highly numerate) are likely to view the drug as relatively risky for Emily, but much safer for John. It's the same information, but a very different reaction can follow. And this innumeracy can lead to all kinds of poor life decisions when it comes to things like cancer screening, vaccine decisions, emergency preparedness, and medicine – any situation where risks and benefits can be described in terms of how often something good happened or could happen or how often something bad happened or could happen.

Numbers are just abstract symbols, which can make them difficult to use in the uncertain grey areas of health where patients' lives can go awry. In a series of well-crafted examples, the authors of this book illustrate that the transparent communication of numeric information can alleviate differences linked to numeracy and culture. Their results suggest that health literacy itself is not solely the responsibility of the individual patient or consumer but it is also the responsibility of health communicators to choose carefully how to present health information. The book presents intriguing insights into how to make health information more transparent and it offers pointed suggestions for where we need to know more. It is an important contribution from current and former members of the renowned Max Planck Institute for Human Development in Berlin, Germany and the University of Granada in Granada, Spain. Results from the book concern central issues in the communication of health risks to patients and the role (and responsibility) of institutions in helping patients to better understand and use critical health information.

Just as it is no longer appropriate for physicians to dictate treatments to patients, it is also no longer appropriate to communicate health information without thought for how people will understand or use it. Although it is a significant challenge to create materials understandable to populations with lower skills, the reality is that "informed" decision making requires it.

Professor of Psychology
The Ohio State University

Ellen Peters

Preface

Today, health organizations and pharmaceutical companies work in a globalized environment. The rise of the Internet and social media means that health information and promotional messages designed for patients in one culture can spread around the world almost instantly. At the same time, the ideals of informed and shared decision making require that patients be able to accurately understand this information to make good decisions about their health. How can we ensure that the same message is accurately understood by people from various cultures who speak different languages?

Emerging research shows that the understanding of medical information across the globe can be improved by using *transparent information formats*. These formats include numerical, visual, and verbal formats that are carefully designed to take into account the fact that most people have only limited risk literacy. This book contains a collection of studies investigating risk understanding and medical decision making in different countries and in patients with different levels of risk literacy and provides a set of guidelines for transparent communication in our globalized world.

We examine the broad theme of risk communication, distinguishing three central topics (1) cultural differences in understanding health-related risks, (2) the use of information formats for enhancing transparent communication of these risks, and (3) methods for overcoming cultural differences in decision making about health. Each of these topics is examined in depth in several chapters analyzing specific problems across different cultures. In turn, each chapter includes a review of the relevant literature, an original empirical study illuminating a specific problem, and a discussion of practical and theoretical implications. Across all these topics, results have converged to demonstrate that many problems associated with risk illiteracy are not simply the result of cognitive biases preventing good decision making. Rather, errors occur because ineffective information formats complicate and mislead adaptive decision makers. Transparent information formats exploit people's inherent capacity to recognize relationships in naturally occurring problems and can dramatically enhance risk comprehension, communication, and recall and foster better decisions about health regardless of culture.

We are grateful for the supportive and inspiring environments of the Max Planck Institute for Human Development, which provided infrastructure and financial support for our studies. This institute is home to scientists from all over the world, fostering projects involving cross-cultural comparisons and multidisciplinary elements. Many of the studies reported in this book also received significant financial support from the Informed Medical Decisions Foundation (formerly the Foundation for Informed Medical Decision Making) in Boston, Massachusetts, including the research project "Helping People With Low Numeracy Understand Medical Information." This is a unique, nonprofit organization dedicated to furthering people's understanding of their medical choices and committed to fostering involvement in personal health decisions. As well, we have received substantial support from the Spanish Ministry for Science and Innovation and the Ministry of Economy (projects "How to Improve Understanding of Risks About Health," PSI2008-02019, and "Helping Doctors and Their Patients Make Decisions About Health," PSI2011-22954), enabling the studies comparing Spanish participants to those of other nations.

We greatly appreciate the helpful and critical comments of Isaac Lipkus and Brian Zikmund-Fisher on initial drafts of this book, and of Edward T. Cokely and other colleagues from the University of Granada, the Center for Adaptive Behavior and Cognition, and the Harding Center for Risk Literacy on various chapters. We are also grateful to Anita Todd and Rona Unrau for language editing, and to Mona Merkert for her help throughout the preparation of the book. Big thanks also to our Springer editors, Janice Stern and Kathryn Hiler, for their careful and kind guidance through the editing process. Finally, we are most grateful to our families for their example and guidance throughout the life. We dedicate this book to them.

Granada, Spain
Berlin, Germany

Rocio Garcia-Retamero
Mirta Galesic

Contents

Contributors

Nicolai Bodemer, Ph.D. Harding Center for Risk Literacy, Center for Adaptive Behavior and Cognition, Max Planck Institute for Human Development, Berlin, Germany

Edward T. Cokely, Ph.D. Department of Cognitive and Learning Sciences, Michigan Technological University, Houghton, MI, USA

Center for Adaptive Behavior and Cognition, Max Planck Institute for Human Development, Berlin, Germany

Mandeep K. Dhami, Ph.D. School of Psychology, University of Surrey, Guildford, UK

Ronald Frank, M.Ed. Gesellschaft für Konsumforschung Association, Nuremberg, Germany

Mirta Galesic, Ph.D. Center for Adaptive Behavior and Cognition, Max Planck Institute for Human Development, Berlin, Germany

Rocio Garcia-Retamero, Ph.D. Departamento de Psicología Experimental, Facultad de Psicología, University of Granada, Granada, Spain

Center for Adaptive Behavior and Cognition, Max Planck Institute for Human Development, Berlin, Germany

Saima Ghazal Department of Cognitive and Learning Sciences, Michigan Technological University, Houghton, MI, USA

Gerd Gigerenzer, Ph.D. Harding Center for Risk Literacy, Center for Adaptive Behavior and Cognition, Max Planck Institute for Human Development, Berlin, Germany

Jutta Mata, Ph.D. University of Basel, Basel, Switzerland

Center for Adaptive Rationality, Max Planck Institute for Human Development, Berlin, Germany

Stephanie M. Müller, Ph.D. Center for Empirical Research in Economics and Behavioral Science (CEREB), University of Erfurt, Erfurt, Germany

Angela Neumeyer-Gromen, M.D., M.P.H, Dr.P.H. Harding Center for Risk Literacy, Center for Adaptive Behavior and Cognition, Max Planck Institute for Human Development, Berlin, Germany

Yasmina Okan Departamento de Psicología Experimental, Facultad de Psicología, University of Granada, Granada, Spain

Eric Schulz Center for Adaptive Behavior and Cognition, Max Planck Institute for Human Development, Berlin, Germany

Cognitive, Perceptual, and Brain Sciences Department, University College London, London, UK

Ellen Peters, Ph.D Psychology Department, The Ohio State University, Columbus, OH, USA

Chapter 1
Introduction: Transparent Communication in a Globalized World

Mirta Galesic and Rocio Garcia-Retamero

Abstract The ideals of informed and shared decision making can only be achieved if patients understand information needed to make good decisions about their health. In today's globalized world, health messages are often aimed at diverse audiences with different cultural and educational backgrounds. However, information about screenings and medical treatments is often presented in nontransparent ways and can deceive even medical professionals. In this chapter, we provide examples of nontransparent information formats and discuss reasons why lack of transparency is today more problematic than ever. We propose a theoretical framework for investigating risk understanding and medical decision making. The framework emphasizes the interplay of information formats, risk literacy of patients, and the underlying cultural context. We introduce a collection of studies using this framework to design and test transparent information formats for communicating health risks in different countries and to patients with different levels of risk literacy.

M. Galesic, Ph.D. (✉)
Center for Adaptive Behavior and Cognition, Max Planck Institute for Human Development, Lentzeallee 94, 14195 Berlin, Germany
e-mail: galesic@mpib-berlin.mpg.de

R. Garcia-Retamero, Ph.D.
Departamento de Psicología Experimental, Facultad de Psicología, University of Granada, Campus Universitario de Cartuja s/n, 18071, Granada, Spain

Center for Adaptive Behavior and Cognition, Max Planck Institute for Human Development, Lentzeallee 94, 14195 Berlin, Germany
e-mail: rretamer@ugr.es

R. Garcia-Retamero and M. Galesic (eds.), *Transparent Communication of Health Risks: Overcoming Cultural Differences*, DOI 10.1007/978-1-4614-4358-2_1,

1.1 The Need for Transparency in Risk Communication

Messages from health professionals and the media are loud and clear: We live in an era of medical wonders. Mammography screenings reduce the risk of dying of breast cancer by 25% (Olsen et al. 2005), prostate-specific antigen (PSA) tests cut deaths of prostate cancer by 20% (Wilde 2009), drugs that lower cholesterol levels reduce the risk of coronary deaths by 42% (Oliver et al. 1995), and genetic tests can predict whether one will develop breast cancer or type I diabetes (Dorman et al. 1999; Nelson et al. 2005). It seems that patients today can simply relax and follow their doctors' advice—medical tests and treatments can stop disease and delay death.

Unfortunately, even though medicine has advanced at an extraordinary rate in the last century, such promises are still overly optimistic. Although all the information presented above is accurate, it is provided in a format that makes medical screenings and treatments seem more beneficial than they actually are. Consider mammography screening. What does 25% reduction in the risk of dying of breast cancer actually mean? Without screening, 4 of 1,000 women will die of breast cancer. In contrast, if 1,000 women participate in regular screening, 3 of them will die (Gigerenzer et al. 2007). The reduction in absolute number of deaths may be even lower than 1 in 1000 (Gøtzsche and Nielsen 2009; Nelson et al. 2009) and in addition, 5 in 1,000 women will receive unnecessary treatment. What about the claim of a 20% reduction in deaths from prostate cancer due to PSA screening? This information is flawed because it masks the fact that the overall mortality remains the same: An equal number of men die with and without the PSA screening, but among those who participate in screening, deaths are more often attributed to causes other than prostate cancer (Schröder et al. 2009). As for the effectiveness of cholesterol-lowering drugs, the impressive 42% reduction in deaths due to coronary disease amounts to an absolute reduction of 3.5% (Skolbekken 1998). Even genetic tests mentioned above are far from being completely certain. For example, not every woman with a mutation on either of two genes that are linked to breast cancer (BRCA1 and BRCA2) will develop this cancer within her lifetime (Hartmann et al. 1999; Nelson et al. 2005). Similarly, the probability of developing insulin-dependent diabetes given the presence of one of the two alleles linked to this disease (DR3 and DR4) is less than 1% because many healthy people also have one of these alleles (Dorman et al. 1999; Gran et al. 1985). As these examples show, medicine is not an exact science. Doctors must make decisions under uncertainty and even the best available medical procedures can be ineffective and potentially harmful. When information about the risks of such procedures is not transparent, both doctors and their patients can make medical decisions that lead to undesirable health outcomes.

Why are benefits of medical screenings and treatments so often presented in a nontransparent way? There are at least four reasons, all stemming from the specific environment in which medical decisions take place.

First, presentation formats that make benefits seem larger and drawbacks smaller promote higher use of treatments and screenings. In fact, this is a key component of pharmaceutical marketing practices, which are designed to cover the enormous costs of developing new drugs (Michaels 2006). Transparent communication that reveals the uncertain and often modest effects of most treatments is not as persuasive (Gigerenzer and Gray 2011). Second, many doctors believe that maintaining an illusion of certainty will increase patients' compliance, reduce their anxiety, and decrease confusion (Gigerenzer 2002). In addition, from the doctors' perspective, it may be more acceptable to over-screen and over-treat their patients rather than risk losing them and being accused of malpractice if an ailment goes undetected or is insufficiently treated (Studdert et al. 2005). Third, there is a lack of awareness that the same information can be presented in different ways leading to different conclusions. The general public lacks basic risk literacy —i.e., the ability to accurately interpret information about risk (Fagerlin et al. 2007; Lipkus et al. 2001; Peters et al. 2006, 2009; Schwartz et al. 1997; see also www.riskliteracy.org). That is, many people do not understand the relationship between the different ways in which probabilistic information can be expressed. For instance, they cannot transform percentages into frequencies and vice versa. In addition, many people do not have much experience with graphical displays and have problems reading even the most basic visual formats, such as simple bar charts (Galesic and Garcia-Retamero 2011b). This is not just a problem for the general population; medical professionals also have trouble recognizing deceptive information formats: Problematic numerical and visual presentations appear even in high-ranking medical journals (Skolbekken 1998). Fourth, many people prefer simply to trust their doctors rather than to attempt to understand information about medical screenings and treatments (Galesic and Garcia-Retamero 2011a; Mechanic and Meyer 2000). "Trust your doctor" is a rule followed even by highly educated patients (Berg et al. 2010; Garcia-Retamero and Galesic 2009). The relationship between patients and physicians has been referred to as the "sacred trust" in classic literature (Starr 1949).

Lack of transparency and insufficient understanding of health-related information is not a new phenomenon. Doctors' incentive to provide an illusion of certainty and patients' desire to believe in the possibility of a cure have been present since the dawn of medicine. Today, however, lack of transparency has become even more problematic than before, for three reasons.

First, doctors have been increasingly encouraged to involve patients in decision making rather than pursuing a paternalistic model in which they make the decisions for their patients (Barry 1999; Frosch and Kaplan 1999; Hanson 2008). To participate in decisions about their health, patients need to be able to understand the complex risks and benefits of different medical treatments and screenings, and doctors need to be able to accurately and transparently communicate these risks and benefits (Brody et al. 1989; Schwartz and Woloshin 2007). Second, the Internet and other media provide an unprecedented amount of information about health and medicine (Murray et al. 2010; Roberts 2010; Xie 2009). Today, many people first consult the Internet about their ailment and then—if at all—their doctor. Numerous websites, forums, and blogs are providing information on all sorts of medical problems and medical treatments ranging from cold remedies to plastic surgery. However, this information is often incomplete or presented in formats that could bias the reader toward certain options (Impiccatore et al. 1997; Jorgensen and Gøtzsche 2004; Schwartz et al. 1999). Patients who lack risk literacy may not understand the many ways in which the same information can be communicated and how these different information formats can bias their judgments and decisions.

Finally, in today's globalized world health risks are often communicated to highly diverse audiences in different countries. Modern social media and communication networks enable remarkably fast dissemination of new health information. A promotional message or a press release designed for and sent to citizens in one particular country can quickly circle the globe. Numerous retellings and translations can easily distort the message's meaning, particularly if it was not transparent to begin with.

Is there a way to achieve transparent communication across cultures? The studies presented in this book show that vague information formats cloud understanding, a problem that is magnified in countries with lower risk literacy. At the same time, these studies show that carefully designed transparent information formats improve understanding in all countries, overcoming cultural differences. These transparent formats include analogies, different visual formats, and specific numerical formats that can be related to everyday experiences. All of these formats exploit the universal human ability to use what individuals already know to understand novel concepts. In addition, these formats do not require advanced numeracy skills, knowledge of graph conventions, or specific medical knowledge.

1.2 Theoretical Framework

When talking about communicating health risks in this book, we refer to informing people about the probability that a medical procedure or a health related behavior has a particular consequence, such as the probability that screening or exercise lead to a decrease in mortality rates. This is just one of the many conceptualizations of risk used in scientific and public discourse (Rohrmann and Renn 2000; see Douglas and Wildawsky 1983; Renn and Rohrmann 2000; Slovic 1999; Taylor-Gooby and Zinn 2006 for other approaches emphasizing the importance of subjective factors). We focus on communicating evidence-based probabilities about different health outcomes, typically derived from randomized trials on population samples. These probabilities are often used as a common currency that enables comparison of different options for pursuing a healthy lifestyle and making informed decisions about one's health. To study how to help patients in different countries to understand health risks and make good decisions, we use a theoretical framework that includes three main factors: patients' risk literacy, formats of risk communication, and the culture in which both the patients and the risk information are immersed (Fig. 1.1).

The first factor, *patients' risk literacy*, can be considered part of the broader concept of health literacy, which encompasses a variety of individual capacities and skills that are essential for navigating the modern health care environment (Baker 2006). Risk literacy includes (a) the skills to understand and manipulate different numerical expressions of probability about health (i.e., numeracy; Chaps. 2 and 3; see also Ancker and Kaufman 2007; Galesic and Garcia-Retamero 2010; Lipkus and Peters 2009; Peters et al. 2007; Reyna et al. 2009), (b) the ability to understand basic graphical representations frequently used to present quantitative health-related information (i.e., graph literacy; Chap. 4; see also Galesic and Garcia-Retamero 2011b), and (c) the knowledge of basic medical facts, such as the benefits and drawbacks of medical treatments and screenings and knowledge of symptoms of diseases

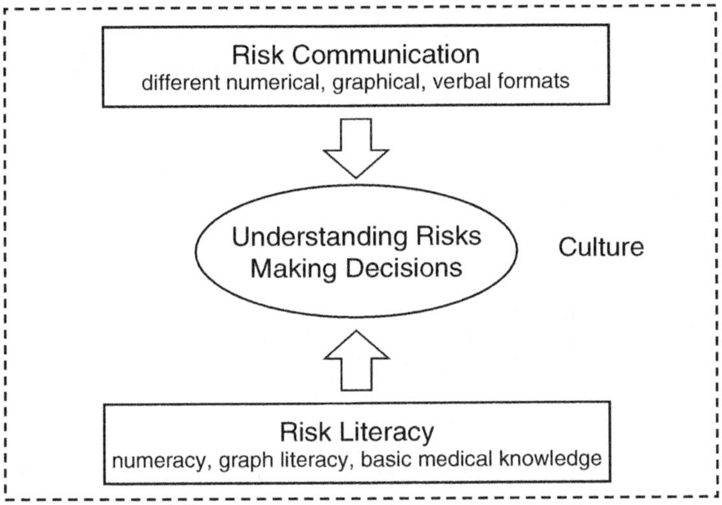

Fig. 1.1 Factors affecting patients' understanding of health risks and medical decision making

(Chaps. 5 and 6; see also Fagerlin et al. 2010). As we will see later in the book, both numeracy and graph literacy skills of the general public are presently low, and patients systematically overestimate the benefits of medical screenings.

The second factor, *formats of risk communication*, is the way medical information is communicated by health professionals, pharmaceutical companies, the government, and the media (Edwards et al. 2002; Lipkus 2007; Lipkus and Hollands 1999). Almost every medical treatment and screening has potential costs and benefits. The way probabilities of benefits and drawbacks are presented has a major influence on both how doctors and patients understand the information (i.e., understanding of health-related risks; see Chaps. 7–11) and the choices they make (i.e., medical decision making; see Chaps. 12 and 13). Studies in this book show that information format is particularly influential for people with low numeracy and graph literacy skills (see also Peters et al. 2006, 2009).

The third factor, the *culture*, moderates the way risk literacy and risk communication affect risk understanding and decision making. By "culture" we mean the relevant aspects of health and educational systems, as well as other historical and contemporary specifics of living in a certain country that can shape people's health-related knowledge and behaviors (see Boyd and Richerson 2005). Most studies collected in this book compared two or more countries, including a number of European and Asian countries and the USA. Other studies investigated the usefulness of different transparent communication formats, already proven to be successful, in new cultural contexts (e.g., in Spain and the UK). All of these countries differ critically in a number of ways, including their health systems, the educational attainment of their citizens, and their media environment. There are also more general cross-cultural differences in customs and beliefs, all of which can affect people's health-related knowledge and behaviors.

Table 1.1 Differences in health systems by country

Indicator	Germany	Spain	USA
Per capita total expenditure on health at average exchange rate (USD)	4,209	2,712	7,285
Total expenditure on health as percentage of gross domestic product	10	9	16
General government expenditure on health as percentage of total expenditure on health	77	72	45
Private expenditure on health as percentage of total expenditure on health	23	28	55
Physicians (per 10,000 inhabitants)	35	38	27
Hospital beds (per 10,000 inhabitants)	83	34	31

Source: World Health Organization (2007)

Table 1.1 shows a comparison of the three countries that are most often investigated in this book: Germany, Spain, and the USA. According to the statistics of the World Health Organization (2007), of the three countries, the USA has the highest per capita expenditure on health but more than half of that expenditure is covered by private funds. In contrast, the majority of health expenditure in Germany and Spain is covered by the government. In addition, although expenditures in the USA are the highest, this country has the lowest density of physicians and the lowest number of hospital beds per 10,000 citizens. There are also large differences in health insurance practices between these countries: Virtually everyone has health insurance in Germany (Statistisches Bundesamt Deutschland 2011) and Spain (Real Decreto Legislativo 1/1994, de 20 de Junio). In contrast, as many as 35% of people living in the USA have inadequate or no health insurance (Schoen et al. 2005). Therefore, they often need to decide about their health on their own, without a doctor, and may be more used to making trade-offs between benefits and drawbacks of different treatment options. At the time of finalizing this book, the USA is going through a major change in its health system that may result in a substantially larger proportion of the population with health insurance. Data presented in this book can serve as a benchmark to study changes in the way Americans decide about medical issues after the new health system is in place.

The three countries also differ in other important aspects of health care. In particular, there are dramatic differences in the way over-the-counter drugs are sold in Germany, Spain, and the USA. While in Germany and Spain patients usually interact with a pharmacist or a doctor who may recommend a particular choice, Americans often choose their over-the-counter drugs directly from the shelves. This requires that they compare different options on their own, without consulting a pharmacist. Accordingly, Americans are less likely to consult doctors when purchasing pain relievers (Hanoch et al. 2007) and are in general more autonomous when making decisions about their health (Galesic and Garcia-Retamero 2011a; Chap. 12). Another factor that may cause differences in patient involvement is direct-to-consumer advertising of prescription drugs, which is allowed in the USA but not in Germany and Spain. For instance, in the USA, the pharmaceutical industry spent 4.3 billion

Table 1.2 Differences in education system by country

Indicator	Germany	Spain	USA
Public expenditure on education[a]			
In billions of euros (2007)	107	51	604
% of gross domestic product (2006)	4.4	4.3	5.5
PISA scores (2006)[b]			
Mathematics	504	480	474
Science	516	488	489
Students' anxiety about mathematics[c]			
All	−0.15	0.08	0.20
Females	−0.05	0.13	0.27
Males	−0.26	0.02	0.13

[a]Eurostat (2010)

[b]PISA (2006)

[c]Index of anxiety is based on five items, including two measuring worry and one each measuring tension, feeling nervous, and feeling helpless. Positive values indicate anxiety and negative confidence (PISA 2006)

dollars on advertising in 2005 alone—almost a fourfold increase compared to 1997 (U.S. Government Accountability Office 2006). Most advertised drugs are prescription drugs for common illnesses such as insomnia, gastrointestinal problems, high cholesterol, and allergies. These advertisements may prompt patients to get more involved in decision making about their health, increasing the likelihood that patients will request specific prescription drugs from their doctors (Kravitz et al. 2005; Zachry et al. 2002).

The educational system in Germany, Spain, and the USA is very different, as well (Table 1.2). Although the USA spends more on education than Germany or Spain, the mathematics performance of its pupils is the worst among the three countries. According to the International Assessment of School Performance of 15-year-olds, conducted within the Programme for International Student Assessment (PISA 2006), German students score substantially better on mathematics and science than Spanish and, in particular, American students. In addition, German students are more confident in their math performance, while Spanish and especially American students show high levels of anxiety about mathematics (Table 1.2). One likely reason for this difference is the greater emphasis on math and science education in early grades in Germany compared to the USA and Spain (Rinderman 2007). Low math achievement and confidence may be related to overall lower levels of risk literacy and consequently to worse understanding of medical risks in the USA and Spain compared to Germany. Thus, we have a paradoxical situation: On the one hand, compared to Germans and Spaniards, Americans—especially those from disadvantaged social strata—are more likely to be required to make medical decisions for themselves. On the other hand, converging evidence indicates that they tend to be the least able to understand the risks involved in such decisions.

1.3 Organization of the Book

Most of the studies in this book were conceived of and conducted by current and former members of the Center for Adaptive Behavior and Cognition (ABC) at the Max Planck Institute for Human Development in Berlin (Germany). We conducted several studies on large, probabilistic national samples using computerized interviewing with more than 2,000 participants in Germany and the USA (see Chaps. 2, 4, 7–11, and 13). The participants were selected using probabilistic sampling methods, enabling the generalization of the results to the population of these countries and the comparison of the two countries. To make the best use of every expensive minute we had with these participants, we carefully planned a number of experiments involving different information formats and tasks. Each experiment was conducted on a random subset of the original sample to ensure the burden on participants was not substantial. The numeracy scale (see Chap. 2) was the only measure administered to all participants. Beyond this large study, chapters in this book describe several studies on other samples: Two studies on probabilistic national samples of nine European countries (Chaps. 5 and 6), studies of online panels in 14 countries, including a number of European and Asian countries and the USA (Chap. 3), paper-and-pencil surveys in groups of patients at high risk (Chaps. 10 and 11), as well as experiments in our laboratories in Germany, Spain, and the USA (Chap. 3).

The book is organized in four parts. In the first part (Chapters 2 to 6), we describe the results of several studies measuring cultural differences in the understanding of health-related risks. In Chaps. 2 and 3 we describe levels of numeracy in the general population and in educated samples across various countries. Chapter 4 is about the development and application of a new measure of health-related graph literacy (see Chap. 15 for the text of all scales in English, German, and Spanish). Chapters 5 and 6 present results of two multinational studies involving nine European countries that explored basic knowledge about benefits of medical screenings and symptoms of diseases in the population.

The second part of the book (Chapters 7 to 11) includes studies investigating the extent to which different information formats improve understanding of risks about health for a wide range of patients, including those with the lowest levels of numeracy and graph literacy. The studies illustrate the promise and challenges of analogies used to explain predictive accuracy in medical screenings (Chap. 7) and of specific numerical formats that can be related to everyday experiences (Chap. 8). As well, we examine the use of different visual aids to enhance risk understanding and risk communication, including the use of bar, pie, and line charts and icon arrays (Chap. 9). We show that simple visual aids can be powerful tools that eliminate biases such as denominator neglect (Chap. 10) and errors induced by message framing (Chap. 11).

The third part of the book (Chapters 12 and 13) includes studies on medical decision making in different countries. Chapter 12 illustrates the lack of transparent information in the media with a prominent example: the coverage of the human papillomavirus (HPV) vaccine. In Chap. 13, we study the relationship between numeracy and patients' willingness to be involved in decision making about health. In the fourth part (Chapter 14), we summarize the findings across all studies to provide some guidelines for transparent communication in our globalized world. The Appendix includes English, German, and Spanish versions of several scales for quick and accurate testing of numeracy and graph literacy. We hope that these scales will be helpful to other researchers who wish to further explore cultural differences in health literacy.

References

Ancker, J. S., & Kaufman, D. (2007). Rethinking health numeracy: A multidisciplinary literature review. *Journal of the American Medical Informatics Association, 14*, 713–721.

Baker, W. D. (2006). The meaning and the measure of health literacy. *Journal of General Internal Medicine, 21*, 878–883.

Barry, M. J. (1999). Involving patients in medical decisions: How can physicians do better? *Journal of the American Medical Association, 282*, 2356–2357.

Berg, N., Biele, G., & Gigerenzer, G. (2010). *Does consistency predict accuracy of beliefs? Economists surveyed about PSA*. MPRA Paper 24976, University Library of Munich, Germany. http://mpra.ub.uni-muenchen.de/24976/1/MPRA_paper_24976.pdf, accessed July 30, 2012.

Boyd, R., & Richerson, P. J. (2005). *The origin and evolution of cultures*. Oxford: Oxford University Press.

Brody, D. S., Miller, S. M., Lerman, C. E., Smith, D. G., Lazaro, C. G., & Blum, M. J. (1989). The relationship between patients' satisfaction with their physicians and perceptions about interventions they desired and received. *Medical Care, 11*, 1027–1035.

Dorman, J. S., McCarthy, B. J., O'Leary, L. A., & Koehler, A. N. (1999). Risk factors for insulin-dependent diabetes. In M. I. Harris, C. C. Cowie, M. P. Stern, E. J. Boyko, G. E. Reiber, & P. H. Bennett (Eds.), *Diabetes in America* (2nd ed., pp. 165–178). Bethesda, MD: National Diabetes Data Group, NIH.

Douglas, M., & Wildawsky, A. (1983). *Risk and culture: An essay on the selection of technological and environmental dangers*. Berkely, CA: University of California Press.

Edwards, A., Elwyn, G., & Mulley, A. (2002). Explaining risks: Turning numerical data into meaningful pictures. *British Medical Journal, 324*, 827–830.

Eurostat (2010). *Europe in figures—Eurostat yearbook 2010: Education (tables and graphs)*. http://epp.eurostat.ec.europa.eu/portal/page/portal/product_details/publication?p_product_code=CH_04_2010_XLS, accessed July 30, 2012.

Fagerlin, A., Sepucha, K. R., Couper, M., Levin, C. A., Singer, E., & Zikmund-Fisher, B. J. (2010). Patients' knowledge about 9 common health conditions: The DECISIONS survey. *Medical Decision Making, 30*, 35S–52S.

Fagerlin, A., Ubel, P. A., Smith, D. M., & Zikmund-Fisher, B. J. (2007). Making numbers matter: Present and future research in risk communication. *American Journal of Health Behavior, 31*, 47–56.

Frosch, D. L., & Kaplan, R. M. (1999). Shared decision making in clinical medicine: Past research and future directions. *American Journal of Preventive Medicine, 17*, 285–294.

Galesic, M., & Garcia-Retamero, R. (2010). Statistical numeracy for health: A cross-cultural comparison with probabilistic national samples. *Archives of Internal Medicine, 170*, 462–468.

Galesic, M., & Garcia-Retamero, R. (2011a). Do low-numeracy people avoid shared decision making? *Health Psychology, 30*, 336–341.

Galesic, M., & Garcia-Retamero, R. (2011b). Graph literacy: A cross-cultural comparison. *Medical Decision Making, 31*, 444–457.

Garcia-Retamero, R., & Galesic, M. (2009). Trust in healthcare. In M. W. Kattan (Ed.), *The encyclopedia of medical decision making* (pp. 1153–1155). Thousand Oaks, CA: Sage.
Gigerenzer, G. (2002). *Calculated risks: How to know when numbers deceive you.* New York: Simon & Schuster.
Gigerenzer, G., Gaissmaier, W., Kurz-Milcke, E., Schwartz, L. M., & Woloshin, S. (2007). Helping doctors and patients make sense of health statistics. *Psychological Science in the Public Interest, 8*, 53–96.
Gigerenzer, G., & Gray, J. A. M. (2011). *Better doctors, better patients, better decisions: Envisioning health care 2020* (Strüngemann Forum Report, Vol. 6). Cambridge, MA: MIT Press.
Gøtzsche, P. C., & Nielsen, M. (2009). Screening for breast cancer with mammography. *Cochrane Database of Systematic Reviews, 4*, Article CD001877.
Gran, J. T., Husby, G., & Thorsby, E. (1985). The prevalence of HLA-DR4 and HLA-DR3 in healthy persons with rheumatoid factor. *Scandinavian Journal of Rheumatology, 14*, 79–82.
Hanoch, Y., Katsikoulos, K. V., Gummerum, M., & Brass, E. P. (2007). American and German students' knowledge, perceptions, and behaviors with respect to over-the-counter pain relievers. *Health Psychology, 26*, 802–806.
Hanson, J. L. (2008). Shared decision making: Have we missed the obvious? *Archives of Internal Medicine, 168*, 1368–1370.
Hartmann, L. C., Schaid, D. J., Woods, J. E., Crotty, T. P., Myers, J. L., Arnold, P. G., et al. (1999). Efficacy of bilateral prophylactic mastectomy in women with a family history of breast cancer. *The New England Journal of Medicine, 340*, 77–84.
Impiccatore, P., Pandolfini, C., Casella, N., & Bonati, M. (1997). Reliability of health information for the public on the World Wide Web: Systemic survey of advice on managing fever in children at home. *British Medical Journal, 314*, 1875–1879.
Jorgensen, K. J., & Gøtzsche, P. C. (2004). Presentation on websites of possible benefits and harms from screening for breast cancer: Cross sectional study. *British Medical Journal, 328*, 148–151.
Kravitz, R. L., Epstein, R. M., Feldman, M. D., Franz, C. E., Azari, R., Wilkes, M. S., et al. (2005). Influence of patients' requests for direct-to-consumer advertised antidepressants: A randomized controlled trial. *Journal of the American Medical Association, 293*, 1995–2002.
Lipkus, I. M. (2007). Numeric, verbal, and visual formats of conveying health risks: Suggested best practices and future recommendations. *Medical Decision Making, 27*, 696–713.
Lipkus, I. M., & Hollands, J. G. (1999). The visual communication of risk. *Journal of the National Cancer Institute. Monographs, 25*, 149–163.
Lipkus, I. M., & Peters, E. (2009). Understanding the role of numeracy in health: Proposed theoretical framework and practical insights. *Health Education and Behavior, 36*, 1065–1081.
Lipkus, I. M., Samsa, G., & Rimer, B. K. (2001). General performance on a numeracy scale among highly educated samples. *Medical Decision Making, 21*, 37–44.
Mechanic, D., & Meyer, S. (2000). Concepts of trust among patients with serious illness. *Social Science and Medicine, 51*, 657–668.
Michaels, D. (2006). Regarding "Phenylpropanolamine and hemorrhagic stroke in the hemorrhagic stroke project": Mercenary epidemiology—Data reanalysis and reinterpretation for sponsors with financial interest in the outcome. *Annals of Epidemiology, 16*, 49–52.
Murray, A. S., Stevenson, E., Kerr, F., & Burns, C. (2010). "A heartbeat moment:" Qualitative study of GP views of patients bringing health information from the internet to a consultation. *British Journal of General Practice, 60*, 88–94.
Nelson, H. D., Hoyt-Huffman, L. H., Fu, R., & Harris, E. L. (2005). Genetic risk assessment and BRCA mutation testing for breast and ovarian cancer susceptibility: Systematic evidence review for the U.S. Preventive Services Task Force. *Annals of Internal Medicine, 143*, 362–379.
Nelson, H. D., Tyne, K., Naik, A., Bougatsos, C., Chan, B. K., & Humphrey, L. (2009). Screening for breast cancer: An update for the U.S. Preventive Services Task Force. *Annals of Internal Medicine, 151*, 727–737.
Oliver, M. F., Poole-Wilson, P., Shepherd, J., & Tikkanen, M. J. (1995). Lower patients' cholesterol now. *British Medical Journal, 310*, 1280–1281.

Olsen, A. H., Njor, S. H., Vejborg, I., Schwartz, W., Dalgaard, P., Jensen, M. B., et al. (2005). Breast cancer mortality in Copenhagen after introduction of mammography screening: Cohort study. *British Medical Journal, 330*, 220–224.

Peters, E., Dieckmann, N. F., Västfjäll, D., Mertz, C. K., Slovic, P., & Hibbard, J. (2009). Bringing meaning to numbers: The impact of evaluative categories on decisions. *Journal of Experimental Psychology: Applied, 15*, 213–227.

Peters, E., Hibbard, J. H., Slovic, P., & Dieckmann, N. F. (2007). Numeracy skill and the communication, comprehension, and use of risk and benefit information. *Health Affairs, 26*, 741–748.

Peters, E., Västfjäll, D., Slovic, P., Mertz, C. K., Mazzocco, K., & Dickert, S. (2006). Numeracy and decision making. *Psychological Science, 17*, 407–413.

Programme for International Student Assessment (PISA) (2006). *PISA country profiles*. http://pisacountry.acer.edu.au/, accessed July 30, 2012.

Real Decreto Legislativo 1/1994, de 20 de Junio, por el que se aprueba el Texto Refundido de la Ley General de la Seguridad Social. *Boletín Oficial del Estado, 154 de 29/6/1994*, 20658–20708.

Renn, O., & Rohrmann, B. (2000). *Cross-cultural risk perception: A survey of empirical studies*. Dordrecht: Kluwer.

Reyna, V. R., Nelson, W. L., Han, P., & Dieckmann, N. F. (2009). How numeracy influences risk comprehension and medical decision making. *Psychological Bulletin, 135*, 943–973.

Rinderman, H. (2007). The g-factor of international cognitive ability comparisons: The homogeneity of results in PISA, TIMSS, PIRLS and IQ-tests across nations. *European Journal of Personality, 21*, 667–706.

Roberts, L. (2010). Health information and the Internet: The 5 Cs website evaluation tool. *British Journal of Nursing, 19*, 322–325.

Rohrmann, B., & Renn, O. (2000). Risk perception research: An introduction. In O. Renn & B. Rohrmann (Eds.), *Cross-cultural risk perception: A survey of empirical studies* (pp. 11–53). Dordrecht: Kluwer.

Schoen, C., Doty, M. M., Collins, S. R., & Holmgren, A. L. (2005). Insured but not protected: How many adults are underinsured? *Health Affairs*, W5-289–W5-302.

Schröder, F. H., Hugosson, J., Roobol, M. J., Tammela, T. L. J., Ciatto, S., Nelen, V., et al. (2009). Screening and prostate-cancer mortality in a randomized European study. *The New England Journal of Medicine, 360*, 1320–1328.

Schwartz, L. M., & Woloshin, S. (2007). Participation in mammography screening: Women should be encouraged to decide what is right for them, rather than being told what to do. *British Medical Journal, 335*, 731–732.

Schwartz, L. M., Woloshin, S., Black, W. C., & Welch, H. G. (1997). The role of numeracy in understanding the benefit of screening mammography. *Annals of Internal Medicine, 127*, 966–972.

Schwartz, L. M., Woloshin, S., & Welch, H. G. (1999). Risk communication in clinical practice: Putting cancer in context. *Journal of the National Cancer Institute Monographs, 25*, 124–133.

Skolbekken, J. A. (1998). Communicating the risk reduction achieved by cholesterol reducing drugs. *British Medical Journal, 316*, 1956–1958.

Slovic, P. (1999). Trust, emotion, sex, politics, and science: Surveying the risk-assessment battlefield. *Risk Analysis, 19*, 689–701.

Starr, P. (1949). *The social transformation of American medicine*. New York, NY: Basic Books.

Statistisches Bundesamt Deutschland (2011). Sozialleistungen Angaben zur Krankenversicherung (Ergebnisse des Mikrozensus) - Fachserie 13 Reihe 1.1 - 2007. https://www.destatis.de/DE/Publikationen/Thematisch/Bevoelkerung/HaushalteMikrozensus/KrankenversicherungMikrozensus2130110079004.html, accessed July 30, 2012.

Studdert, D. M., Mello, M. M., Sage, W. M., DesRoches, C. M., Peugh, J., Zapert, K., et al. (2005). Defensive medicine among high-risk specialist physicians in a volatile malpractice environment. *Journal of the American Medical Association, 293*, 2660–2662.

Taylor-Gooby, P., & Zinn, J. O. (2006). Current directions in risk research: New developments in psychology and sociology. *Risk Analysis, 26*, 397–411.

U. S. Government Accountability Office (2006). *Prescription drugs: Improvements needed in FDA's oversight of direct-to-consumer advertising* (GAO Report No. GAO-07-54). http://www.gao.gov/htext/d0754.html, accessed July 30, 2012.

Wilde, J. (2009, 18 March). *PSA screening cuts deaths by 20%, says world's largest prostate cancer study* (ERSPC Press Office, Carver Wilde Communications). http://www.erspc-media.org/psa-screening-cuts-deaths-by-20-says-worlds-largest-prostate-cancer-study/, accessed July 30, 2012.

World Health Organization (WHO) (2007). *Global health observatory*. http://apps.who.int/ghodata/, accessed July 30, 2012.

Xie, B. (2009). Older adults' health information wants in the Internet age: Implications for patient-provider relationships. *Journal of Health Communication, 14*, 510–524.

Zachry, W. M., Shepherd, M. D., Hinich, M. J., Wilson, J. P., Brown, C. M., & Lawson, K. A. (2002). Relationship between direct-to-consumer advertising and physician diagnosing and prescribing. *American Journal of Health Systems Pharmacy, 59*, 42–49.

Part I
Cultural Differences in Health Literacy and the Understanding of Health-Related Risks

Chapter 2
Statistical Numeracy for Health*

Mirta Galesic and Rocio Garcia-Retamero

Abstract Statistical numeracy is essential for understanding health-related risks and making informed medical decisions. However, this concept has not been investigated on the level of the general population or compared cross-culturally. In this chapter, we describe research that sought (1) to investigate differences in the level of statistical numeracy between two countries with different education and medical systems—the United States and Germany; (2) to study the relationship between statistical numeracy and demographic characteristics such as age, sex, and education; and (3) to test whether a subjective measure of numeracy is a valid indicator of objective measures. In a survey of probabilistic national samples in the United States and Germany, participants answered about two-thirds of the items testing objective numeracy. German participants had somewhat higher numeracy skills than participants in the USA. There was a large gap in numeracy skills between people with lower and higher educational levels, particularly in the USA. Subjective estimates of numeracy were a good indicator of the objective measures. Physicians should be aware that many patients may not understand all information relevant to making an informed decision.

*In this chapter, we partially reproduced the article Galesic, M., & Garcia-Retamero, R. (2010). Statistical numeracy for health: A cross-cultural comparison with probabilistic national samples. *Archives of Internal Medicine*, *170*, 462–468.

M. Galesic, Ph.D. (✉)
Center for Adaptive Behavior and Cognition, Max Planck Institute for Human Development, Lentzeallee 94, Berlin 14195, Germany
e-mail: galesic@mpib-berlin.mpg.de

R. Garcia-Retamero, Ph.D.
Departamento de Psicología Experimental, Facultad de Psicología, University of Granada, Campus Universitario de Cartuja s/n, Granada 18071, Spain

Center for Adaptive Behavior and Cognition, Max Planck Institute for Human Development, Lentzeallee 94, Berlin 14195, Germany
e-mail: rretamer@ugr.es

R. Garcia-Retamero and M. Galesic (eds.), *Transparent Communication of Health Risks: Overcoming Cultural Differences*, DOI 10.1007/978-1-4614-4358-2_2,

2.1 Introduction and Background

What percentage is 20 of 100? For most readers of this book, the answer is straightforward. Many patients, however, have difficulties grasping this and other basic statistical concepts (Davids et al. 2004; Lipkus et al. 2001; Schwartz et al. 1997; Woloshin et al. 2001). Statistical numeracy is part of a more general concept of quantitative or mathematic literacy (Golbeck et al. 2005; Speros 2005) and includes understanding the concept of a random toss and knowing how to perform elementary calculations with percentages (Davids et al. 2004; Lipkus et al. 2001). This knowledge is essential for understanding risks associated with different diseases, medical screenings, and treatments, and, consequently, for making informed decisions about health (Cokely and Kelley 2009; Estrada et al. 2004; Nelson et al. 2008; Peters et al. 2006; Reyna and Brainerd 2007; Rothman et al. 2006). This chapter describes a cross-cultural study investigating three important unanswered questions about statistical numeracy in the health context.

First, are there differences in the level of statistical numeracy between countries with different educational and medical systems—such as the USA and Germany? Several large national and international studies have included items that measure a broader concept of quantitative literacy, for example, the Programme for International Student Assessment (PISA 2003), the Trends in International Mathematics and Science Study (TIMSS; Gonzales et al. 2004), the National Assessment of Adult Literacy (NAAL; Kutner et al. 2006), and the International Adult Literacy Survey (IALS; Tuijnman 2000). Most of these studies, however, are limited to student populations and/or do not deal specifically with statistical numeracy—in particular not in the context of health. Given a stronger emphasis on mathematics and science education in the early grades in Germany compared with the USA (Rindermann 2007), it is possible that statistical numeracy is higher in Germany. However, the opposite could also be true. Because most health expenditure in the USA is privately based (55%) (see Chap. 1; World Health Organization 2012) and because patient-targeted advertising of prescription drugs is allowed, US residents may have more experience in dealing with information about medical risks, and consequently have higher statistical numeracy than the residents of Germany—where only 23% of health expenditure is privately based.

Second, what is the relationship between statistical numeracy and demographic characteristics such as age, sex, and education? To promote the ideal of informed and shared medical decision making (Barry 1999; Frosch and Kaplan 1999; Hanson 2008), it is essential to identify low-numeracy groups and to educate them in using quantitative statistical information or communicate information about health using nonquantitative formats such as visual displays and analogies (Edwards 2003; Galesic and Garcia-Retamero in press; Galesic et al. 2009; Garcia-Retamero and Galesic 2009), see Chaps. 7 and 9–11. However, all of the extant studies of statistical numeracy in health used nonprobabilistic samples of patients and students. Although informative about the numeracy skills of certain narrow groups, these studies do not allow for generalizations to any broader population. Consequently, they do not allow us to draw conclusions about the relationship between numeracy and demographic characteristics such as sex, age, and education.

Third, are objective measures of statistical numeracy equivalent to recently proposed subjective measures of this concept (Fagerlin et al. 2007)? In studies of convenience samples of patients and an Internet population, subjective measures were found to be less burdensome for the participants, at the same time approaching predictive validity of the objective measures of statistical numeracy (Zikmund-Fisher et al. 2007). Subjective measures of numeracy, however, have not yet been administered to probabilistic national samples that would enable researchers to study the relationship between objective and subjective numeracy in different demographic subgroups or to conduct cross-cultural comparisons.

To answer these questions, we conducted two studies on probabilistic national samples in the USA and Germany. This enabled us to compare statistical numeracy skills of adult population in these countries and in different sociodemographic groups within the countries.

2.2 Study 1: Investigating Objective Statistical Numeracy in Probabilistic National Samples

In Study 1, conducted on probabilistic national samples in the USA and Germany, we investigated whether there are differences between the two countries in the level of objective statistical numeracy and sought to determine the relationship between numeracy and demographic characteristics.

2.2.1 Method

2.2.1.1 Participants

Study 1 was conducted from July 10 through 24, 2008, on probabilistic national samples in the USA ($n = 1{,}009$) and Germany ($n = 1{,}001$), using panels of households selected through probabilistic random digit dial telephone surveys and afterward supplied with equipment that enabled them to complete computerized questionnaires. Thus, existing Internet access or lack thereof did not affect households' ability to become panel members. The panels—built and maintained by the online research panel Knowledge Networks in the USA [http://www.knowledgenetworks.com; 43,000 households (16% of those in the initial sample)] and the market research institute Forsa in Germany [http://www.forsa.de; 20,000 households (11% of those in the initial sample)]—allow for statistical inference to the general population. These panels were already used successfully in a number of studies in the areas of health, medicine, political and social sciences, economics, and public policy (Baker et al. 2003; Jacoby 2006; Lerner et al. 2003; Miller et al. 2006; Schlenger et al. 2002). Methodological studies have shown that data from such panels are comparable to the results obtained through traditional probabilistic surveys

(Chang and Krosnick 2009). The possibility of using computerized questionnaires enabled us to ask relatively complex questions involving numerical and visual information about medical treatments on a nationally representative sample.

Of the panel members who were invited to participate in the study, 54% in the USA and 52% in Germany completed the questionnaire. This is a good response rate for this survey mode (Vehovar et al. 2002). The sample structure is shown in Table 2.1. According to official statistics, the percentage of population with less education is much higher in Germany than in the USA, so we oversampled the less-educated population in the USA to ensure equivalent sample sizes of less-educated participants in both countries. To adjust for this and for minor discrepancies due to nonresponse, we used design (in the USA) and poststratification (in both countries) survey weights to bring the sample proportions in line with the population proportions. The goal of such weighting adjustments is to correct for known differences between sample and population in the hope of providing unbiased survey estimates (Bethlehem 2002; Gelman and Carlin 2002). Standard errors in all analyses were estimated using the Taylor series linearization method for estimating population characteristics from complex sample survey data, by means of commercially available software (SPSS Complex Samples procedures, SPSS version 17.0.1 (SPSS, Inc, Chicago, IL) and SUDAAN [RTI International, Research Triangle Park, North Carolina]; Siller and Tompkins 2006).

2.2.1.2 Stimuli and Procedure

Statistical numeracy was measured on a scale including three items developed by Schwartz et al. (1997), and six items developed by Lipkus et al. (2001), for a maximum score of 9 (see Table 2.2). The questions were translated into German by a native German speaker with excellent knowledge of English, back-translated into English by another person with equivalent language skills, and compared with the original English version. Any inconsistencies were resolved by a native German speaker and an excellent English speaker familiar with the research objectives. Finally, the English and German versions were compared and edited by a bilingual English and German speaker Chap. 15. When programming the questionnaire, special care was taken to ensure that the interface looked the same in the English and German versions. In sum, we believe that the materials in English and German were comparable. The Ethics Committee of the Max Planck Institute for Human Development approved the method used herein, and all participants consented to participation through an online consent form at the beginning of the survey.

2.2.2 Results

The statistical numeracy scale has satisfactory internal consistency: Cronbach alpha was 0.80 in the USA and 0.73 in Germany. Percent of correct answers to each of the

Table 2.1 Structure of the sample of participants in Study 1 in terms of gender, age, and education[a]

	USA			Germany		
	Sample size (unweighted)	Sample % (weighted)	Population %[b]	Sample size (unweighted)	Sample % (weighted)	Population %[c]
Total	1,009	100%	100%	1,001	100%	100%
Gender						
Male	480	48.2	49.2	526	50.3	49.9
Female	529	51.8	50.8	475	49.7	50.1
Age						
25–39	242	33.0	35.7	270	31.4	32.5
40–54	394	39.2	38.3	410	38.9	39.9
55–69	373	27.8	26.1	321	29.7	27.7
Education[d]						
Less than high school	114	12.2	13.4	401	42.9	41.0
High school	599	31.8	31.2	346	31.1	31.7
Some college	145	26.1	26.0	102	11.0	11.5
College or higher	151	29.9	29.4	152	15.0	15.7

[a]Percentages have been rounded and may not total 100

[b]From Statistisches Bundesamt Deutschland, Microcensus (2007) https://www-genesis.destatis.de/genesis/online

[c]From the US Census Bureau, Current Population Survey (2008) Annual Social and Economic Supplement (http://www.census.gov/cps/)

[d]In Germany, less than high school includes participants who finished *Hauptschule*; high school, those who finished *Realschule*; and some college, those who obtained *Abitur*

Table 2.2 Percent correct answers for each item of the numeracy scale by country in Study 1 (see also Chap. 15)

	% Correct	
	USA	Germany
1. Imagine that we flip a fair coin 1,000 times. What is your best guess about how many times the coin will come up heads in 1,000 flips? ____ times out of 1,000	73.2	72.6
2. In the Bingo Lottery, the chance of winning a $10 prize is 1%. What is your best guess about how many people would win a $10 prize if 1,000 people each buy a single ticket to Bingo Lottery? ____ person(s) out of 1,000	57.7	67.6
3. In the Daily Times Sweepstakes, the chance of winning a car is 1 in 1,000. What percent of tickets to Daily Times Sweepstakes win a car? ____ % of tickets	23.5	46.3
4. Imagine that we roll a fair, six-sided die 1,000 times. Out of 1,000 rolls, how many times do you think the die would come up even (2, 4, or 6)? ____ times out of 1,000	57.1	63.5
5. Which of the following numbers represents the biggest risk of getting a disease? 1 in 10, 1 in 100, or 1 in 1,000?	75.3	71.8
6. Which of the following represents the biggest risk of getting a disease? 1, 5, or 10%?	83.1	78.6
7. If the chance of getting a disease is 10%, how many people would be expected to get the disease out of 1,000? ____ people	83.1	88.8
8. If the chance of getting a disease is 20 out of 100, this would be the same as having a ____% chance of getting the disease.	70.3	72.8
9. If Person A's chance of getting a disease is 1 in 100 in ten years, and Person B's risk is double that of A, what is B's risk?	57.3	54.5

items is presented in Table 2.2. For further analysis, we transformed the original scores ranging from 0 to 9 to a scale of 0 to 100%, indicating the percentage of the nine items that were answered correctly.

As shown in Table 2.3, German participants had higher numeracy skills than those in the USA: On average 69 vs. 65% of the items were answered correctly. This difference remains after controlling for differences in sex, age, education, and income between the two countries.

On the level of each country, sex, age, and education are all related to the numeracy score. In both countries, men had higher scores than women. Numeracy skills dropped with age (r=–0.12 [–0.19, –0.05] in the USA, and r=–0.13, 95% CI [–0.20, –0.06] in Germany) and increased with education (r=0.50 [0.44, 0.56] in the USA, and r=0.28 [0.21, 0.35] in Germany) and income (r=0.32 [0.25, 0.39] in the USA, and r=0.20 [0.13, 0.27] in Germany). When we enter sex, age, education, and income together in a regression model, all four show independent effects in Germany, but in the USA only sex, education, and income explain differences in numeracy scores, while the effect of age was no longer present.

Table 2.3 Average percentage of correctly answered items on the objective numeracy scale by country and demographic groups in Study 1

	USA ($n = 1{,}009$)		Germany ($n = 1{,}001$)	
	% correct	(SE)	% correct	(SE)
Overall	64.5	(1.3)	68.5	(1.1)
Gender				
Male	69.1	(2.0)	74.1	(1.6)
Female	60.2	(1.7)	62.9	(1.6)
Age				
25–39	66.5	(2.6)	72.8	(2.0)
40–54	67.5	(2.0)	68.3	(1.8)
55–69	57.9	(2.0)	64.3	(2.1)
Education[a]				
Less than high school	39.9	(3.1)	62.3	(1.7)
High school	56.4	(1.4)	67.3	(2.0)
Some college	64.5	(2.8)	79.2	(2.8)
College or higher	83.1	(1.8)	80.7	(2.5)
Household income[b]				
Lower third (up to ~$30,000)	55.3	(2.2)	60.6	(2.3)
Middle third (~$30–60,000)	60.8	(2.3)	70	(1.7)
Upper third (more than ~$60,000)	76.5	(2.0)	74.1	(2.1)

[a] In Germany, "less than high school" includes participants who finished Hauptschule; "high school"—Realschule; and "some college"—Abitur

[b] In Germany, the categories are up to 18,000€, 18–36,000€, and more than 36,000€. To compare incomes, we used the average exchange rate for the 12 months preceding the interviews, cf. http://www.federalreserve.gov/releases/h10/Hist/dat00_eu.txt

The inequality in numeracy skills was larger in the USA than in Germany, as reflected in the ratio between the scores in the 90th and 10th percentile of the participants ordered by their scores: This ratio was 4.5 in the USA vs. 3.0 in Germany. The inequality is visible, in particular, in average scores of people with low educational attainment vs. highly educated people in the USA: 40 vs. 83% correct, compared to 62 vs. 81% in Germany (see Table 2.3). We discuss the implications of these results in Sect. 2.4.

2.3 Study 2: Investigating Subjective Statistical Numeracy in Probabilistic National Samples

In Study 2, we investigated whether subjective measures of statistical numeracy (Fagerlin et al. 2007) correspond to objective measures (Lipkus et al. 2001; Schwartz et al. 1997) in general populations of the USA and Germany. If a subjective numeracy scale can differentiate between people with objectively low and high numeracy skills across different demographic groups, this would speak to its wide applicability. In addition, we tested whether the subjective perceptions of one's numeracy are

Table 2.4 Structure of the sample of participants in Study 2 in terms of numeracy, gender, age, and education

	USA ($n=238$)		Germany ($n=260$)	
	Low-numeracy group ($n=117$)	High-numeracy group ($n=121$)	Low-numeracy group ($n=127$)	High-numeracy group ($n=133$)
Mean numeracy	35.6	90.9	37.2	95.5
Female (%)	58.1	45.6	60.6	40.2
Mean age (years)	44.3	45.1	49.9	43.3
High educational levels (%)[a]	44.4	72.8	9.3	41.3

[a]Indicates some college and college or higher, as defined in Table 2.1.

dependent on the context in which they are measured, namely, before or after answering several difficult numerical questions. If the scale is sensitive to context, this would limit its applicability because the results in clinical practice would depend on patients' recent experiences with quantitative information.

2.3.1 *Method*

2.3.1.1 Participants

Study 1 participants were ordered by their objective numeracy scores, and those with the highest and lowest scores were invited to participate in Study 2, conducted 3 weeks after Study 1 (August 1–15, 2008), resulting in a sample of 498 participants. Basic demographic characteristics of the sample are given in Table 2.4. This sample enables us to compare low- and high-numeracy groups within each country, as well as each of those groups between countries.

In the USA, 65.8% of all participants in Study 1 completed Study 2, and in Germany, 83.1%. The response rates among high- and low-numeracy participants were similar in both countries (i.e., it was not the case that the low-numeracy group had lower response rates). The low- and high-numeracy groups in Germany represent, respectively, approximately the bottom and top third of the population sorted by numeracy scores. Because of lower response rates in the USA, the low- and high-numeracy groups represent, respectively, approximately the bottom and top 40% of the population. Nevertheless, the average numeracy scores in both groups were still somewhat lower in the USA (Table 2.4).

2.3.1.2 Stimuli and Procedure

Subjective numeracy was measured with seven of the eight items developed by Fagerlin et al. (2007; see also Zikmund-Fisher et al. 2007). The items were answered on a six-point scale, where higher values indicate higher perceived numeracy.

We excluded the item "How good are you at calculating a 15% tip?" because it is culturally specific to the USA (see Table 2.5; see Chap. 15 for the translation of the items into German). Chapter 15 lists all of the items used. The questionnaire was developed in the same way as that for Study 1. Half of the participants were randomly assigned to complete these items before a set of questions involving relatively demanding numerical calculations of risk reductions and the remaining half completed the items after answering the questions (for more details on these questions, see Garcia-Retamero and Galesic 2009; see also Chap. 10).

2.3.2 *Results*

To compare the scores on the subjective numeracy scale with the objective numeracy data, we recoded each item—originally answered on a scale of 1 to 6—to be 0 when the answer was 3 or less, or 1 when the answer was 4 or higher. Mean and standard deviation of answers to each of the items are presented in Table 2.5. For further analyses, we summed the recoded answers to the seven items and transformed the resulting scores to a scale of 0–100%, indicating the percentage of answers to the seven items that reflected high subjective numeracy.

The subjective numeracy scale has satisfactory internal consistency. The Cronbach's alpha ranged from 0.75 to 0.87 across the two countries and groups with high vs. low objective numeracy skills. The scores on the scale were not sensitive to context: They were similar when the items were positioned before or after the tasks involving difficult calculations (average before/after difference = 2.8, 95% CI [−5.4, 11.0]); this was so for high- and low-numeracy groups in both countries.

How well does the subjective numeracy scale differentiate between participants who are very high vs. very low in terms of their objective numeracy skills (as determined in Study 1)? The average subjective numeracy scores for these two extreme groups were 38.9 (SE = 4.4) and 79.0 (SE = 2.5) in the USA, and 45.5 (SE = 3.7) and 80.0 (SE = 2.7) in Germany. These differences were stable across gender, age, education, and income groups. However, compared to the differences in objective numeracy scores between the two extreme groups ($M = 35.6$, SE = 2.8 vs. $M = 90.9$, SE = 1.1 in the USA, and $M = 37.2$, SE = 2.0 vs. $M = 95.6$, SE = 0.7 in Germany; see Table 2.4), the differences in subjective numeracy scores were smaller.

How well does the subjective numeracy scale differentiate between participants who are very high vs. very low in terms of their objective numeracy skills (as determined in study 1)? The mean (SE) subjective numeracy scores for these two extreme groups were 38.9 (4.4) and 79.0 (2.5) in the USA, and 45.5 (3.7) and 80.0 (2.7) in Germany. These differences were stable across sex, age, education, and income groups. However, compared with the differences in objective numeracy scores between the two extreme groups (mean [SE], 35.6 [2.8] vs. 90.9 [1.1] in the USA, and 37.2 [2.0] vs. 95.5 [0.7] in Germany; Table 2.4), the differences in subjective numeracy scores were smaller.

Table 2.5 Mean ratings of items in the subjective numeracy scale by country and numeracy in Study 2

	Mean (SD)			
	USA		Germany	
	Low numeracy	High numeracy	Low numeracy	High numeracy
1. How good are you at working with fractions? Not at all good–extremely good (*six-point scale*)	2.4 (1.2)	3.9 (1.3)	2.8 (1.2)	4.2 (1.2)
2. How good are you at working with percentages? Not at all good–extremely good (*six-point scale*)	2.4 (1.2)	4.1 (1.3)	3.3 (1.3)	4.6 (1)
3. How good are you at figuring out how much a shirt will cost if it is 25% off? Not at all good–extremely good (*six-point scale*)	3.5 (1.4)	4.9 (1.0)	4.1 (1.3)	5.0 (0.9)
4. When reading the newspaper, how helpful do you find tables and graphs that are parts of a story? Not at all–extremely (*six-point scale*)	3.3 (1.4)	4.5 (1.2)	3.2 (1.5)	4.7 (1.1)
5. When people tell you the chance of something happening, do you prefer that they use words ("it rarely happens") or numbers ("there's a 1% chance")? Always prefer words–always prefer numbers (*six-point scale*)	2.6 (1.7)	4.2 (1.7)	3.0 (1.8)	4.3 (1.6)
6. When you hear a weather forecast, do you prefer predictions using percentages (e.g., "there will be a 20% chance of rain today") or predictions using only words (e.g., "there is a small chance of rain today")? Always prefer words–always prefer percentages (*six-point scale*)	4.2 (1.5)	5.0 (1.2)	3.0 (1.8)	4.0 (1.7)
7. How often do you find numerical information to be useful? Never–very often (*six-point scale*)	3.3 (1.3)	5.0 (1.1)	3.9 (1.4)	4.9 (1)

2.4 Discussion and Conclusions

An average citizen of the USA and Germany could answer only two-thirds of nine relatively simple items testing basic statistical numeracy skills (Table 2.3). Statistical numeracy was somewhat lower for women than for men, and it dropped slightly with age but only in Germany. Across most demographic groups, German participants achieved somewhat higher scores than did US participants. An exception was the group with the highest education, in which US participants fared somewhat better. Differences in education systems—in particular the stronger focus on mathematics and science education in Germany from an early age (Stigler et al. 1999; Tuijnman 2000)—are likely to be the main factor underlying the differences in statistical numeracy between countries.

The inequality between people with more or less education in the USA was much larger than in Germany. Although a college-educated American could answer 83.1% of items correctly, those with less than a high school diploma could do so for only 39.9% of the items. Even for those who had a high school education the average percentage of correct answers in the USA was only 56.4%, lower than the average for German participants who had not completed a high school education (62.3%; Table 2.3).

The large differences in numeracy between persons with lower and higher educational levels have varying consequences in different medical systems. For instance—at least before the new health care reform—less educated US residents are particularly likely to be in a position to have to decide about their medical care. Although 99.7% of Germans have health insurance (see Chap. 1; see also Statistisches Bundesamt Deutschland 2011), 35% of US residents—in particular, those of lower socioeconomic status—had no health insurance or insufficient coverage (Schoen et al. 2005) and had to decide whether to pay for various medical treatments and screenings (Schoen et al. 2007). Given their low statistical numeracy, they might have had difficulty making good decisions.

The present chapter, to the best of our knowledge, describes the first study investigating statistical numeracy skills in probabilistic national samples in the USA and Germany, allowing comparison of different demographic groups within each country as well as comparison between the two countries. It also describes the first cross-cultural comparison of objective and subjective measures of statistical numeracy.

At the same time, a limitation of the studies is that levels of numeracy in the general population could be even lower than our results suggest. To become members of the national panels from which our samples were selected, participants had to accept having a computer or special TV set with Internet access installed in their homes. It is possible that people with low numeracy refused this more often than did those with high numeracy skills. On the other hand, our sample represents accurately the overall population in terms of education. Furthermore, there is no particular reason to expect that numeracy but not general educational level would be related to higher rates of refusal.

Our findings have clear implications for medical practice. Physicians should not assume that all patients can understand simple statistical indicators that are often used to express risks and benefits of medical screenings and treatments. For example, approximately 20% of the participants in both Germany and the USA could not say which of the following numbers represents the biggest risk of getting a disease: 1, 5, or 10%. Ratios were even more difficult—almost 30% could not answer whether 1 in 10, 1 in 100, or 1 in 1,000 represents the largest risk. Similarly, almost 30% of the study participants in both countries could not state what percentage 20 of 100 is, and most (76.5% and 53.7% of the participants in the USA and Germany, respectively) could not transform 1 of 1,000 to a percentage. Furthermore, many participants lacked the understanding of the concept of random toss. When asked how many times a fair coin would come up heads in 1,000 flips, more than one-fourth of the study participants in both countries gave answers that were obviously incorrect (less than 400 or more than 600 times).

Given the low levels of statistical numeracy of many patients, physicians could use items from the subjective numeracy scale to identify patients who may have problems understanding numerical information. If they have such a patient, physicians could communicate risks and benefits of treatments by means of formats that do not require high levels of numeracy, such as visual displays (see Chaps. 9, 10, and 11; see also Hanson 2008; Galesic et al. 2009; Lipkus 2007; Lipkus and Hollands 1999) and analogies (see Chap. 7; see also Garcia-Retamero and Galesic 2009; Galesic and Garcia-Retamero 2012), rather than numerical expressions. In this way, patients with low numeracy skills could understand statistical information and make better decisions about their health.

References

Baker, L., Wagner, T. H., Singer, S., & Bundorf, M. K. (2003). Use of the Internet and email for health care information: Results from a national survey. *Journal of the American Medical Association, 289*, 2400–2406.

Barry, M. J. (1999). Involving patients in medical decisions: How can physicians do better? *Journal of the American Medical Association, 282*, 2356–2357.

Bethlehem, J. G. (2002). Weighting nonresponse adjustments based on auxiliary information. In R. M. Groves, D. A. Dillman, J. L. Eltinge, & R. J. A. Little (Eds.), *Survey nonresponse* (pp. 275–288). New York: Wiley.

Chang, L., & Krosnick, J. A. (2009). National surveys via RDD telephone interviewing versus the Internet: Comparing sample representativeness and response quality. *Public Opinion Quarterly, 73*, 641–678.

Cokely, E. T., & Kelley, C. M. (2009). Cognitive abilities and superior decision making under risk: A protocol analysis and process model evaluation. *Judgment and Decision Making, 4*, 20–33.

Davids, S. L., Schapira, M. M., McAuliffe, T. L., & Nattinger, A. B. (2004). Predictors of pessimistic breast cancer risk perceptions in a primary care population. *Journal of General Internal Medicine, 19*, 310–315.

Edwards, A. (2003). Communicating risks through analogies. *British Medical Journal, 327*, 749.

Estrada, C. A., Martin-Hryniewicz, M., Peek, B. T., Collins, C., & Byrd, J. C. (2004). Literacy and numeracy skills and anticoagulation control. *The American Journal of the Medical Sciences, 328*, 88–93.

Fagerlin, A., Zikmund-Fisher, B. J., Ubel, P. A., Jankovic, A., Derry, H. A., & Smith, D. M. (2007). Measuring numeracy without a Math test: Development of the subjective numeracy scale. *Medical Decision Making, 27*, 672–680.

Frosch, D. L., & Kaplan, R. M. (1999). Shared decision making in clinical medicine: Past research and future directions. *American Journal of Preventive Medicine, 17*, 285–294.

Galesic, M. & Garcia-Retamero, R. (2012). Using analogies to communicate information about health risks. *Applied Cognitive Psychology*. doi: 10.1002/acp.2866

Galesic, M., Garcia-Retamero, R., & Gigerenzer, G. (2009). Using icon arrays to communicate medical risks: overcoming low numeracy. *Health Psychology, 28*, 210–216.

Garcia-Retamero, R., & Galesic, M. (2009). Communicating treatment risk reduction to people with low numeracy skills: A cross-cultural comparison. *American Journal of Public Health, 99*, 2196–2202.

Gelman, A., & Carlin, J. B. (2002). Poststratification and weighting adjustments. In R. M. Groves, D. A. Dillman, J. L. Eltinge, & R. J. A. Little (Eds.), *Survey nonresponse* (pp. 289–302). New York: Wiley.

Golbeck, A. L., Ahlers-Schmidt, C. R., Paschal, A. M., & Dismuke, S. E. (2005). A definition and operational framework for health numeracy. *American Journal of Preventive Medicine, 29*, 375–376.

Gonzales, P., Guzmán, J. C., Partelow, L., Pahlke, E., Jocelyn, L., Kastberg, D., et al. (2004). *Highlights from the trends in international mathematics and science study (TIMSS) 2003*. U.S. Department of Education, National Center for Education Statistics. Washington, DC: U.S. Government Printing Office.

Hanson, J. L. (2008). Shared decision making: Have we missed the obvious? *Archives of Internal Medicine, 168*, 1368–1370.

Jacoby, W. G. (2006). Value choices and American public opinion. *American Journal of Political Science, 50*, 706–723.

Kutner, M., Greenberg, E., Jin, Y., & Paulsen, C. (2006). *The health literacy of America's adults: results from the 2003 national assessment of adult literacy (NALS)*. U.S. Department of Education, National Center for Education Statistics. Washington, DC: U.S. Government Printing Office.

Lerner, J. S., Gonzalez, R. M., Small, D. A., & Fischhoff, B. (2003). Effects of fear and anger on perceived risks of terrorism: A national field experiment. *Psychological Science, 14*, 144–150.

Lipkus, I. M. (2007). Numeric, verbal, and visual formats of conveying health risks: Suggested best practices and future recommendations. *Medical Decision Making, 27*, 696–713.

Lipkus, I. M., & Hollands, J. G. (1999). The visual communication of risk. *Journal of the National Cancer Institute. Monographs, 25*, 149–163.

Lipkus, I. M., Samsa, G., & Rimer, B. K. (2001). General performance on a numeracy scale among highly educated samples. *Medical Decision Making, 21*, 37–44.

Miller, J. D., Scott, E. C., & Okamoto, S. (2006). Public acceptance of evolution. *Science, 313*, 765–766.

Nelson, W., Reyna, V. F., Fagerlin, A., Lipkus, I., & Peters, E. (2008). Clinical implications of numeracy: Theory and practice. *Annals of Behavioral Medicine, 35*, 261–274.

Peters, E., Vastfjall, D., Slovic, P., Mertz, C. K., Mazzocco, K., & Dickert, S. (2006). Numeracy and decision making. *Psychological Science, 17*, 407–413.

Programme for International Student Assessment (PISA). (2003). *The PISA 2003 assessment framework—Mathematics, reading, science, and problem solving knowledge and skills*. Paris: OECD.

Reyna, V. F., & Brainerd, C. J. (2007). The importance of mathematics in health and human judgment: Numeracy, risk communication, and medical decision making. *Learning and Individual Differences, 17*, 147–159.

Rindermann, H. (2007). The g-factor of international cognitive ability comparisons: The homogeneity of results in PISA, TIMSS, PIRLS and IQ-tests across nations. *European Journal of Personality, 21*, 667–706.

Rothman, R. L., Housam, R., Weiss, H., Davis, D., Gregory, R., Gebretsadik, T., et al. (2006). Patient understanding of food labels—The role of literacy and numeracy. *American Journal of Preventive Medicine, 31*, 391–398.

Schlenger, W. E., Caddell, J. M., Ebert, L., Jordan, B. K., Rourke, K. M., Wilson, D., et al. (2002). Psychological reactions to terrorist attacks—Findings from the national study of Americans' reactions to September 11. *Journal of the American Medical Association, 288*, 581–588.

Schoen, C., Doty, M. M., Collins, S. R., & Holmgren, A. L. (2005). Insured but not protected: how many adults are underinsured? *Health Affairs*, W5-289–W5-302.

Schoen, C., Osborn, R., Doty, M. M., Bishop, M., Peugh, J., & Murukutla, N. (2007). Toward higher-performance health systems: Adults' health care experiences in seven countries, 2007. *Health Affairs, 26*, W717–W734.

Schwartz, L. M., Woloshin, S., Black, W. C., & Welch, H. G. (1997). The role of numeracy in understanding the benefit of screening mammography. *Annals of Internal Medicine, 127*, 966–972.

Siller, A. B., & Tompkins, L. (2006). *The Big Four: Analyzing complex sample survey data using SAS, SPSS, STATA, and SUDAAN*. Paper presented at the SAS Users Group International conference (SUGI) 31, San Francisco, CA. http://www.nesug.org/proceedings/nesug05/pos/pos3.pdf, accessed July 30, 2012.

Speros, C. (2005). Health literacy: Concept analysis. *Journal of Advanced Nursing, 50*, 633–640.

Statistisches Bundesamt Deutschland (2011). Sozialleistungen Angaben zur Krankenversicherung (Ergebnisse des Mikrozensus) - Fachserie 13 Reihe 1.1 - 2007. https https://www.destatis.de/DE/Publikationen/Thematisch/Bevoelkerung/HaushalteMikrozensus/KrankenversicherungMikrozensus2130110079004.html, accessed July 30, 2012.

Stigler, J. W., Gonzales, P., Kawanaka, T., Knoll, S., & Serrano, A. (1999). *The TIMSS videotape classroom study: Methods and findings from an exploratory research project on eighth-grade mathematics instruction in Germany, Japan, and the United States*. U.S. Department of Education, National Center for Education Statistics. Washington, DC: U.S. Government Printing Office.

Tuijnman, A. (2000). *Benchmarking adult literacy in America: An international comparative study: International adult literacy survey (IALS)*. Washington, DC: Department of Education, OVAE.

Vehovar, V., Batagelj, Z., Lozar Manfreda, K., & Zaletel, M. (2002). Nonresponse in Web surveys. In R. M. Groves, D. A. Dillman, J. L. Eltinge, & R. J. A. Little (Eds.), *Survey nonresponse* (pp. 229–242). New York: Wiley.

Woloshin, S., Schwartz, L. M., Moncur, M., Gabriel, S., & Tosteson, A. N. A. (2001). Assessing values for health: Numeracy matters. *Medical Decision Making, 21*, 382–390.

World Health Organization (2012). *World Health Statistics* 2012. http://www.who.int/gho/publications/world_health_statistics/2012/en/, accessed July 30, 2012.

Zikmund-Fisher, B. J., Smith, D. M., Ubel, P. A., & Fagerlin, A. (2007). Validation of the subjective numeracy scale: Effects of low numeracy on comprehension of risk communications and utility elicitations. *Medical Decision Making, 27*, 663–671.

Chapter 3
How to Measure Risk Comprehension in Educated Samples*

Edward T. Cokely, Saima Ghazal, Mirta Galesic, Rocio Garcia-Retamero, and Eric Schulz

Abstract The Berlin Numeracy Test is a psychometrically sound instrument designed to quickly assess statistical numeracy and risk comprehension in educated samples (e.g., college students or medical and business professionals). The test is available in multiple languages and formats including an online adaptive test that automatically scores data (http://www.riskliteracy.org). In this chapter, we review results of a validation study (n = 300) documenting convergent (e.g., cognitive

---

*In this chapter, we partially reproduced the article Cokely, E.T., Galesic, M. Schulz, E., Ghazal, S., & Garcia-Retamero, R. (2012). Measuring risk literacy: The Berlin Numeracy Test. *Judgment and Decision Making, 7*, 25–47.

E.T. Cokely, Ph.D. (✉)
Department of Cognitive and Learning Sciences, Michigan Technological University, 212 Meese Center, Houghton, MI, USA

Center for Adaptive Behavior and Cognition, Max Planck Institute for Human Development, Lentzeallee 94, Berlin 14195, Germany
e-mail: ecokely@mtu.edu

S. Ghazal
Department of Cognitive and Learning Sciences, Michigan Technological University, 212 Meese Center, Houghton, MI, USA
e-mail: sghazal@mtu.edu

M. Galesic, Ph.D.
Center for Adaptive Behavior and Cognition, Max Planck Institute for Human Development, Lentzeallee 94, Berlin 14195, Germany
e-mail: galesic@mpib-berlin.mpg.de

R. Garcia-Retamero, Ph.D.
Departamento de Psicología Experimental, Facultad de Psicología, University of Granada, Campus Universitario de Cartuja s/n, Granada 18071, Spain

Center for Adaptive Behavior and Cognition, Max Planck Institute for Human Development, Lentzeallee 94, Berlin 14195, Germany
e-mail: rretamer@ugr.es

R. Garcia-Retamero and M. Galesic (eds.), *Transparent Communication of Health Risks: Overcoming Cultural Differences*, DOI 10.1007/978-1-4614-4358-2_3,

ability, numeracy), discriminant (e.g., personality, life satisfaction), and predictive validity (e.g., numerical and non-numerical risky choices). The Berlin Numeracy Test was found to be the strongest predictor of a battery of everyday risky decisions (e.g., evaluating claims about medical treatments, consumer goods, and interpreting forecasts), providing more than twice the predictive power of other numeracy instruments. The Berlin Numeracy Test also accounted for unique variance beyond other related cognitive tests (e.g., cognitive reflection, working memory, and intelligence). Twenty additional validation studies (n = 5,036) indicated that the Berlin Numeracy Test maintained psychometric discriminability across 15 countries (e.g., China, England, Germany, Japan, India, Pakistan, Spain, Sweden, and the USA) and various samples (i.e., community samples, Mechanical Turk web panels, medical professionals). Discussion centers on construct validity and the benefits and limits of adaptive testing.

3.1 Introduction and Background

Efforts to measure individual differences in statistical numeracy come primarily in three forms. Some research examines risky decisions in relation to individual differences in overall educational attainment, cognitive abilities, or cognitive styles (Frederick 2005; Stanovich and West 2000, 2008). Other research primarily focusing on clinical and health domains has developed a valid subjective instrument for self-reported estimations of statistical numeracy (Zikmund-Fisher et al. 2007). Most common, however, is the use of direct performance measures of numeracy—i.e., psychometric tests (for a list of tests see Reyna et al. 2009; see also Black et al. 1995; Galesic and Garcia-Retamero 2010; Lipkus et al. 2001; Peters et al. 2006; Schwartz et al. 1997; Weller et al. 2012).

In this chapter, we describe the most widely used statistical numeracy instruments (Lipkus et al. 2001; Schwartz et al. 1997; see also Chaps. 2 and 15), examining their successes and psychometric limits. We then introduce a new test of statistical numeracy for risk literacy: the Berlin Numeracy Test.[1] This test can be

[1] The Berlin Numeracy Test is named to reflect the international, interdisciplinary development effort initiated in 2007 at Center for Adaptive Behavior and Cognition in the Max Planck Institute for Human Development. For additional discussion and similar public outreach efforts concerning expertise, ethics, and philosophical judgment see philosophicalcharacter.org (Feltz and Cokely 2009, 2012; Schulz et al. 2011).

E. Schulz
Cognitive, Perceptual, and Brain Sciences Department, University College London, 26 Bedford Way, London WC1H 0AP, UK

Center for Adaptive Behavior and Cognition, Max Planck Institute for Human Development, Lentzeallee 94, 14195, Berlin, Germany
e-mail: hanshalbe@googlemail.com

used in multiple formats (i.e., computer-adaptive, paper-and-pencil, single-item median-split, multiple-choice) and provides a fast, valid, and reliable tool for research, assessment, and public outreach. We show that the new test offers unique predictive validity for everyday risky decisions beyond other cognitive ability (e.g., cognitive reflection, working memory span, and fluid intelligence) and numeracy tests. Further, we show that the Berlin Numeracy Test dramatically improves psychometric discriminability among highly educated individuals (e.g., college students, graduates, and medical professionals) and across diverse cultures and different languages. We close the chapter with a discussion of implications of the current results for construct validity as well as discussion of the merits of fast and accurate measurement of numeracy (e.g., custom-tailored interactive risk communication).

3.2 Numeracy in Educated Samples

In 2001, Lipkus et al. published the numeracy test for highly educated samples, which was an extension of previous work by Schwartz et al. (1997). Lipkus et al. (2001) conducted a series of four studies ($n=463$) on community samples of well-educated adult participants (at least 40 years of age) in North Carolina. Among other tasks, all participants answered 11 numeracy questions including (a) one practice question, (b) three numeracy questions taken from the work of Schwartz et al. (1997), and (c) seven other questions (one of which had two parts) that were framed in the health domain (e.g., if the chance of getting a disease is 10% how many people would be expected to get the disease: (a) Out of 100, (b) Out of 1,000; see also Chaps. 2 and 15). Two questions had multiple-choice options while all others were open-ended. All questions were scored (0 or 1) with data aggregated across several studies and entered into a factor analysis. The analysis showed that a one factor solution was appropriate. Overall, results indicated that the refined test of Lipkus et al. (2001) was a reliable and internally consistent measure of western high-school and college educated individuals' statistical numeracy.

The results of Lipkus et al. (2001) were interesting for a number of reasons. First, they provided additional evidence that even among highly educated US community samples some sizable proportion of individuals was likely to be statistically innumerate (e.g., 20% failed simple questions dealing with risk magnitude). Such findings were and continue to be important as many efforts designed to support informed and shared decision-making rest on an erroneous assumption that decision-makers are numerate (or at least sufficiently statistically numerate, see Chap. 13; see also Guadagnoli and Ward 1998 and Schwartz et al. 1997). Second, results indicated that domain framing (e.g., medical vs. financial vs. abstract gambles) did not necessarily differentially affect test performance or comprehension. This finding suggests that various domain-specific items (e.g., items framed in terms of financial or medical or gambling risks) can provide a reasonable basis for the assessment of general statistical numeracy skills that can transfer across domains. Overall, for nearly a decade, the Lipkus et al. (2001) test, and its predecessor from Schwartz et al. (1997) have provided relatively short, reliable, and valuable instruments that have been used in more than 100 studies on topics such as medical decision making, shared decision making, trust, patient education, sexual behavior, stock evaluations, credit-card usage, graphical communication, and insurance decisions, among many others (see Lipkus and Peters 2009).

3.3 Psychometric Limits of Previous Measures of Numeracy

Despite its many successes and its influential role in advancing risky decision research, as anticipated by Lipkus et al. (2001), a growing body of data suggests some ways that the current numeracy instrument could be improved (for an item response theory based analysis see Schapira et al. 2009; see also Weller et al. 2012). For example, one major concern is that the Lipkus et al. (2001) test is not hard enough to adequately differentiate among the higher-performing, highly educated individuals who are often studied (e.g., convenience samples from major research universities). To illustrate, in one study of college students at Florida State University (a public research university in the USA), data indicated that the Lipkus et al. (2001) test was a significant predictor of risky decisions. The test, however, showed extensive negative skew with scores approaching the measurement ceiling (e.g., most participants answered more than 80% of items correctly, see Cokely and Kelley 2009; for similar results see also Peters et al. 2006, 2007a, 2008, and Schapira et al. 2009; for similar findings in physicians-in-training see Hanoch et al. 2010). Another recent study by Galesic and Garcia-Retamero (2010) using large probabilistic national samples of the whole populations of two countries (i.e., the USA and Germany) revealed negative skew in numeracy scores even among participants from the general population (see also Chap. 2).

A second psychometric concern is that there is relatively little known about the relations between either the Lipkus et al. (2001) or Schwartz et al. (1997) numeracy test and other individual differences, such as basic cognitive abilities (Liberali et al. 2012). To illustrate, one might argue that statistical numeracy is a useful predictor of risky choice simply because it serves as a proxy for fluid intelligence. It is well known that tests of general intelligence, particularly those designed to measure fluid intelligence, are valid and reliable predictors of a wide variety of socially desirable cognitive, behavioral, occupational, and health-related outcomes (Neisser et al. 1996).[2] Fluid intelligence tests such as Raven's Standard or Advanced Progressive Matrixes tend to be more time consuming yet also confer considerable benefits in terms of psychometric rigor and cross-cultural fairness (Raven 2000). To date,

[2] The underlying cognitive mechanisms that give rise to these effects are debated and remain unclear (Cokely et al. 2006; Ericsson et al. 2007; Fox et al. 2009; Neisser et al. 1996).

however, there are few tests that have investigated the extent to which the Lipkus et al. (2001) or Schwartz et al. (1997) instruments provide unique predictive power beyond other cognitive ability instruments either within or across cultures (see Chaps. 2, 9 and 11; see also Cokely and Kelley 2009; Galesic and Garcia-Retamero 2010; Garcia-Retamero and Galesic 2010a, 2010b; Liberali et al. 2012; Okan et al. 2012).

A third psychometric concern is that even if numeracy is compared with other abilities, the observed measurement skew and ceiling effects will complicate comparative evaluations (e.g., intelligence vs. statistical numeracy). Consider a recent study designed to investigate the extent to which each of several individual differences (e.g., executive functioning, cognitive impulsivity, and numeracy) influenced decision-making competence (Del Missier et al. 2010, 2012). The study found that numeracy was less related to some decision-making competencies as compared to measures of executive functioning or cognitive impulsivity, measured by the cognitive reflection test (Frederick 2005). However, it is possible that, at least in part, some negative skew in numeracy scores among the college student sample could have limited differentiation of those individuals with the highest levels of numeracy. In contrast, both executive functioning and the cognitive reflection tests are known to prove discrimination even among highly educated individuals. To be clear, our reading of the individual differences study by Del Missier et al. (2012) is that it represents precise and careful research using many of the best available methods and tools. However, the potential psychometric limits inherent in the now 10-year-old numeracy test leave open important questions. To the extent that a numeracy instrument does not adequately or accurately estimate variation in the sub-populations of interest it is not an efficient basis for theory development or policy evaluations.

3.4 Development and Validation of the Berlin Numeracy Test

Building on the work of Lipkus et al. (2001) and Schwartz et al. (1997), we endeavored to develop a new psychometrically sound statistical numeracy test that could be used with highly educated, high-ability samples. Here, our goal was not to develop a high-fidelity comprehensive test of statistical numeracy or of its sub-skills. Rather, the goal was to develop a brief, valid, and easy-to-use instrument, with improved discriminability. The development of the Berlin Numeracy Test began with pre-testing on a pool of items including all items from both the Lipkus et al. (2001) and Schwartz et al. (1997) tests along with other items that were internally generated. Following a protocol analysis in which participants solved all numeracy items while thinking aloud (see also Fox et al. 2011), we analyzed responses and selected 28 candidate questions for inclusion in the next stage of test development (i.e., 12 original items plus 16 new items).

3.4.1 Participants

We tested a community sample of 300 participants (57% women) from Berlin, Germany at the Max Planck Institute for Human Development. Participants were primarily current or former undergraduate or graduate students from the Humboldt, Free, and Technical Universities of Berlin. The mean participant age was approximately 26 years old (i.e., 25.9, SD = 4.0; range = 18–44). Each participant completed about 6 hours of testing over the course of 2–3 weeks in exchange for 40€ (ca. $55).

3.4.2 Stimuli and Procedure

A number of different instruments were used to provide convergent, discriminant, and predictive validity for the Berlin Numeracy Test. All comparative instruments are listed and described in Table 3.1. Participants were tested in three separate phases. In phase 1, all participants were tested individually via computer and/or with the assistance of a laboratory technician as required by the particular instrument. The first testing session lasted for approximately 2 hours and consisted primarily of cognitive ability instruments and cognitive performance tasks, including assessment of all candidate numeracy items. During this session calculators were not allowed; however, participants were provided with paper and pens/pencils for notes. In phase 2, participants completed an online assessment from their home including a variety of self-report personality and other survey instruments. All participants agreed to complete the online portion of the study in one session in which they sat alone, in a quiet room. In phase 3, participants returned about 2 weeks after phase 1 and completed another 2 hours of testing. All participants were again tested individually via computer and/or with the assistance of a laboratory technician as required by the particular instrument/task. The final 2 hours of testing involved new cognitive performance tasks including a battery of everyday risky decision-making questions that served as a means of assessing predictive validity.

3.4.3 Test Construction and Test Items

Our goal was to create a brief test that would score each participant on a 1–4 point interval scale corresponding to that participant's quartile rank relative to other highly educated individuals (i.e., higher scores are associated with higher quartiles). Performance quartiles for all participants were assessed according to performance on all 28 candidate statistical numeracy questions. A subset of five questions with a four-level tree structure was identified using the decision tree (i.e., categorization tree) application from the predictive modeling and forecasting software DTREG (Sherrod 2003). The tree structure was constructed such that participants arriving at each branch of the tree had approximately a 50% probability of answering correctly/

Table 3.1 Descriptions and references for tests used to establish psychometric validity of the Berlin Numeracy Test

Measure	Description	Reference
Fluid intelligence (RAPM)	Short form Raven's Advanced Progressive Matrices—a 12 item test of fluid intelligence	Bors and Stokes (1998)
Cognitive reflection (CRT)	The Cognitive Reflection Test uses 3 math questions to assess cognitive impulsivity	Frederick (2005)
Crystallized intelligence (vocabulary)	A 37 item "spot-a-word" German vocabulary test	Lindenberger et al. (1993)
Working memory capacity (span)	A multi-item performance measure of one's ability to control attention when simultaneously solving math operations and remember words	Turner and Engle (1989)
Understanding everyday risks	A multi-item test of one's understanding of information about consumer products, medical treatments, and weather forecasts	Cokely et al. (2012)
Maximizing–satisficing	A 13 item scale measuring one's tendency to maximize vs. satisfice during decision making	Schwartz et al. (2002)
Persistence	The Grit-S is an 8 item brief measure designed to assess persistence in the face of adversity	Duckworth et al. (2011)
Achievement motivation	The AMS-R is a 10 item trait assessment of one's general achievement motivation (e.g., one's desire to achieve good grades or performance evaluations)	Lang and Fries (2006)
Self-efficacy	A10 item self-report measure of one's general sense of self-efficacy	Schwarzer and Jerusalem (1995)
Personality	A 10 item assessment of the Big Five personality traits	Gosling et al. (2003)
Test anxiety	The TAI-G is a 20 item assessment of test-taking anxiety	Hodapp and Benson (1997)
Implicit theories	A 4 item measurement of the extent to which one believes that intelligence is stable vs. changeable	Blackwell et al. (2007)
Satisfaction with life	A 5 item instrument measuring self-reported levels of one's satisfaction with life	Diener et al. (1985)

incorrectly. The test's tree structure was subjected to cross-validation and showed less than 10% misclassification.[3] Subsequent analyses indicated that reducing the four-level solution to a simpler three-level solution (i.e., removing one problem) did not affect test classification performance or validity yet reduced test-taking time

[3] Although some misclassification is unavoidable, the algorithm rarely misclassified a participant by more than one quartile. The assessment is similar to an item response theory analysis, in that it identifies items with maximal discriminability across the range of item difficulty, with a guessing parameter of zero.

(i.e., 10% reduction), increased test format flexibility (i.e., simplified the paper-and-pencil format), and provided improved discriminability among new samples (see Sect. 3.6). All final Berlin Numeracy Test formats are based on the four questions used for the optimal three-level categorization tree as follows (see also Chap. 15):

1. Out of 1,000 people in a small town 500 are members of a choir. Out of these 500 members in a choir 100 are men. Out of the 500 inhabitants that are not in a choir 300 are men. What is the probability that a randomly drawn man is a member of the choir? Please indicate the probability in percent. ______ (*correct answer*: 25%)

2a. Imagine we are throwing a five-sided die 50 times. On average, out of these 50 throws how many times would this five-sided die show an odd number (1, 3 or 5)? ____ out of 50 throws (*correct answer*: 30)

2b. Imagine we are throwing a loaded die (6 sides). The probability that the die shows a 6 is twice as high as the probability of each of the other numbers. On average, out of these 70 throws how many times would the die show the number 6? ______out of 70 throws (*correct answer*: 20)

3. In a forest 20% of mushrooms are red, 50% brown, and 30% white. A red mushroom is poisonous with a probability of 20%. A mushroom that is not red is poisonous with a probability of 5%. What is the probability that a poisonous mushroom in the forest is red? ______ (*correct answer*: 50%)

3.4.4 Test Formats and Scoring

Different research environments have different constraints on factors such as computer-access, group-testing options, data-security requirements, etc. Accordingly, we designed the test to be flexible by offering multiple formats.

3.4.4.1 Computer-Adaptive Test Format

In this format, 2–3 questions (of 4 possible questions) are asked to participants. Questions are adaptively selected based on participants' past success in answering previous questions using an adaptive scoring algorithm (see Fig. 3.1 for test structure). The adaptive structure means that all questions have about a 50% probability of being answered correctly with subsequent questions adjusted on the basis of participants' prior answers. If an answer is correct/incorrect then a harder/easier question is automatically provided that again has a 50% probability of being right/wrong. A participant's skill-level can then be determined from answers to only 2–3 questions in roughly half the time normally required for the Lipkus et al. (2001) numeracy test (less than 3 min; see Table 3.2). To facilitate access, the computer-adaptive Berlin Numeracy Test is available online in a format that automatic scores participants' responses and reports data to researchers in terms of estimated partici-

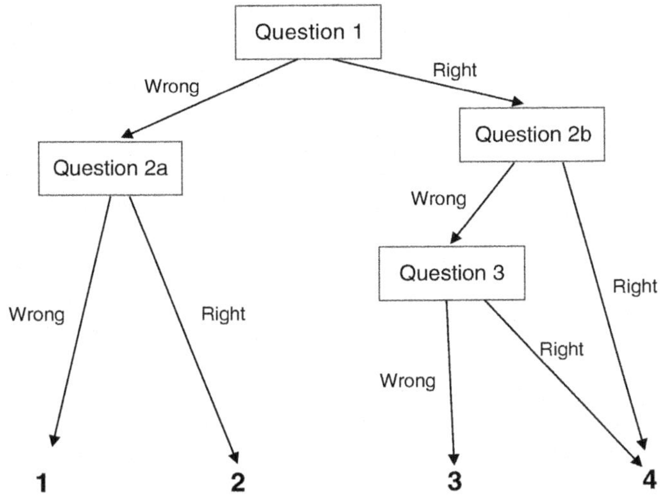

Fig. 3.1 The structure of the computer-adaptive Berlin Numeracy Test. Each question has a 50% probability of being right/wrong. If a question is answered right/wrong a harder/easier question is provided that again has a 50% probability of being right/wrong

pant quartile scores. This version of the test can also be accessed via internet ready hand-held devices (e.g., smart phones) for work in clinics or in the field. The online forum provides an option for the public to complete the test and receive feedback on their performance along with information about potential challenges they may face when making risky decisions. The test can be accessed at the following internet address: http://www.riskliteracy.org. Before completing any test items, the portal seamlessly redirects participants to a secure online location. Online data collection is managed and hosted via the unipark survey software system designed for academic research (unipark.de). We recommend that researchers use the computer-adaptive Berlin Numeracy Test whenever possible as this format provides an efficient balance between speed and psychometric accuracy, and allows us to continue to collect data to further refine the test.

3.4.4.2 Traditional (Paper-and-Pencil) Format

The alternative, traditional format requires that participants answer all four questions of the Berlin Numeracy Test in sequence. Scoring involves totaling all correct answers (i.e., 0–4 points possible). In this format, the structure of the adaptive test is ignored, although the adaptive scoring algorithm can be applied following data collection as might be useful for comparison with other samples. This alternative standard format may be useful when computerized testing is impractical (e.g., group

Table 3.2 Psychometric properties of the numeracy tests: Basic attributes, reliability, and discriminability

	Schwartz et al. (1997) 3 items	Lipkus et al. (2001) 11 items	Berlin Numeracy Test (Cokely et al. 2012) Computer-adaptive test format	Paper-and-pencil format	Single-item format
Basic attributes					
Range of possible scores	0–3	0–11	1–4	0–4	0–1
Range of achieved scores	0–3	5–11	1–4	0–4	0–1
Average score					
Mean	2.4	9.7	2.6	1.6	0.52
Median	3	10	3	2	1
Standard deviation	0.82	1.38	1.13	1.21	0.50
Length					
Number of items	3	11	2–3	4	1
Mean duration in minutes	1.2	4.5	2.6	4.3	1.1
Reliability					
Cronbach's alpha	0.52	0.54	–[a]	0.59	–[a]
Discriminability					
Item % correct (mean)	0.82	0.89	–[b]	0.41	0.52
Mean score of					
1st quartile	0.8	7.3	1.0	0.0	0.0
2nd quartile	2.0	9.0	2.0	1.0	
3rd quartile	3.0	10.0	3.0	2.0	1.0
4th quartile	3.0	11.0	4.0	3.3	

[a] Cronbach's alpha cannot be computed
[b] Approximately 50%, conditional on previous responses

testing, limited computer access). Testing requires about as long as the original Lipkus et al. (2001) numeracy test (i.e., less than 5 min).

3.4.4.3 Single-Item (Median) Format

When time is extremely limited, it is possible to use only the first item of the test (question 1; see Sect. 3.4.3) as a means of estimating median splits. Those who answer the question right are estimated to belong to the top half of highly educated participants while all others are assigned the bottom half. Note that the use of median splits can be problematic. Therefore, given the relatively small time savings over the adaptive format, we recommend this option be avoided whenever practical. Generally, this test format takes about as long as the Schwartz et al. (1997) instrument (i.e., about 1 min).

3.5 Results and Discussion

3.5.1 Psychometric Properties

Results of psychometric analyses are presented in Tables 3.2, 3.3, 3.4 and 3.5. The three formats of the Berlin Numeracy Test (i.e., computer-adaptive, paper-and-pencil, and single-item) are compared with the standard numeracy test by Lipkus et al. (2001) as well as with the brief three-item test by Schwartz et al. (1997).

Table 3.3 Psychometric properties of the numeracy tests: Convergent and discriminant validity

			Berlin Numeracy Test (Cokely et al. 2012)		
	Schwartz et al. (1997) 3 items	Lipkus et al. (2001) 11 items	Computer-adaptive test format	Paper-and-pencil format	Single-item format
Convergent validity					
Numeracy tests					
Lipkus et al. 11 items	0.75**				
Berlin Numeracy (computer-adaptive)	0.45**	0.49**			
Berlin Numeracy (paper-and-pencil)	0.50**	0.50**	0.91**		
Berlin Numeracy (single-item)	0.39**	0.42**	0.90**	0.75**	
Cognitive abilities/styles					
Fluid intelligence	0.41**	0.37**	0.48**	0.53**	0.41**
Cognitive reflection	0.40**	0.41**	0.51**	0.56**	0.41**
Crystallized intelligence	0.25**	0.21**	0.24**	0.25**	0.22**
Working memory span	0.14*	0.11	0.21**	0.20**	0.16**
Discriminant validity					
Motivation measures					
Maximizing–satisficing	0.01	0.04	0.05	0.04	0.05
Persistence (Grit-S)	0.02.	0.03	−0.05	−0.07	−0.03
Achievement motivation	−0.08	−0.10	−0.02	0.00	−0.01
Self-efficacy	0.00	−0.01	−0.01	0.02	0.03
Personality traits					
Emotional stability	−0.10	−0.05	0.01	0.05	−0.02
Conscientiousness	−0.09	−0.04	−0.09	−0.08	−0.06
Agreeableness	−0.03	−0.07	−0.14*	−0.08	−0.17**
Extraversion	−0.07	−0.06	−0.05	−0.05	−0.06
Openness to experience	−0.14*	−0.16**	−0.18**	−0.14*	−0.16**
Other measures					
Test anxiety	−0.15*	−0.16*	−0.12	−0.16*	−0.09
Implicit theories	−0.15*	−0.13**	−0.07	−0.10*	−0.04
Satisfaction with life	0.14*	0.08	0.12	0.16	0.07

*$p<0.05$; **$p<0.01$

Table 3.4 Psychometric properties of the numeracy tests: Predictive validity

			Berlin Numeracy Test (Cokely et al. 2012)		
	Schwartz et al. (1997) 3 items	Lipkus et al. (2001) 11 items	Computer-adaptive test format	Paper-and-pencil format	Single-item format
Predictive validity					
Understanding everyday risks	0.20**	0.18**	0.27**	0.31**	0.23**
Mean proportion correct of					
1st quartile	0.72	0.68	0.68	0.66	0.70
2nd quartile	0.74	0.66	0.70	0.70	
3rd quartile	0.78	0.78	0.74	0.78	0.78
4th quartile	0.78	0.78	0.84	0.84	

$^{**}p<0.01$

Table 3.5 Explanatory value of the numeracy tests over and above Raven Advanced Progressive Matrixes and cognitive reflection test scores (beta coefficients from hierarchical regression analyses)

			Berlin Numeracy Test (Cokely et al. 2012)		
	Schwartz et al. (1997) 3 items	Lipkus et al. (2001) 11 items	Computer-adaptive test format	Paper-and-pencil format	Single-item format
As single predictor	0.20**	0.20	0.29**	0.34**	0.25**
With CRT	0.09	0.08	0.17**	0.23**	0.14*
With Raven	0.14*	0.15*	0.24**	0.31**	0.19**

$^{*}p<0.05$; $^{**}p<0.01$

3.5.2 Basic Attributes

In our highly educated sample, scores on the standard Lipkus et al. (2001) numeracy scale show dramatic negative skew (see Table 3.2). Although possible scores range from 0 to 11, the lowest observed score was 5 (45% correct). Both the mean and median are close to the measurement ceiling (i.e., 88% and 91% correct, respectively). Similar levels of skew are observed for the Schwartz et al. (1997) test. In contrast, scores on the Berlin Numeracy Test are distributed evenly across the whole range of possible scores regardless of format. In addition, all Berlin Numeracy Test formats typically take less time to complete than the standard Lipkus et al. (2001) numeracy scale.

3.5.3 Convergent and Discriminant Validity

If the Berlin Numeracy Test is successful in assessing levels of statistical numeracy, it should correlate with other numeracy tests and with measures of cognitive ability (i.e., convergent validity). Moreover, to the extent the Berlin Numeracy Test primarily measures statistical numeracy it should not correlate with essentially unrelated constructs, such as motivation, personality, beliefs, or attitudes (i.e., discriminant validity). As Table 3.3 shows, both requirements—high correlations with related constructs and low with unrelated constructs—are satisfied for all three forms of Berlin Numeracy Test.

3.5.4 *Predictive Validity*

One of the intended purposes of the Berlin Numeracy Test is predicting people's understanding of risks in everyday contexts. To investigate the predictive validity of the Berlin Numeracy Test, we administered a short battery of items dealing with information about risks related to common consumer, health, and medical choices (e.g., evaluating toothpastes, cancer screenings), as well as information about probabilities typically used in forecasts (see Chap. 7; Galesic and Garcia-Retamero in press). Table 3.4 shows correlations of the different numeracy tests with the overall accuracy of answers to these items. All formats of the Berlin Numeracy Test were superior to the previous numeracy tests, essentially doubling the predictive resolution.

We further investigated the extent to which the Berlin Numeracy Test explained additional variance in risk understanding after controlling for the strongest alternative predictors of performance (i.e., fluid intelligence and cognitive reflection). As Table 3.5 shows, all formats of the Berlin Numeracy Test explain a substantial portion of additional variance after these others tests are included in a hierarchical regression model. In contrast, both the standard numeracy test by Lipkus et al. (in press) and the brief three-item test by Schwartz et al. (1997) lose most (or all) of their predictive power when intelligence or cognitive reflection tests are included. Overall, results indicate that the Berlin Numeracy Test is a reliable and valid test of statistical numeracy offering higher levels of discriminability and overcoming key psychometric limitations of previous numeracy tests.

3.6 Cross-Cultural Validation Studies

The initial validation of the Berlin Numeracy Test was completed on a sample of highly educated people living in a major metropolitan city in Germany. As a means of out-of-sample validation, we sought to assess the extent to which the test generalized to other highly educated samples from different cultures, presented in different languages. Specifically, we examined test performance in studies conducted in 14 different countries with diverse cultural backgrounds. Studies were conducted by different research groups, examining college-student samples at research-active universities, primarily drawn from introduction to psychology participant pools. Studies were conducted in China (Tsinghua University), Japan (University of Tokyo), India (Thapar University), Pakistan (University of Punjab), Norway (University of Oslo),[4] Sweden (Uppsala University), England (University College London), France (Universite de Lausanne), Germany (Max Planck Institute for Human Development), Switzerland (University of Basel), Poland (Wroclaw University), Portugal (University of Porto),[5] Spain (University of Granada), and the USA (Michigan Technological University).[6] In total, data from 2,379 college students was examined. All reported data are scored via the adaptive Berlin Numeracy Test algorithm, where 2–3 questions (out of 4) are used to estimate statistical numeracy quartiles for each participant.[7]

Overall results show that the test generally discriminated within desirable tolerances (i.e., ±10%) for each quartile (see Table 3.6). Aggregating across all samples, the mean test score was 51.7% correct, which closely approximated the ideal score of 50%. This score indicates that on average, across all countries, the first question of the Berlin Numeracy Test achieved the intended 50% discriminability. Across all countries, we also observed modest underestimation of the third quartile and commensurate overestimation in the top quartile (i.e., the fourth quartile). In part, higher top quartile scores may reflect the fact that several of our samples were collected from some elite, highly selective universities (e.g., University College London; Tsinghua University in China). Visual inspection reveals some positive and negative skewing of scores across various countries.[8] For example, Spain, Pakistan, and India all show positive skew. In contrast, the sample from China was the highest performing group, showing extreme negative skew. Overall, however, when all groups were averaged together differences approximated the intended quartiles. The observed distributions indicate that with only 2–3 statistical numeracy questions the Berlin Numeracy Test achieves good discriminability across most countries even when presented in different languages or when used at elite or technological/engineering universities.

---

[4] Data collection in Norway used a standard rather than adaptive form of the Berlin Numeracy Test. Data reported in the table are calculated using the adaptive scoring algorithm, which was highly correlated with overall score, $r_{154} = 0.90$. In the standard format the average score was 62% correct showing modest skew (0.29).

[5] Data collection in Portugal used a modified Berlin Numeracy Test. Therefore, data were only available for the single-item test and are not presented in Table 3.6. Overall 46.4% of participants ($n = 306$) from Portugal answered the first question right (theoretical ideal test score = 50%).

[6] We thank Nicolai Bodemer, Siegfried Dewitte, Stefan Herzog, Marcus Lindskog, Hitashi Lomash, Yasmina Okan, Jing Qian, Samantha Simon, Helena Szrek, Masanori Takezawa, Karl Teigen, Jan Woike, and Tomek Wysocki for assistance with cross cultural data collection.

[7] Translation involved iterative cycles of back-translation with revision.

[8] The Berlin Numeracy Test estimates quartiles and so caution is required when interpreting standard assessments of skew.

Table 3.6 Percentage of people in each quartile from 14 different countries estimated by the computer-adaptive test format of the Berlin Numeracy Test. Countries are ordered by their percentage of top quartile scores

Country	Language	*N*	1st quartile	2nd quartile	3rd quartile	4th quartile
China	English	166	0.04	0.07	0.14	0.75
Poland	Polish	205	0.14	0.20	0.22	0.44
England	English	420	0.20	0.31	0.14	0.35
Japan	Japanese	63	0.06	0.36	0.24	0.34
Sweden	Swedish	47	0.21	0.28	0.17	0.34
France	French	86	0.30	0.13	0.23	0.34
USA	English	55	0.20	0.29	0.20	0.31
Switzerland	German	503	0.26	0.23	0.23	0.28
Germany	German	173	0.29	0.21	0.22	0.28
Norway	Norwegian	156	0.25	0.24	0.25	0.26
Belgium	Dutch	50	0.30	0.30	0.16	0.24
India	English	83	0.19	0.52	0.08	0.21
Pakistan	English	114	0.29	0.41	0.19	0.11
Spain	Spanish	258	0.48	0.41	0.07	0.04
Total		2,379	0.23	0.28	0.18	0.31

3.7 Validation Across Different Populations

3.7.1 Numeracy in Physician Assistants

One goal for the Berlin Numeracy Test is to offer an instrument that can quickly assess statistical numeracy in working professionals. Of particular interest are those professionals who commonly make risky decisions and communicate risks. One such group in the USA is physician assistants. Physician assistants are independently licensed medical professionals who diagnose and treat patients, and provide care similar to that provided by a physician across all medical subspecialties (e.g., emergency medicine, family practice, surgery). Physician assistants' training typically involves 2 or 3 years of postgraduate study and clinical rotations, usually leading to a terminal master's degree.

As noted, previous studies of physicians-in-training in the UK (Hanoch et al. 2010) revealed dramatic skew in responses to the Lipkus et al. (2001) test. Specifically, in one sample of physician-in-training, Hanoch and colleagues found that the average Lipkus et al. (2001) test score was 95% correct, with 64% of participants answering all questions correctly. Here, we assessed performance of the Berlin Numeracy Test by administering the paper-and-pencil format to a group of physician assistant students ($n=51$) who were completing their final semester of training at the University of Oklahoma.[9] Results of the study indicated that the mean test score was 44.3% correct, which reasonably approximated the ideal score of

[9] We thank Robert Hamm for data collection.

Table 3.7 Percentage of people in each quartile from three different samples estimated by the computer-adaptive test format of the Berlin Numeracy Test

Sample	*N*	1st quartile	2nd quartile	3rd quartile	4th quartile
Graduating US physician assistants	51	0.16	0.39	0.29	0.16
General population of Sweden	213	0.20	0.36	0.24	0.20
USA web-panel sample (M-Turk)	1,612	0.49	0.27	0.12	0.13
Total	1,876	0.28	0.34	0.22	0.16

50%. Results also revealed very modest positive skew (0.16) indicating the test was generally well calibrated. A similar distribution was observed when the adaptive scoring algorithm was applied (Table 3.7). Note that in contrast to other highly educated samples, these data show slightly more central clustering of scores. To the extent this pattern generalizes, it suggests physician assistants are somewhat less likely to have either very low or high levels of statistical numeracy. Overall, results indicate that the Berlin Numeracy Test is well suited for use with these and other professionals and individuals with post-graduate educations. Ongoing research is assessing test performance among other professional groups (e.g., judges, lawyers, physicians, dieticians, financial advisors).

3.7.2 *Numeracy in the General Population*

The Berlin Numeracy Test was designed for, and normed with, highly educated individuals. However, considering the observed skew in scores from the Lipkus et al. (2001) test, the Berlin Numeracy Test may also be suitable for use with some well-educated general populations. As part of a larger validation and translation study, data were collected from 213 adults in Sweden who were sampled to be representative of the general population (see Lindskog et al. 2012).[10] The test was presented in Swedish and was administered using the computer-adaptive test format. Results show that the average test score was 48.8% correct, which closely approximated the theoretically ideal score of 50%. Distributions of estimated quartiles were somewhat concentrated around the middle quartiles, particularly the second quartile (see Table 3.7). This suggests that compared to other highly educated groups of individuals, there are moderately fewer people in Sweden with either very low or very high levels of statistical numeracy.

In addition, participants in this study also completed the Lipkus et al. (2001) test. As expected, results showed rather profound skew in scores with an average score

[10] This research was financed by the Swedish Research Council. We thank Marcus Lindskog and colleauges for these data.

of 83.5% correct and clear negative skew (−1.94). We compared the scores in the Lipkus et al. (2001) test in this study with those in the study of Galesic and Garcia-Retamero (2010) using probabilistic national samples in the USA and Germany (see Chap. 2). Results indicate that Swedish residents' scores showed considerably more negative skew reflecting significantly higher levels of numeracy compared to the populations in Germany, $t_{1,209}=9.29$, $p=0.001$, skew=−0.55, and the USA, $t_{1,375}=13.51$, $p=0.001$, skew=−0.33.

Overall, results indicate that the Berlin Numeracy Test is well suited for estimating numeracy among the general population of Sweden and other similar highly numerate countries. However, because the general population of Sweden is more numerate than that of either the USA or Germany, we can expect positive skew in general population samples from the USA, Germany, and other similar countries. Accordingly, when assessing statistical numeracy in most general populations we suggest including at least one other test in addition to the Berlin Numeracy Test (e.g., Weller et al. 2012). One promising strategy that adds only about 1 min in testing time is to combine the three-item Schwartz et al. (1997) test with the Berlin Numeracy Test data (for an example see Sect. 3.7.3). Ongoing studies are examining this potential strategy along with performance of the Berlin Numeracy Test in probabilistic national samples of residents in the USA.

3.7.3 Numeracy in Web-Panel Data

Behavioral scientists are increasingly using paid web panels for data collection and hypothesis testing. One popular option for data collection is Amazon.com's Mechanical Turk web panel (for a review see Paolacci et al. 2010). The first published study to assess numeracy among participants from Mechanical Turk was published in 2010. In this study, Paolacci et al. (2010) assessed numeracy using a subjective numeracy scale (see Chaps. 2 and 15; see also Fagerlin et al. 2007), which is known to correlate with the Lipkus et al. (2001) test. Results revealed an average subjective numeracy score of 4.4 (i.e., about 67% of maximum), which is in line with previously reported scores (e.g., participants recruited from a university hospital with a modest skew of −0.3; see Fagerlin et al. 2007). Similarly, we recently investigated numeracy using the Schwartz et al. (1997) test on a convenience sample using Mechanical Turk ($n=250$; Okan et al. 2012). Consistent with results from the subjective numeracy test, results showed an average score of 2.1 (i.e., 70% correct), which revealed moderate negative skew (−1.2). A total of 42% of the sample also answered 100% of the questions correct.

To evaluate the performance of web panelists on the Berlin Numeracy Test, we administered the computer-adaptive test format to a large Mechanical Turk web-panel convenience sample ($n=1{,}612$). All reported data were scored via the adaptive algorithm, where 2–3 questions (out of 4) are used to estimate statistical numeracy quartiles for each participant. As anticipated, we observed positive

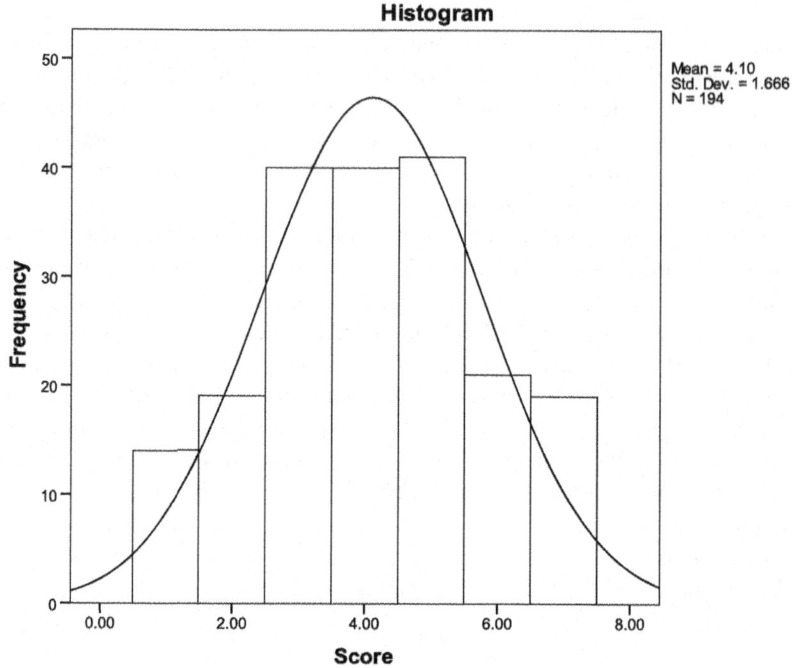

Fig. 3.2 Distribution of combined scores (Mechanical Turk web-panel sample) on the Berlin Numeracy Test and the Schwartz et al. (1997) three numeracy items

skew (0.90) in the sample scores indicating that the test was somewhat too difficult (see Table 3.7).[11] This finding of positive skew is not surprising given that the Berlin Numeracy Test was designed to measure numeracy among highly educated samples.

In the web-panel studies we mentioned above, we observed positive skew for the Berlin Numeracy Test and negative skew for the Schwartz et al. (1997) test. It stands to reason that combining the two tests would yield a better distribution, providing increased discriminability. Therefore, we conducted a new study including both the Schwartz et al. (1997) test and the Berlin Numeracy Test with a convenience sample of participants on Mechanical Turk ($n = 206$). When scored separately, we replicated the negative (−0.62) and positive (0.48) skewing of scores on the two tests. However, simply adding the two scores together yielded a normal distribution with no evidence of skew (−0.016; Fig. 3.2). In summary, combining the Berlin Numeracy Test with the Schwartz et al. (1997) test provides a very fast assessment (<4 min) with

[11] To the extent our data generalize, results suggest that our single question 2a (see Sect. 3.4.3) may allow for a rough approximation of a median split among Mechanical Turk participants. This question is simpler/easier than question 1 (see Sect. 3.4.4.3), and therefore was a good approximation of a median split in less highly educated samples.

good discriminability that is well suited for use with Mechanical Turk. In addition, combining both tests should also be appropriate for measuring numeracy in other general samples (e.g., older adults).

3.8 A Multiple-Choice Format

In some cases researchers may require more flexibility than the current Berlin Numeracy Test formats provide. For example, many psychometric tests are given in a multiple-choice format. Unfortunately, providing potential answers to participants increases the benefits of simple guessing. With four options, guessing would be expected to yield a score of approximately 25% correct. In contrast, in all other "fill in the blank" formats of the Berlin Numeracy Test, the contribution of a guessing parameter is essentially zero. To address this issue, we developed a multiple-choice format of the test, which began with an analysis of patterns of incorrect responses to previous tests from participants in the aforementioned Mechanical Turk study ($n=1{,}612$). For each question, we selected the most frequently listed incorrect options (recorded in 8–20% of incorrect answers). We then included the correct answer, the two highest frequency incorrect answers, and a "none of the above" option.

Next, we collected data from participants at the Michigan Technological University ($n=269$). Participants included convenience samples primarily from Departments of Psychology, Mechanical Engineering, and Computer Science. The majority of participants were undergraduate students, with a small proportion of the sample composed of either graduate students or faculty. Participants were either sent a link asking them to complete a survey via internal listservs or tests were administered in classes. Participants were presented with one of the two versions of the multiple-choice format differing only in the wording of question 1 (see Sect. 3.4.3).[12] This manipulation was conducted because we received feedback that some professional groups may be more willing to participate if questions seemed related to their areas of expertise (e.g., some medical doctors will see more face validity in questions about genetic mutations as compared to choir membership). Accurate responses to the new ($M=0.56$) vs. old ($M=0.60$) question did not reliably differ $\chi_1^2=0.26$. Distributions of scores did not significantly differ between tests either, $t_{267}=1.38$, $p=0.17$, and so data sets were combined for subsequent analyses. Overall, the mean multiple-choice test score was 55% correct, which reasonably approximated the ideal score of 50%. Analysis of distributions of responses indicated that the multiple-choice format showed no skew (−0.01). Results indicate that the multiple-choice format provided good discriminability and remained well balanced even when used with highly numerate individuals (e.g., computer science students).

[12] The exact wording of the alternative question is as follows: "Out of 1,000 people in a small town, 500 have a minor genetic mutation. Out of these 500 who have the genetic mutation, 100 are men. Out of the 500 inhabitants who do not have the genetic mutation, 300 are men. What is the probability that a randomly drawn man has the genetic mutation?"

3.9 Discussion and Conclusions

Over the last decade, the Schwartz et al. (1997) and Lipkus et al. (2001) numeracy tests have proven useful and even essential for some aspects of theory development, as well as for applications in risk communication. However, as anticipated by Lipkus et al. (2001), in the 10 years since publication of their test, research has identified a number of limitations and opportunities for improvement in measures of statistical numeracy. Building on the work of Lipkus et al. (2001), Schwartz et al. (1997), and many others (e.g., Peters et al. 2006, 2007b; Reyna et al. 2009), we developed and validated a flexible, multi-format test of statistical numeracy for risk literacy in educated samples: The Berlin Numeracy Test, which measures the range of statistical numeracy skill that is important for accurately interpreting and acting on information about risk. With the help of colleagues from around the world, we conducted 21 validation studies showing that a very short, adaptive format of the Berlin Numeracy Test provides sound assessment with dramatically improved discriminability across diverse populations, cultures, education levels, and languages. Content validity is clear in the types of questions included in the test—i.e., math questions involving ratio concepts and probabilities. Convergent validity was documented by showing high intercorrelations with other numeracy tests, as well as with other assessments of general cognitive abilities, cognitive styles, and education. Discriminant validity was documented by showing that the test was unrelated to common personality and motivation measures (e.g., uncorrelated with emotional stability). Predictive validity was documented by showing that the Berlin Numeracy Test provided unique predictive validity for both numeric and non-numeric everyday risky decision-making. This unique predictive validity held when statistically controlling for all the existing numeracy tests and other general ability and cognitive-style instruments. Taken together, results converge and contribute to our evolving understanding of the construct validity of numeracy.[13]

Going forward, more research is needed to document the causal linkages between numeracy and risky decision making (for a detailed discussion see Cokely et al. 2012). Theoretically, improving some types of math skills will improve risk literacy and risky decision making. However, the evidence of such benefits along with quantification of the magnitudes of benefits is surprisingly limited (e.g., how much study time is required to improve decisions). As well, despite the utility of current theoretical frameworks, our theoretical understanding underlying mechanisms is underspecified. Research is likely to benefit by more closely aligning with current research in mathematics and general literacy education, as well as research on mathematics development (e.g., Siegler 1988), mathematics expertise, and training

[13]According to Cronbach and Meehl's (1955) review of construct validity "a construct is some postulated attribute of people, assumed to be reflected in test performance." Similarly, contemporary views hold that construct validity "…is not a property of the test or assessment as such, but rather of the meaning of the test scores" which is established by integrating and evaluating multiple lines of evidence (Messick 1995).

for transfer. Additionally, there is a need for validated tests that provide larger item pools and parallel forms that can be administered multiple times to assess learning. Related development efforts are currently underway for the Berlin Numeracy Test.

It is important to again note that the Berlin Numeracy Test is designed specifically for educated samples (e.g., college students, business, medical, and legal professionals). Discriminability will be reduced when assessing individuals who have lower levels of educational attainment or when administered to groups that come from considerably less selective universities (i.e., the Berlin Numeracy Test will show some positive skew in less educated samples). When this is a concern, researchers can include an additional instrument such as the fast three-item test by Schwartz et al. (1997). The results of our Mechanical Turk's web-panel study (see Sect. 3.7.3) show that this strategy can produce excellent discriminability with virtually no skew providing a 4-min assessment that is sensitive to both low and high levels of statistical numeracy.

Because the Berlin Numeracy Test provides a broad estimate of variation in statistical numeracy it is not able to provide detailed assessment of differences in specific numeracy skills, such as identifying deficits in reasoning about probability as compared to proportions or multiplication. As noted, factor analytic research by Liberali et al. (2012) indicates that, at least with respect to some risky decisions and judgments, component numeracy skills (e.g., multiplication vs. probability) may be differentially beneficial.[14] We also currently do not have any theoretical account systematically linking component numeracy skills and competencies with the many various types of risky decisions people commonly face. There is a need for larger scale cognitive process tracing and factor analytic assessments to be conducted across all aspects of numeracy, risk literacy, and risky decision making. Initial studies may benefit by examining relations between established numeracy tests, component math skills, and other established instruments such as the advanced decision-making competency tests (Bruine de Bruin et al. 2007; Parker and Fischhoff 2005).

Future research will need to use methods that provide details about the ecological frequencies of problematic risky decisions related to numeracy, including techniques like representative sampling (Dhami et al. 2004). This type of epidemiological data could then be used to start to quantify the economic, personal, and social impact of specific weaknesses in numeracy and risk literacy (e.g., is denominator neglect a dangerous factor in high-stakes risky decisions and to what extent does numeracy inoculate? For related discussion see Chap. 10; see also Garcia-Retamero et al. 2012). This ecological approach would provide essential input for relative prioritization of different interventions (i.e., which kind of problems do the most harm and which kinds of interventions will produced the biggest benefits). Unfortunately, because there may be many numeracy skills a test of all component skills may turn out to be very long. In this case, and perhaps even if a comprehensive test is not particularly long, adaptive testing is likely to offer many benefits (Thompson and Weiss 2011).

[14] The factor structures varied across two studies, which complicate interpretation. Nevertheless, the results are suggestive.

Research on all these topics is ongoing in our laboratories. As new tools, interactive activities, and improved tests become available they will be added to the content on http://www.riskliteracy.org (for other individual difference measures see also Appelt et al. 2011; http://www.sjdm.org/dmidi/).

References

Appelt, K. C., Milch, K. F., Handgraaf, M. J. J., & Weber, E. U. (2011). The decision making individual differences inventory and guidelines for the study of individual differences in judgment and decision-making research. *Judgment and Decision Making, 6*, 252–262.

Black, W. C. W., Nease, R. F. R., & Tosteson, A. N. A. (1995). Perceptions of breast cancer risk and screening effectiveness in women younger than 50 years of age. *Journal of the National Cancer Institute, 87*, 720–731.

Blackwell, L., Trzesniewski, K., & Dweck, C. S. (2007). Implicit theories of intelligence predict achievement across an adolescent transition: A longitudinal study and an intervention. *Child Development, 78*, 246–263.

Bors, D. A., & Stokes, T. L. (1998). Raven's advanced progressive matrices: Norms for first-year university students and the development of a short form. *Educational and Psychological Measurement, 58*, 382–398.

Bruine de Bruin, W. B., Parker, A. M., & Fischhoff, B. (2007). Individual differences in adult decision-making competence. *Journal of Personality and Social Psychology, 92*, 938–956.

Cokely, E. T., Galesic, M., Schulz, E., Ghazal, S., & Garcia-Retamero, R. (2012). Measuring risk literacy: The Berlin Numeracy Test. *Judgment and Decision Making, 7*, 25–47.

Cokely, E. T., & Kelley, C. M. (2009). Cognitive abilities and superior decision making under risk: A protocol analysis and process model evaluation. *Judgment and Decision Making, 4*, 20–33.

Cokely, E. T., Kelley, C. M., & Gilchrist, A. H. (2006). Sources of individual differences in working memory: Contributions of strategy to capacity. *Psychonomic Bulletin and Review, 13*, 991–997.

Cronbach, L. J., & Meehl, P. E. (1955). Construct validity in psychological tests. *Psychological Bulletin, 52*, 281–302.

Del Missier, F., Mäntylä, T., & Bruine de Bruin, W. (2010). Executive functionions in decision making: An individual differences approach. *Thinking and Reasoning, 16*, 69–97.

Del Missier, F. T., Mäntylä, T., & Bruine de Bruin, W. (2012). Decision-making competence, executive functioning, and general cognitive abilities. *Journal of Behavioral Decision Making*. doi: 10.1002/bdm.731

Dhami, M. K., Hertwig, R., & Hoffrage, U. (2004). The role of representative design in an ecological approach to cognition. *Psychological Bulletin, 130*, 959–988.

Diener, E., Emmons, R. A., Larsen, R., & Griffin, S. (1985). The satisfaction with life scale. *Journal of Personality Assessment, 49*, 71–75.

Duckworth, A. L., Quinn, P. D., Lynam, D. R., Loeber, R., & Stouthamer-Loeber, M. (2011). Role of test motivation in intelligence testing. *Proceedings of the National Academy of Sciences, 108*, 7716–7720.

Ericsson, A., Prietula, M. J., & Cokely, E. T. (2007). The making of an expert. *Harvard Business Review, 85*, 114–121.

Fagerlin, A., Zikmund-Fisher, B., Ubel, P. A., Jankovic, A., Derry, H. A., & Smith, D. M. (2007). Measuring numeracy without a math test: Development of the subjective numeracy scale. *Medical Decision Making, 27*, 672–680.

Feltz, A., & Cokely, E. T. (2009). Do judgments about freedom and responsibility depend on who you are? Personality differences in intuitions about compatibilism and incompatibilism. *Consciousness and Cognition, 18*, 342–350.

Feltz, A., & Cokely, E. T. (2012). The philosophical personality argument. *Philosophical Studies*. doi: 10.1007/s11098-011-9731-4

Fox, M. C., Ericsson, K. A., & Best, R. (2011). Do procedures for verbal reporting of thinking have to be reactive? A meta-analysis and recommendations for best reporting methods. *Psychological Bulletin, 137*, 316–344.

Fox, M. C., Roring, R., & Mitchum, A. L. (2009). Reversing the speed-IQ correlation: Intra-individual variability and attentional control in the inspection time paradigm. *Intelligence, 37*, 76–80.

Frederick, S. (2005). Cognitive reflection and decision making. *Journal of Economic Perspectives, 19*, 25–42.

Galesic, M., & Garcia-Retamero, R. (2010). Statistical numeracy for health: A cross-cultural comparison with probabilistic national samples. *Archives of Internal Medicine, 170*, 462–468.

Galesic, M., & Garcia-Retamero, R. (in press). Using analogies to communicate information about health risks. Applied Cognitive Psychology. doi: 10.1002/acp.2866.

Garcia-Retamero, R., & Galesic, M. (2010a). How to reduce the effect of framing on messages about health. *Journal of General Internal Medicine, 25*, 1323–1329.

Garcia-Retamero, R., & Galesic, M. (2010b). Who profits from visual aids: Overcoming challenges in people's understanding of risks. *Social Science and Medicine, 70*, 1019–1025.

Garcia-Retamero, R., Okan, Y., & Cokely, E. T. (2012). Using visual aids to improve communication of risks about health: A review. *The Scientific World Journal*. Article ID 562637. Doi:10.1100/2012/562637

Gosling, S. D., Rentfrow, P. J., & Swann, W. B. (2003). A very brief measure of the big-five personality domains. *Journal of Research in Personality, 37*, 504–528.

Guadagnoli, E., & Ward, P. (1998). Patient participation in decision-making. *Social Science and Medicine, 47*, 329–339.

Hanoch, Y., Miron-Shatz, T., Cole, H., Himmelstein, M., & Federman, A. D. (2010). Choice, numeracy and physicians-in-training performance: The case of Medicare part D. *Health Psychology, 29*, 454–459.

Hodapp, V., & Benson, J. (1997). The multidimensionality of test anxiety: A test of different models. *Anxiety, Stress, and Coping, 10*, 219–244.

Lang, J. W. B., & Fries, S. (2006). A revised 10-item version of the Achievement Motives Scale: Psychometric properties in German-speaking samples. *European Journal of Psychological Assessment, 22*, 216–224.

Liberali, J. M., Reyna, V. F., Furlan, S., Stein, L. M., & Pardo, S. T. (2012). Individual differences in numeracy and cognitive reflection, with implications for biases and fallacies in probability judgment. *Journal of Behavioral Decision Making*. doi: 10.1002/bdm.752

Lindenberger, U., Mayr, U., & Kliegl, R. (1993). Speed and intelligence in old age. *Psychology and Aging, 8*, 207–220.

Lindskog, M., Kerimi, N., Winman, A., & Juslin, P. (2012). A Swedish validation study of the Berlin Advanced Numeracy Test (manuscript in preparation).

Lipkus, I. M., & Peters, E. (2009). Understanding the role of numeracy in health: Proposed theoretical insights. *Health Education & Behavior, 36*, 1065–1081.

Lipkus, I. M., Samsa, G., & Rimer, B. K. (2001). General performance on a numeracy scale among highly-educated samples. *Medical Decision Making, 21*, 37–44.

Messick, S. (1995). Validity of psychological assessment: Validation of inferences from persons responses and performances as scientific inquiry into score meaning. *The American Psychologist, 50*, 741–749.

Neisser, U., Boodoo, G., Bouchard, T. J., Boykin, A. W., Brody, N., Ceci, S. J., et al. (1996). Intelligence: Knowns and unknowns. *The American Psychologist, 51*, 77–101.

Okan, Y., Garcia-Retamero, R., Cokely, E. T., & Maldonado, A. (2012). Individual differences in graph literacy: Overcoming denominator neglect in risk comprehension. *Journal of Behavioral Decision Making*. doi: 10.1002/bdm.751

Paolacci, G., Chandler, J., & Ipeirotis, P. G. (2010). Running experiments on Amazon Mechanical Turk. *Judgment and Decision Making, 5*, 411–419.

Parker, A. M., & Fischhoff, B. (2005). Decision-making competence: External validation through an individual differences approach. *Journal of Behavioral Decision Making, 18*, 1–27.

Peters, E., Dieckmann, N. F., Dixon, A., Slovic, P., Mertz, C. K., & Hibbard, J. H. (2007a). Less is more in presenting quality information to consumers. *Medical Care Research and Review, 64*, 169–190.

Peters, E., Hibbard, J. H., Slovic, P., & Dieckmann, N. F. (2007b). Numeracy skill and the communication, comprehension, and use of risk and benefit information. *Health Affairs, 26*, 741–748.

Peters, E., Slovic, P., Västfjäll, D., & Mertz, C. K. (2008). Intuitive numbers guide decisions. *Judgment and Decision Making, 3*, 619–635.

Peters, E., Västfjäll, D., Slovic, P., Mertz, C. K., Mazzocco, K., & Dickert, S. (2006). Numeracy and decision making. *Psychological Science, 17*, 407–413.

Raven, J. (2000). The Raven's progressive matrices: Change and stability over culture and time. *Cognitive Psychology, 41*, 1–48.

Reyna, V. F., Nelson, W. L., Han, P. K., & Dieckmann, N. F. (2009). How numeracy influences risk comprehension and medical decision making. *Psychological Bulletin, 135*, 943–973.

Schapira, M. M., Walker, C. M., & Sedivy, S. K. (2009). Evaluating existing measures of health numeracy using item response theory. *Patient Educational and Counseling, 75*, 308–314.

Schulz, E., Cokely, E. T., & Feltz, A. (2011). Persistent bias in expert judgments about free will and moral responsibility: A test of the expertise defense. *Consciousness and Cognition, 20*, 1722–1731.

Schwartz, B., Ward, A., Monterosso, J., Lyubomirsky, S., White, K., & Lehman, D. R. (2002). Maximizing versus satisficing: Happiness is a matter of choice. *Journal of Personality and Social Psychology, 83*, 1178–1197.

Schwartz, L. M. L., Woloshin, S. S., Black, W. C. W., & Welch, H. G. H. (1997). The role of numeracy in understanding the benefit of screening mammography. *Annals of Internal Medicine, 127*, 966–972.

Schwarzer, R., & Jerusalem, M. (1995). Generalized self-efficacy scale. In J. Weinman, S. Wright, & M. Johnston (Eds.), *Measures in health psychology: A user's portfolio* (pp. 35–37). Windsor: Nfer-Nelson.

Sherrod, P. H. (2003). *DTREG: Predictive Modeling Software*. http://www.dtreg.com, accessed June 30, 2012.

Siegler, R. S. (1988). Strategy choice procedures and the development of multiplication skill. *Journal of Experimental Psychology: General, 117*, 258–275.

Stanovich, K. E., & West, R. F. (2000). Advancing the rationality debate. *The Behavioral and Brain Sciences, 23*, 701–726.

Stanovich, K. E., & West, R. F. (2008). On the relative independence of thinking biases and cognitive ability. *Journal of Personality and Social Psychology, 94*, 672–695.

Thompson, N. A., & Weiss, D. J. (2011). A framework for the development of computerized adaptive tests. *Practical Assessment, Research, and Evaluation, 16*, 1–9.

Turner, M. L., & Engle, R. W. (1989). Is working memory capacity task dependent? *Journal of Memory and Language, 28*, 127–154.

Weller, J. A., Dieckmann, N., Tusler, M., Mertz, C. K., Burns, W., & Peters, E. (2012). Development and testing of an abbreviated numeracy scale: A rasch analysis approach Journal of Behavioral Decision Making. doi: 10.1002/bdm.1751

Zikmund-Fisher, B., Smith, D. M., Ubel, P. A., & Fagerlin, A. (2007). Validation of the subjective numeracy scale: Effects of low numeracy on comprehension of risk communications and utility elicitations. *Medical Decision Making, 27*, 663–671.

Chapter 4
Graph Literacy for Health*

Mirta Galesic and Rocio Garcia-Retamero

Abstract Visual displays are often used to facilitate communication of important medical information to patients. However, even the simplest graphs are not understood by everyone. In this chapter, we develop and test a scale to measure health-related graph literacy and investigate the level of graph literacy in the USA and Germany. The scale was developed in the laboratory and tested on national samples in the two countries. The graph literacy scale predicted which patients can benefit from visual aids and had promising measurement properties. Results showed that approximately one-third of the population in the USA and Germany had both low-graph literacy and low-numeracy skills.

4.1 Introduction and Background

Graph literacy, or the ability to understand graphically presented information, is essential in everyday life: graphs are ubiquitous in newspapers and magazines, on television, and the Internet. Graphs often provide important information for medical,

*In this chapter, we partially reproduced the article Galesic, M., & Garcia-Retamero, R. (2011). Graph literacy: A cross-cultural comparison. *Medical Decision Making*, *31*, 444–457.

M. Galesic, Ph.D. (✉)
Center for Adaptive Behavior and Cognition, Max Planck Institute for Human Development, Lentzeallee 94, Berlin 14195, Germany
e-mail: galesic@mpib-berlin.mpg.de

R. Garcia-Retamero, Ph.D.
Departamento de Psicología Experimental, Facultad de Psicología, University of Granada, Campus Universitario de Cartuja s/n, Granada 18071, Spain

Center for Adaptive Behavior and Cognition, Max Planck Institute for Human Development, Lentzeallee 94, Berlin 14195, Germany
e-mail: rretamer@ugr.es

R. Garcia-Retamero and M. Galesic (eds.), *Transparent Communication of Health Risks: Overcoming Cultural Differences*, DOI 10.1007/978-1-4614-4358-2_4,

financial, nutritional, and political choices. Recent studies have shown that graphical displays—bar charts, pie charts, line plots, and icon arrays—can improve understanding of the risks and benefits associated with medical treatments, screenings, and life-styles (see Chaps. 9–11; Ancker et al. 2006; Lipkus 2007; Lipkus and Hollands 1999).

However, even the simplest graphs may be difficult to understand for many people. Bar charts, pie charts, and line plots were first used in the late eighteenth and early nineteenth century. William Playfair, an economist and author of *Commercial and Political Atlas* (1786) and *Statistical Breviary* (1801), first used those graphical formats (Friel et al. 2001; Spence 2005). Icon arrays are even more recent: they began to be widely used only in the early twentieth century, when Otto Neurath (1882–1945), a philosopher, economist, and a prominent member of the Vienna Circle, used them to explain complex social and economic statistics to uneducated Viennese (Neurath 1936). In other words, in most of human history there were no graphical representations of statistical information—at least not in the formats that are ubiquitous today. Therefore, there is no immediate reason that people should understand such graphs intuitively. For example, although pie charts are used very frequently to communicate various statistical facts, the scientific evidence about their usefulness is equivocal (Feldman-Stewart et al. 2000; Spence 2005; Spence and Lewandowsky 1991).

The work described in this chapter has two aims. The first aim is to develop a scale that can be used to assess the graph literacy skills needed to understand risks in the health domain. To date, graph understanding has not been assessed by any health literacy instrument (Ancker and Kaufman 2007). Within national assessments of literacy (Kutner et al. 2006), only a few document literacy questions investigate selected aspects of graph comprehension, but most of these items are relatively complex and require an advanced understanding of graphs. In a similar vein, Kramarski and Mevarech (2003) developed a 36-item Graph Interpretation Test to investigate the effects of different instructional methods on the ability of eighth-grade students to interpret graphs in general. However, their test is not embedded in the health domain, is too long to be used in clinical practice, is focused mostly on line graphs, and involves questions that require relatively advanced graph interpretation skills. Therefore, we have constructed a new graph literacy scale that (a) investigates both basic graph-reading skills and more advanced graph comprehension, (b) involves examples of different types of graphs, (c) is embedded in the context of medical decisions, and (d) is brief enough for use in everyday clinical practice.

The second aim is to investigate the extent and distribution of graph (il)literacy on probabilistic national samples in the USA and Germany—two countries with very different educational and medical systems. It is known that a significant part of the general population has problems understanding numerically presented statistical data, in particular lower educated people (see Chap. 2; see also Galesic and Garcia-Retamero 2010; Schwartz et al. 1997). The same may hold for understanding of graphs. Indeed, a portion of the population may have problems with understanding *both* numerically and graphically presented information. To promote informed medical decision making, it is important to identify these people and either train them to understand existing forms of graphs, or offer them representations that can be understood without training.

In what follows, we first describe the development and evaluation of the new graph literacy scale. We then report on the level of graph literacy in the USA and Germany.

4.2 Study 1: Development of the Graph Literacy Scale

To determine which items to include in our graph literacy scale, we started from the traditional division of graph comprehension skills on three levels (Friel et al. 2001). On the first level, one should have the ability to *read the data*, that is, to find specific information in a graph. For example, one should be able to read the height of a particular bar within a bar chart or the number of icons of a particular type in an icon array. On the second level, one should be able to *read between the data*, that is, to find relationships in the data as shown on a graph. For instance, one should be able to read the difference between two bars or sets of icons or sum up several slices on a pie chart. The highest level of graph comprehension is reflected in the ability to *read beyond the data* or make inferences and predictions from the data. For example, one should be able to project a future trend from a line chart, understand the importance of attending to scale ranges and scale labels when comparing two charts, and use the existing labels to interpolate scale labels that are missing. For examples of items measuring each of the three skills, see Fig. 4.1.

Following this classification, we developed the 42 items included in the initial scale. In creating these items, we were guided by several principles. First, we embedded all graphs in a medical context—each presented data that patients could realistically encounter when making health-related decisions. For example, we included tasks dealing with the communication of medical risks, treatment efficiencies, prevalence of diseases, etc. Second, we designed items to cover four frequently used graph types—line plots, bar charts, pies, and icon arrays (Ancker et al. 2006; Lipkus 2007; Lipkus and Hollands 1999; Spence and Lewandowsky 1991). Third, we varied the complexity of graphs by changing the number of data series displayed on the same graph (one, two, or three), and whether the data were uni-dimensional or bi-dimensional.

4.2.1 Method

4.2.1.1 Participants

We pretested the initial version of the scale on convenience samples of 60 German students (33 women, mean age 24.8 years) and 60 German older adults (31 women,

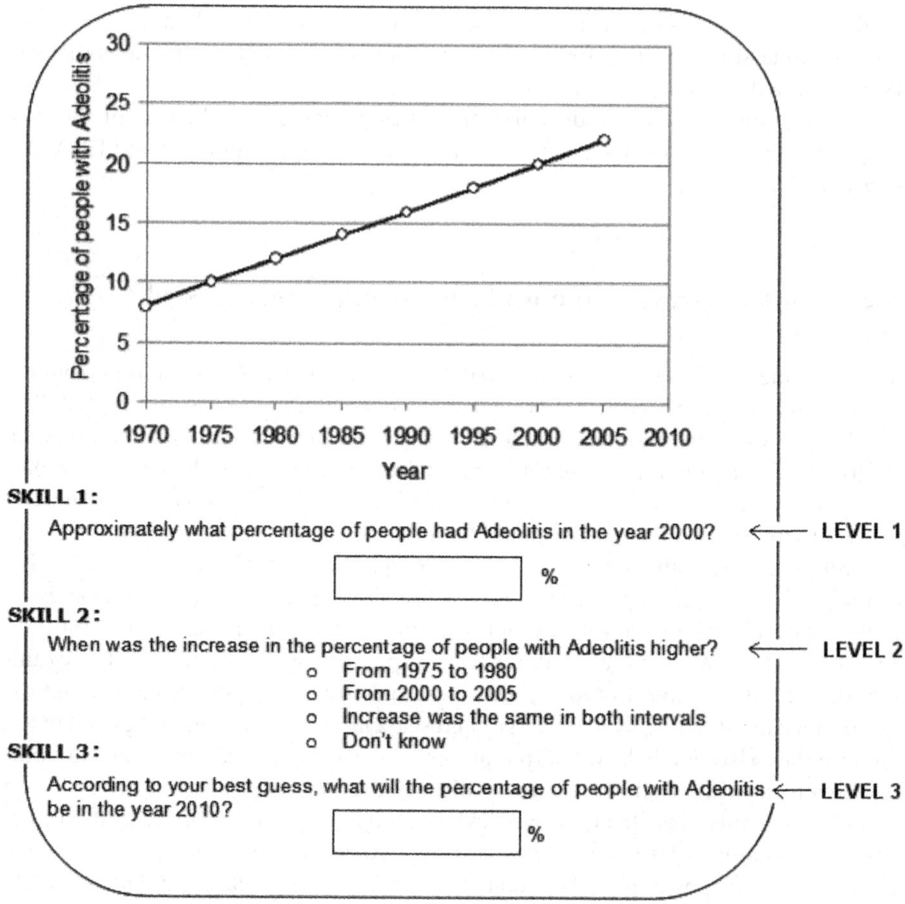

Fig. 4.1 Examples of tasks measuring three levels of graph comprehension. Level 1 is the ability to read the data. Level 2 is the ability to read between the data. Level 3 is the ability to read beyond the data

mean age 67.0 years, 31 with high school and 29 with college education), recruited from the pool of participants maintained by the Max Planck Institute for Human Development in Berlin. Participants were compensated at 10 Euros per hour.

4.2.1.2 Stimuli and Procedure

The scale was administered on computers in our laboratory. Besides the newly developed, 42-item graph literacy scale, we also administered several previously developed items to evaluate convergent validity. These items investigated several aspects of graph comprehension, including reading the data, reading between the data, and reading beyond the data (Friel et al. 2001). We selected items from the International Adult Literacy Survey (IALS; Tuijnman 2000), the National Assessment of Adult Literacy (NAAL; National Center for Education Statistics 1985), and the Program for International Student Assessment (PISA 2003). We also included two items from Kramarski and Mevarech's (2003) Graph Interpretation Test and an additional unpublished item kindly shared with us by those authors. This last item measured the ability to recognize which of several graphs depicts the relationship between time and distance of a car traveling from one place to another and back.

Participants completed two additional measures that served to establish the divergent validity of the new graph literacy scale. First, they completed three of the four items from the numeracy part of the short form of the Test of Functional Health Literacy (Baker et al. 1999). The excluded item (understanding the information on an appointment slip for a diabetic clinic) was judged to be too culturally and content-specific. Second, participants completed four numeracy items selected from Schwartz et al. (1997) and Lipkus et al. (2001; see Chaps. 2 and 15). Both scales included items designed to measure the basic numerical skills needed to understand statistical information.

4.2.2 Results

We evaluated the scale on several criteria: duration, discriminability (i.e., the ability to differentiate between those taking the test; Kline 1998), reliability, and validity.

Duration. The initial version of the graph literacy scale took on average 21 min to complete (SD=8.0; median: 19 min). Older people took significantly longer to complete the scale compared to the students (M=27, SD=7.0 vs. M=16, SD=4.1 min, respectively).

Discriminability. Participants completed from 10 to 41 items correctly, with an overall mean of 34 correct items (students: 36 items; older adults: 31 items). The probability of answering individual items correctly ranged from 10% to 99%, with a mean of 80%. The discriminability of items was higher among the older adults than among the students.

Reliability. The correlations between individual items and the total score ranged from 0.07 to 0.63, with a mean of 0.38. Cronbach's alpha was 0.85, indicating a satisfactory level of internal consistency.

Validity. The average correlation of the total score with the graph comprehension items taken from the existing literacy questionnaires was 0.44, indicating a satisfactory convergent validity. As for the divergent validity, the correlation with the test of functional literacy was 0.19, suggesting that it measures a different type of skill. The correlation with the numeracy scale was relatively high at 0.51, suggesting that the same meta-cognitive abilities that lead to high numeracy scores also foster good graph literacy skills. We discuss the implications of these results in Sect. 4.5.

4.3 Study 2: Evaluation of the Graph Literacy Scale

Based on the pretest results, we selected 13 items to be included in the refined version of the scale. The items were chosen according to the following criteria (1) discriminability (percent correct lower than 90%), (2) item-total correlation of at least 0.3, (3) correlation with existing graph comprehension items of at least 0.3, (4) representation of the three levels of graph comprehension (reading the data, reading between the data, and reading beyond the data) and of different types of graphs (bar, pie, and line charts, as well as icon arrays), and (5) the scale had to be short—ideally not longer than 10 min—and efficient, with each item measuring a somewhat different aspect of graph literacy. The items included in the complete scale in English, German, and Spanish are shown in Chap. 15.

4.3.1 Method

4.3.1.1 Participants

The final version of the scale was administered on probabilistic national samples in the USA and Germany as part of the project "Helping people with low numeracy understand medical information," funded by the Foundation for Informed Medical Decision Making. The project involved a survey that gathered data for a number of studies related to understanding and communicating risks (see also Chaps. 2, 7–11, and 13), using large national samples of participants ($n = 1{,}009$ in the USA and $n = 1{,}001$ in Germany for the overarching project). Randomly selected groups of 492 participants in the USA and of 495 in Germany were asked to answer the questions presented in this study. The sample structure is shown in Table 4.1 (see Chap. 2 for more details about the sample and the methodology of the survey).

4.3.1.2 Stimuli and Procedure

The questionnaire was administered through the Web. Some respondents (62% in the USA and 64% in Germany) completed the questionnaire via personal computers, while the rest used Web TV with infrared keyboards. We checked whether this variable affected the results but did not find any differences between the two groups in either country.

We put special effort into making the English and German versions of the questionnaire comparable. All questions were developed in English and edited by a native English speaker, translated into German by a native German speaker with excellent knowledge of English, back-translated into English by another person of equivalent language skills, and compared with the original English version (see Chap. 2 for more details about the translation of the materials and the programmed questionnaire). The Ethics Committee of the Max Planck Institute for Human Development approved the methodology, and all participants consented to participation through an online consent form at the beginning of the survey.

Table 4.1 Structure of the sample of participants in study 2 in terms of gender, age, and education

	USA			Germany		
	Sample size (unweighted)	Sample % (weighted)	Population %[a]	Sample size (unweighted)	Sample % (weighted)	Population %[b]
Total	492	100	100	495	100	100
Gender						
Male	236	48.4	49.2	254	50.3	49.9
Female	256	51.6	50.8	241	49.7	50.1
Age						
25–39	120	31.2	35.7	125	31.4	32.5
40–54	194	40.6	38.3	210	39.0	39.9
55–69	178	28.2	26.1	160	29.6	27.7
Education						
High school or less	356	44.5	44.6	393	74.1	72.3
Some college or more[c]	136	55.5	55.4	102	25.9	27.7

[a] Statistisches Bundesamt Deutschland, Microcensus (2007) (http://www-genesis.destatis.de/genesis/online)

[b] US Census Bureau, Current Population Survey (2008) Annual Social and Economic Supplement (http://www.census.gov/cps/)

[c] In Germany, this category includes people with Abitur

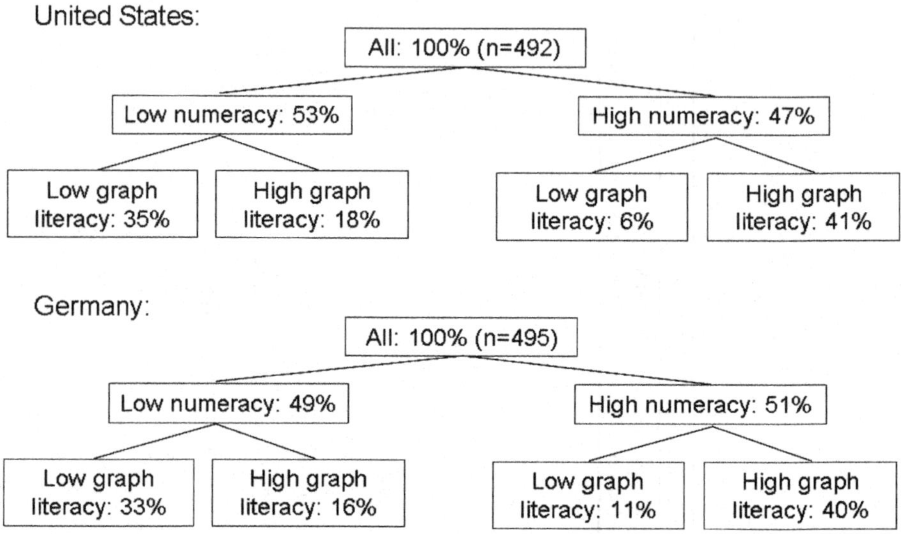

Fig. 4.2 Graph literacy skills among people with low- and high-numeracy skills, in the USA and Germany in Study 2. Groups are defined by median split (for numeracy: 6, for graph literacy: 9 correct answers)

4.3.2 Results

The final version of the graph literacy scale took 9–10 min to complete ($M=10.1$, SD=5.7 in the USA, and $M=9.2$, SD=5.7 in Germany) and had good measurement properties. When calculating participants' results, we required exactly correct answers to all questions except for question Q7, where we allowed as correct all answers that fell between 23 and 25, and for question Q3 and Q4, where we allowed as correct all answers between 24 and 26.

Reliability. Cronbach's alpha was 0.79 in the USA and 0.74 in Germany, and average item–total correlations were 0.42 and 0.37 in the USA and Germany, respectively, indicating a satisfactory level of internal consistency. Average correlations between individual items were 0.23 in the USA and 0.19 in Germany, indicating that each item measured a somewhat distinctive aspect of graph literacy. This is reflected in relatively low internal consistencies of items testing each skill: 0.62, 0.48, and 0.45, for the ability of "reading the data," "reading between the data," and "reading beyond the data," respectively.

Validity. The average correlation of the total score with education level was 0.54 in the USA and 0.29 in Germany. As shown in Fig. 4.2, the correlation with numeracy was also substantial (0.55 in the USA and 0.47 in Germany). Correlation with the graph comprehension items from the existing literacy questionnaires was 0.50 in the USA and 0.32 in Germany, indicating satisfactory convergent validity. The existing items correlated most highly with items testing basic and moderately advanced graph literacy skills ("reading the data" and "reading between the data"; average correlation 0.36). The correlation with items testing more advanced graph literacy skills ("reading beyond the data") was a lower but nevertheless substantial (0.33).

4.4 Extent of Graph Literacy in the USA and Germany

Participants in both countries completed approximately 9 of 13 items correctly (M=9.3, SD=2.9 in the USA, and M=9.4, SD=2.6 in Germany). Table 4.2 shows percentage of correct responses to each of the items. The items testing the ability of "reading the data" were answered correctly by large majority of participants in both countries. The items testing the two more advanced skills—"reading between the data" and "reading beyond the data"—were more difficult. The most difficult item was the one that required noticing that it is not possible to compare the effectiveness of two different drug treatments when the data are displayed on different charts with unlabeled axes (Q11; see Chap. 15). Only 20% of participants in the USA and 16% in Germany knew this. A similar item (Q10), testing the ability to notice that two

Table 4.2 Percentage of correct responses to items included in the final scale in study 2

	Overall % correct responses	
Items	USA (n=492)	Germany (n=495)
Reading the data		
Q1. Reading off a point on a bar chart	84.6	82.7
Q3. Knowing what a quarter of a pie is in %	83.5	87.7
Q5. Reading off a point on a line chart	84.8	81.7
Q8. Reading off number of icons	90.3	88.6
Average	85.8	85.2
Reading between the data		
Q2. Determining difference between two bars	69.6	67.1
Q4. Summing slices within a quarter of a pie	77.6	74.2
Q6. Comparing slopes of a line at two intervals	61.6	82.1
Q9. Determining difference between two groups of icons	58.1	51.0
Average	66.7	68.6
Reading beyond the data		
Q7. Projecting future trend from a line chart	79.2	81.8
Q10. Comparing two bar charts: Attending to scale range	66.1	62.8
Q11. Comparing two line charts: Attending to scale labels	19.3	15.5
Q12. Differentiating slope and height of a line	77.5	86.1
Q13. Reading off a point on a bar chart when bar falls between two labels	75.2	80.1
Average	63.5	65.3
Mean number of correct answers (SE); Max=13	9.3 (0.18)	9.4 (0.17)

See Chap. 15 for the complete scale

different graphs present the same data but use different scale ranges, produced a higher but still troubling level of accuracy, with 66% of participants in the USA and 63% in Germany giving the correct answer.

Of particular concern for health communicators is that a significant portion of both populations has both low numeracy and low graph literacy skills. As Fig. 4.2 shows, approximately one-third of people in both countries are likely to have problems understanding both numerically presented information and standard visual displays.

4.5 Discussion and Conclusions

We developed and evaluated a graph literacy scale to identify people who have problems understanding graphically presented information related to health issues. The scale has promising psychometric properties and may be suitable for use in many clinical and research circumstances. The scale successfully identified people for whom graphically presented information may be very useful, and also those who are less likely to profit from visual aids. Among people with low-numeracy skills, who are disadvantaged when it comes to grasping a host of numerical concepts that are prerequisites for understanding health-relevant risk communications (Fagerlin et al. 2007), a significant portion (approximately one-third) can be aided by means of standard visual displays. However, a large percentage of low-numeracy people also have low-graph literacy skills and they may require either specially designed information formats that are undemanding in terms of both numeracy and graph literacy, such as analogies (see Chap. 7; see also Edwards 2003; Galesic and Garcia-Retamero 2012; Chap. 7 or natural frequencies (Galesic et al. 2009a, b), and/or additional training in use of standard graphs.

We administered the scale on probabilistic national samples in the USA and Germany. In both countries, the scores were highest on items designed to measure the most basic graph comprehension skill: "reading the data." On average, 86% of people in the USA and 85% in Germany answered these questions correctly. The two more advanced skills had significantly lower average scores: About two-thirds of people in each country were able to answer these questions. Although these percentages may seem high, it is important to note that there are still significant parts of the population that cannot perform elementary tasks involving very simple graphs. For example, 16% of Americans (12% of Germans) do not know what a quarter of a pie chart is in percentages (Q3; see Chap. 15). Similarly, 15% of people in the USA (17% in Germany) cannot read the height of a bar chart with fully labeled axes and gridlines as an additional help (Q1). These percentages translate into rather striking numbers when expanded to the total adult population 25–69 years of age in both countries. In addition, we found that graph literacy correlates with education in both the USA and Germany. This result suggests that understanding graphs is not entirely intuitive but requires a certain level of meta-knowledge about graphs acquired through formal education. The correlation of graph literacy and education was stronger in the USA than in Germany. This may be the result of differences in education systems, in particular the stronger focus on math and science education in Germany from an early age (Stigler et al. 1999).

By design, internal consistency and inter-item correlations among graph items demonstrated considerable heterogeneity and the internal consistencies of items testing each skill were low. In order to make the best use of the short time available for completing the scale, we designed an instrument that captured different aspects of graph literacy and contained no redundant items. On each skill level, we intentionally included items involving very different visual displays: bars, pies, lines, and icon arrays.

Although we designed items reflecting different levels of graph literacy, we did not aspire to design a Guttman scale (Kline 1998), because we wanted to keep the scale short and broad in scope. Understanding graphs includes a number of loosely related processes, from perceptual and interpretative to integrative processes (Carpenter and Shah 1998; Shah and Hoeffner 2002). It would be difficult to systematically test these processes on each skill level and for different types of graphs in the time available in most clinical and research settings. Therefore, we used the framework of different skill levels in order to select a diverse set of items rather than to systematically test all processes involved in each skill. Nevertheless, the majority of participants who answered more difficult items correctly (the skill of "reading beyond the data") also answered the less difficult items well. For example, on average, of those who answered correctly an item on the third level of difficulty ("reading beyond the data"), 90% answered correctly items on the first level ("reading the data"), compared to only 73% of those who did not answer the level 3 items correctly. Similarly, of those who gave a correct answer to items on the second level of difficulty ("read between the data"), 92% answered items on the first level correctly, compared to only 72% of those who did not answer the level 2 items correctly.

People with low-graph literacy often have low levels of numeracy skills (Fig. 4.2). In fact, elementary graph literacy measured by our test correlates more highly with elementary statistical numeracy than with more advanced graph comprehension items (see Sect. 4.2). Nevertheless, as we will show in Chap. 9 (see also Garcia-Retamero and Galesic 2010), graph literacy predicts how helpful graphs are to people independently of numeracy. Graphs help low-numeracy people with relatively high-graph literacy, but they do not help to those with low-graph literacy. Furthermore, as Fig. 4.2 shows, about a third of people who are below the median of the population in numeracy have above median values for graph literacy. This relatively large proportion is not surprising given that most of our items do not require any calculation, with the exception of two questions that require fairly simple deduction of two integers (45–30 in Q1 and 60–40 in Q9). It is more likely that both numeracy and graph literacy skills require a certain level of meta-knowledge about statistics and the meaning of statistical indicators. Our research shows that to some people this knowledge is more accessible in visual rather than numeric formats, and also that a large segment of the population simply does not know enough statistics to be helped by any of the standard formats.

To the best of our knowledge, the present chapter describes the first effort to develop a graph literacy scale that can identify people who have problems understanding graphically presented medical information. At the same time, it leaves several questions open. For instance, one avenue for future research could be to test the scale on physicians. Recent research on numeracy in health decision making has shown that not only patients but also their physicians have difficulty in grasping numerical concepts that are prerequisites for understanding health-relevant risk communications (Gigerenzer et al. 2007). Another open question relates to the generalizability of our scale. As we mentioned above, our aim was to develop an instrument that could be used to assess graph literacy in the health domain. To what extent is our scale useful to evaluate graph literacy in general or in other important domains such as finance, nutrition, or education? Although our studies enabled us to draw clear conclusions and demonstrate the generalizability of our results, it is possible that there are substantial differences between domains. Furthermore, we used a computerized questionnaire, and equivalence of results obtained using paper and pencil should be checked. Finally, the present version of the graph literacy scale focuses on understanding of simple bar, line, and pie charts, and icon arrays. Further research on understanding of more complex graphs, such as survival curves, is needed.

Our research suggests that understanding of both numerical and standard graphical representations of statistical information requires a certain level of statistical thinking. However, unlike reading and writing, statistical thinking is not routinely taught in schools. As a result, a large part of the population is insufficiently prepared to cope with many novel risks and uncertainties of the modern world. The goal of informed decision making hinges on educating the general public to understand statistical information about medical treatments, and on finding alternative, more intuitive formats for communicating risks.

References

Ancker, J. S., & Kaufman, D. (2007). Rethinking health numeracy: A multidisciplinary literature review. *Journal of the American Medical Informatics Association, 14*, 713–721.

Ancker, J. S., Senathirajah, Y., Kukafka, R., & Starren, J. B. (2006). Design features of graphs in health risk communication: A systematic review. *Journal of the American Medical Informatics Association, 13*, 608–618.

Baker, D. W., Williams, M. V., Parker, R. M., Gazmararian, J. A., & Nurss, J. (1999). Development of a brief test to measure functional health literacy. *Patient Education and Counseling, 38*, 33–42.

Carpenter, P. A., & Shah, P. (1998). A model of the perceptual and conceptual processes in graph comprehension. *Journal of Experimental Psychology: Applied, 4*, 75–100.

Edwards, A. (2003). Communicating risks through analogies. *British Medical Journal, 327*, 749.

Fagerlin, A., Ubel, P. A., Smith, D. M., & Zikmund-Fisher, B. J. (2007). Making numbers matter: Present and future research in risk communication. *American Journal of Health Behavior, 31*, 47–56.

Feldman-Stewart, D., Kocovski, N., McConnell, B. A., Brundage, M. D., & Mackillop, W. J. (2000). Perception of quantitative information for treatment decisions. *Medical Decision Making, 20*, 228–238.

Friel, S. N., Curcio, F. R., & Bright, G. W. (2001). Making sense of graphs: Critical factors influencing comprehension and instructional implications. *Journal for Research in Mathematics Education, 32*, 124–158.
Galesic, M., & Garcia-Retamero, R. (2010). Statistical numeracy for health: A cross-cultural comparison with probabilistic national samples. *Archives of Internal Medicine, 170*, 462–468.
Galesic, M. & Garcia-Retamero, R. (2012). Using analogies to communicate information about health risks. *Applied Cognitive Psychology*. doi: 10.1002/acp.2866
Galesic, M., Garcia-Retamero, R., & Gigerenzer, G. (2009a). Using icon arrays to communicate medical risks: Overcoming low numeracy. *Health Psychology, 28*, 210–216.
Galesic, M., Gigerenzer, G., & Straubinger, N. (2009b). Natural frequencies help older adults and people with low numeracy to evaluate medical screening tests. *Medical Decision Making, 29*, 368–371.
Garcia-Retamero, R., & Galesic, M. (2010). Who profits from visual aids: Overcoming challenges in people's understanding of risks. *Social Science and Medicine, 70*, 1019–1025.
Gigerenzer, G., Gaissmaier, W., Kurz-Milcke, E., Schwartz, L. M., & Woloshin, S. (2007). Helping doctors and patients make sense of health statistics. *Psychological Science in the Public Interest, 8*, 53–96.
Kline, P. (1998). *The new psychometrics: Science, psychology, and measurement*. London: Routledge.
Kramarski, B., & Mevarech, Z. R. (2003). Enhancing mathematical reasoning in the classroom: The effects of cooperative learning and metacognitive training. *American Educational Research Journal, 40*, 281–310.
Kutner, M., Greenberg, E., Jin, Y., & Paulsen, C. (2006). *The health literacy of America's adults: Results from the 2003 national assessment of adult literacy (NALS)*. Washington, DC: U.S. Department of Education, National Center for Education Statistics.
Lipkus, I. M. (2007). Numeric, verbal, and visual formats of conveying health risks: Suggested best practices and future recommendations. *Medical Decision Making, 27*, 696–713.
Lipkus, I. M., & Hollands, J. G. (1999). The visual communication of risk. *Journal of the National Cancer Institute Monographs, 25*, 149–163.
Lipkus, I. M., Samsa, G., & Rimer, B. K. (2001). General performance on a numeracy scale among highly educated samples. *Medical Decision Making, 21*, 37–44.
National Center for Education Statistics (1985). National Assessment of Adult Literacy (NAAL): Sample Questions 1985. http://nces.ed.gov/NAAL/sample_items.asp, accessed July 30, 2012.
Neurath, O. (1936). *International picture language*. London: Kegan Paul.
Programme for International Student Assessment (PISA). (2003). *The PISA 2003 assessment framework—Mathematics, reading, science, and problem solving knowledge and skills*. Paris: OECD.
Schwartz, L. M., Woloshin, S., Black, W. C., & Welch, H. G. (1997). The role of numeracy in understanding the benefit of screening mammography. *Annals of Internal Medicine, 127*, 966–972.
Shah, P., & Hoeffner, J. (2002). Review of graph comprehension research: Implications for instruction. *Educational Psychology Review, 14*, 47–69.
Spence, I. (2005). No humble pie: The origins and usage of a statistical chart. *Journal of Educational and Behavioral Statistics, 30*, 353–368.
Spence, I., & Lewandowsky, S. (1991). Displaying proportions and percentages. *Applied Cognitive Psychology, 5*, 61–77.
Stigler, J. W., Gonzales, P., Kawanaka, T., Knoll, S., & Serrano, A. (1999). *The TIMSS videotape classroom study: Methods and findings from an exploratory research project on eighth-grade mathematics instruction in Germany, Japan, and the United States*. Washington, DC: U.S. Department of Education. National Center for Education Statistics.
Tuijnman, A. (2000). *Benchmarking adult literacy in America: An international comparative study: International adult literacy survey (IALS)*. Washington, DC: Department of Education, OVAE.

Chapter 5
Public Knowledge of Benefits of Breast and Prostate Cancer Screening*

Gerd Gigerenzer, Jutta Mata, and Ronald Frank

Abstract Given the harms that can ensue from cancer screening procedures, people's decisions as to whether to undergo cancer screening should be based on a realistic knowledge of its benefits. In this chapter, we described a study conducted among a representative sample of men and women in nine European countries. Participants were asked to choose among estimates of the number of fewer cancer-specific deaths (per 1,000 individuals screened) by prostate-specific antigen (PSA) and mammography screening, respectively. Participants were also queried as to their sources of medical information. The study reported found dramatic (by an order of magnitude or more) overestimation of the benefits (absolute cancer-specific mortality reduction) of mammography and PSA testing in the vast majority of women and men, respectively, in all countries surveyed. Frequent consultation of sources of medical information (including physicians) was not associated with more realistic knowledge of the benefits of screening. A basis for informed decisions by people about participation in screening for breast and prostate cancer is largely non-existent in Europe, suggesting inadequacies in the information made available to the public.

---

* In this chapter, we partially reproduced the article Gigerenzer, G., Mata, J., & Frank, R. (2009). Public knowledge of benefits of breast and prostate cancer screening in Europe. *Journal of the National Cancer Institute, 101*, 1216–1220.

G. Gigerenzer, Ph.D. (✉)
Harding Center for Risk Literacy, Center for Adaptive Behavior and Cognition,
Max Planck Institute for Human Development, Lentzeallee 94, Berlin 14195, Germany
e-mail: gigerenzer@mpib-berlin.mpg.de

J. Mata, Ph.D.
University of Basel, Missionsstrasse 62a, Basel 4055, Switzerland
e-mail: jutta.mata@unibas.ch

R. Frank, M.Ed.
Gesellschaft für Konsumforschung Association, Nordwestring 101,
Nuremberg 90419, Germany
e-mail: ronald.frank@gfk-verein.org

R. Garcia-Retamero and M. Galesic (eds.), *Transparent Communication of Health Risks: Overcoming Cultural Differences*, DOI 10.1007/978-1-4614-4358-2_5,

5.1 Introduction and Background

Women and men in countries with modern health systems are confronted with the question of whether to participate in screening for breast cancer and prostate cancer. Yet, because screening can also lead to harms such as overtreatment, they need to understand the potential benefits of these screening programmes before they can make informed decisions about participating. Ideally, physicians, health pamphlets and other information sources should assist in clarifying the actual size of benefits (see also Chap. 1).

Screening for breast cancer with mammography is widely encouraged by governmental programmes in both the European Union (E.U.) and the USA under the assumption that the screening programmes save lives. In the case of breast cancer, there is some evidence of such a benefit: an analysis of randomised trials with some 247,000 women aged 40–74 years showed that for every 1,000 women who participated in screening, 3.9 died with the diagnosis breast cancer, compared to 5.0 among those who did not participate (Nystrom et al. 2002). The follow-up time ranged between 5.8 and 20.2 years. Thus, the absolute risk reduction was on the order of 1 in 1,000 (Humphrey et al. 2002). The authors of a recent review of six trials involving half a million women estimated the absolute risk reduction to be about 1 in 2,000 (Gøtzsche and Nielsen 2006). Note that this benefit relates to fewer breast-cancer deaths; no reduction in mortality from all cancers or other causes was found. Whether the potential of breast cancer screening to reduce mortality outweighs the harms of overdiagnosis and overtreatment is still under discussion (Elmore et al. 1998; Gøtzsche and Nielsen 2006; Schwartz et al. 2004; Welch 2004).

Screening for prostate cancer with prostate-specific antigen (PSA) tests, although often encouraged by physicians and health information pamphlets, is not part of governmental screening programmes and is recommended by few medical organisations. The evidence for any benefit of screening is limited. The U.S. Preventive Services Task Force (2002) reviewed the available studies and concluded that it was unclear whether increased detection of prostate cancer from screening would reduce mortality and morbidity, and a nested case–control study concluded that it did not (Concato et al. 2006). A European randomised trial reported a prostate cancer-specific mortality reduction of about 1 in 1,400 after 9 years (Schroeder et al. 2009), but a randomised trial in the USA found no reduction after 7 or 10 years (Andriole et al. 2009). Thus, the best estimate seems to be a reduction of death from prostate cancer of 0 or 1 for every 1,000 men screened, and the evidence is insufficient to determine whether the benefits outweigh the harms, such as incontinence through overtreatment of non-progressive cancers.

5.2 Study: Measuring Knowledge of Benefits of Breast and Prostate Cancer Screening in Women and Men

This study addresses two main questions: (1) Do women and men have realistic knowledge about the benefits of mammography and PSA screening, respectively? (2) What information sources do they rely on? Here, we also addressed a related question: Does the frequency of consulting a given source improve understanding of benefits? To our knowledge, the study reported in this chapter is the first European survey of women's and men's perceptions of the benefits of mammography and PSA screening, and the information sources that they rely on, with representative samples of the general population.

5.2.1 Method

5.2.1.1 Participants

We conducted a survey of the public's knowledge of the benefits of screening in eight countries of the E.U. and the European part of Russia. The eight E.U. countries include about 75% of people in the 27 E.U. countries and have a total population of about 500 million. The European part of Russia has a population of about 106 million out of a total of 143 million Russians. The percentage of women who have had mammography is 57 in Germany, 78 in France, 76 in Austria, 85 in the Netherlands, 66 in Italy, 75 in the UK, 52 in Spain, 47 in Poland (for women aged 45–54) and 19 in Russia (Binkowska and Debski 2005; World Health Organisation 2008). PSA screening programmes do not exist in the nine countries, apart from a regional state-funded programme in Tyrol, Austria. National health systems are predominantly financed by taxes in the UK, Italy, and Poland and by contributions to social health insurance in Austria, France, Germany, and the Netherlands.

The data were collected as part of the European Consumer Study 2007 conducted between September and December 2006 by the GfK-Nürnberg Group (GfK-Nürnberg e.V. and Frank 2007). Participants within each country were selected according to a quota method based on the official statistics concerning five variables: region, size of household, sex, profession, and age (Särndal et al. 1992). The population in each country was first segmented into subgroups based on these five criteria, and within each subgroup, subjects were sampled in proportion to their distribution in the entire country. Initial contacts were made by telephone; the interviews were conducted in the participants' homes. Consistent with earlier representative quota sampling surveys conducted by the GfK Group, across all countries, about 60% of initial phone contacts resulted in a complete interview; in the remaining cases, sampling was continued until the quotas were met. Across all countries, the age distribution of participants was as follows: 14–19 years (8.4%), 20–29 years (16.6%), 30–39 years (18.0%), 40–49 years (18.4%), 50–59 years (15.2%), 60–69 years (11.8%), and 70 years and older (11.5%). The total number of interviews was 10,228, with 2,054 in Germany and 2,019 in Russia (the countries with the largest populations); 1,005 in France, 1,042 in the UK, 1,007 in Italy, 1,019 in Poland and 1,024 in Spain; and 501 in Austria and 557 in the Netherlands (the two countries with the smallest populations). Table 5.1 shows the sample frame (taken from Frank 2007).

5.2.1.2 Stimuli and Procedure

Participants were questioned in face-to-face interviews with computer assistance, except in Russia, where for security reasons, interviewers used paper and pencil. Using personal interviews avoided some of the problems of telephone interview methods, such as excluding poorer households without telephones and hence introducing a bias in comparisons between countries. The Ethics Committee of the Max Planck Institute for Human Development approved the methodology, and all participants consented to participation at the beginning of the survey.

As a measure of the perceived benefit of mammography screening, we focussed on cancer-specific mortality reduction, because this is the endpoint typically communicated to the public (as opposed to total mortality reduction, for example). Women were questioned as follows: "1,000 women age 40 and older from the general population participate every 2 years in screening for breast cancer with mammography. After 10 years, the benefit is measured. Please estimate how many fewer women die from breast cancer in the group who participate in screening compared to women who do not participate in screening." The response alternatives were 0, 1, 10, 50, 100, 200 (out of 1,000), and "I don't know." For the perceived benefit of PSA screening, men were questioned similarly: "1,000 men age 50 and older from the general population participate every 2 years in screening for prostate cancer with PSA tests. After 10 years, the benefit is measured. Please estimate how many fewer men die from prostate cancer in the group who participate in screening compared to men who do not participate in screening." The response alternatives were the same as those used for breast cancer screening.

To measure the frequency of information sources used, we asked participants how often they used each of 14 sources that were divided into four categories as follows: family and/or friends (considered both a source and a category), experts (general practitioner and pharmacist), general media (television, popular magazines, daily newspaper, and radio), and health-specific sources (pamphlets by health organisations, reference books, health insurance, Internet, consumer counselling, patient counselling, and self-help organisations). The response alternatives were never, rarely, sometimes, frequently, and don't know.

We calculated the proportion of best estimates of screening benefits for all countries, all age groups, and for the group of citizens aged 50–60 years who are targeted by the screening campaigns. The proportion of participants reporting use of sources of health information was calculated for all countries, all age groups, and all of the 14 sources. Correlation coefficients between frequency of use of particular sources of health information and estimates of screening benefits were calculated.

Table 5.1 Sampling frame of the study

		Germany	France	Spain	Austria	Poland	Italy	Netherlands	UK	Russia
Sex	Male	48.0	48.0	48.6	48.2	47.8	48.1	48.2	48.0	46.7
	Female	52.0	52.0	51.4	51.8	52.2	51.9	51.8	52.0	53.3
Age	14–19	7.8	9.1	8.2	7.2	8.9	7.2	6.8	7.0	9.9
	20–29	12.0	15.8	18.9	15.0	20.0	14.7	15.5	15.0	20.0
	30–39	18.2	17.3	18.7	19.8	16.0	18.5	20.4	21.0	16.7
	40–49	17.4	17.9	15.9	18.4	17.2	16.9	18.7	17.0	21.7
	50–59	14.7	15.7	13.1	14.4	17.1	14.8	16.4	15.0	15.6
	60–69	15.6	10.4	11.2	12.0	10.3	12.4	10.9	11.0	10.8
	70+	14.4	13.9	14.0	13.2	10.4	15.5	11.2	14.0	5.3
Occupation	Employed	47.9	42.8	49.2	58.2	41.2	46.3	55.7	58.0	58.6
	Unemployed	7.5	7.7	6.6	2.9	12.2	4.1	4.2	6.3	5.8
	Retired	27.6	24.6	19.9	24.7	29.1	25.6	17.1	22.5	19.9
	Student	10.1	11.3	10.1	5.4	13.3	11.0	7.5	4.3	10.2
	Housewife/-husband	7.0	13.7	14.1	8.7	4.2	12.9	12.3	8.4	5.0
Education	Low	41.5	26.8	11.3	20.2	55.1	46.2	26.1	51.4	16.9
	Medium	36.1	46.9	66.5	56.5	35.2	44.6	46.1	29.1	58.1
	High	18.3	25.8	21.8	23.2	9.7	8.8	27.4	19.5	24.6
Household size	1 person	19.9	15.4	15.7	15.8	8.6	12.2	17.4	17.9	8.1
	2 persons	36.7	30.7	26.9	28.2	16.2	26.0	37.1	33.3	20.2
	3 persons	19.4	21.3	23.8	20.8	20.8	25.8	17.3	19.5	26.1
	4 persons	18.2	18.8	23.6	20.6	25.2	26.4	19.5	17.4	25.1
	5 or more	5.8	13.8	10	14.6	29.2	9.6	8.7	11.9	20.5

Table 5.2 Estimated reduction of breast cancer mortality through regular participation in mammography screening (women only)

Reduction	Percentage of responders								
out of 1,000?	Mean	Germany	France	Austria	Netherlands	Italy	UK	Spain	Poland	Russia
None	6.4	1.4	0.8	2.4	0.7	5.3	2.0	3.9	4.2	16.1
1	1.5	0.8	1.3	2.9	1.4	1.3	1.9	2.7	0.8	1.7
10	11.7	12.8	15.7	11.0	10.7	10.6	10.3	6.9	9.7	12.4
50	18.9	21.3	21.7	22.1	22.6	17.4	13.9	11.7	20.5	20.1
100	15.0	16.8	21.5	20.8	22.5	13.9	17.0	11.3	14.8	10.8
200	15.2	13.7	23.7	11.0	20.1	15.2	26.9	15.7	17.1	6.8
Don't know	31.4	33.1	15.3	29.8	22.1	36.3	28.0	48.0	32.9	32.1

The question was "How many fewer women die from breast cancer in the group who participate in screening, compared to women who do not participate in screening?" Mean across all nine countries is weighted by sample size

For mammography screening, overestimation of benefit was defined as the difference between the estimated benefit (expressed in X out of 1,000 women) and 1 out of 1,000. For instance, if the estimate was 50 in 1,000, the overestimation was 49 in 1,000. A positive correlation means the higher the reported frequency of use, the larger the overestimation. For PSA screening, the same procedure was used except that estimates of 0 were not scored as underestimation, but 0 and 1 in 1,000 were considered equally accurate. The correlations between overestimation and frequency of use of particular sources did not include participants who answered the question concerning the benefit of screening with "don't know" (Table 5.2 shows the frequency of these responses).

5.2.2 *Results*

Do women and men have realistic knowledge about the benefits of mammography and PSA screening? Among all participants, only 1.5% of women (range across different countries 0.8–2.9%) chose the best estimate for reduction in mortality due to breast cancer screening, that is, one woman saved for every 1,000 screened (Table 5.2). Four times as many women answered that the benefit was zero, and 92.1% overestimated the benefit by at least one order of magnitude or answered that they didn't know; this proportion was higher (95.9%) in the eight E.U. countries due to the large proportion of no-benefit estimates in Russia. The greatest overestimation was observed in France, the Netherlands, and the UK, where more than 40% of the women answered that the reduction in mortality was 100 or 200 women per 1,000 screened; in the UK, almost 27% chose the highest figure. These three countries also had high participation rates in mammography screening. In Russia, where the availability of mammography equipment is limited (Rozhkova and Kochetova 2005), the percentage of women who exhibited overestimation or did not know was the lowest of the countries surveyed, 82%.

Table 5.3 Estimated reduction of prostate cancer mortality through regular participation in PSA screening (men only)

Reduction	Percentage of responders									
out of 1,000?	Mean	Germany	France	Austria	Netherlands	Italy	UK	Spain	Poland	Russia
None	8.3	3.8	1.6	4.1	3.0	5.7	0.5	9.3	5.0	20.3
1	2.4	2.3	2.7	3.5	2.2	1.8	0.9	4.3	0.7	2.9
10	14.4	17.7	16.9	24.4	11.5	11.9	15.9	17.0	13.9	10.7
50	19.3	23.0	21.6	27.1	20.2	18.5	17.3	25.1	17.9	15.0
100	14.0	17.2	21.1	20.8	20.3	9.2	15.6	18.8	14.5	7.3
200	11.8	9.7	20.2	14.2	14.2	12.2	19.5	17.9	11.3	3.4
Don't know	29.8	26.3	15.9	5.9	28.5	40.6	30.2	7.6	36.7	40.4

The question was "How many fewer men die from prostate cancer in the group who participate in screening, compared to men who do not participate in screening?" Mean across all nine countries is weighted by sample size

Some of the women included in our study were younger than women targeted by screening programmes and may have had little motivation to inform themselves about screening. However, in every country, the percentage of women who gave the best estimate was lower among those aged 50–69 and thus targeted by screening programmes than among women younger than 50. Furthermore, in every country but Russia, 50-69-year-old women gave worse estimates than all other age groups.

In all countries surveyed, only 10.7% of men made reasonable estimates of the benefits of prostate cancer screening (i.e., deaths from prostate cancer prevented for every 1,000 men screened were less than or equal to 1, Table 5.3); 89.3% overestimated or answered that they didn't know. Like their female counterparts, more than 40% of the French men estimated that screening would save 100 or 200 men from dying from prostate cancer per 1,000 screened. Men in Austria, the Netherlands, Spain, and the UK made similar overestimates. As observed for women, the percentage of Russian men who overestimated the benefits or did not know was the lowest among the nine countries surveyed, 77%.

Similar to what was observed in women, the distribution of estimates by men between the ages of 50 and 69 made was not more accurate than what was observed overall. The percentage of men who estimated zero and one life saved decreased from 8.3 to 2.4%, respectively, in all age groups to 7.3 and 1.9%, respectively, among men aged 50–69 years.

Does frequent consulting of information sources improve understanding of benefits of mammography and PSA screening? Most (59%) of women reported using one or more sources frequently, compared with 47% of men. In every country, older citizens searched for more information than younger ones.

Within the general categories of health information sources, family and friends, experts, general media and health-specific sources, the correlations between the frequencies of use of two sources were consistently high (correlation coefficients >0.5), whereas the correlations between sources from different categories were consistently lower. The sources of health-related information reported most often were family and/or friends, followed in descending order by experts (general practitioner and pharmacist), general media (television was the most reported source in this category), and health-specific sources (among all participants, the seven sources in this category were the least used among the 14 sources).

Individual trends according to country were observed with respect to sources of health information (Table 5.4). In Poland and Russia, family and/or friends were by far the most often reported source of information. In Austria, France, Germany, Italy, and Spain, the general practitioner was the primary source of information, and, except for family and friends, little use was made of other sources in these countries. The Netherlands had the most even distribution of reported information sources. In the UK, the frequency of reported consultation of most sources of information was generally low. For only two sources did British citizens report higher than average frequencies.

Frequent consulting of sources was not associated with an increase in understanding of the benefits of screening, but instead was often associated with overestimation. For the women in Austria, France, Germany, Poland, Russia, Spain, and the UK, there was no single source of information whose frequent use was associated with more accurate understanding of the benefits. By contrast, German women who more often consulted leaflets and pamphlets from medical organisations (41% of Germans use this source; Table 5.4) tended to overestimate the benefit of mammography screening ($r=0.15$, 95% confidence interval (CI)$=0.07$–0.23), as did French women ($r=0.12$, 95% CI$=0.04$–0.29). The German women who more often consulted a general practitioner ($r=0.10$, 95% CI$=0.02$–0.18) or a pharmacist ($r=0.11$, 95% CI$=0.03$–0.19) for health information also had less accurate understanding of benefits.

The only sources associated with improved knowledge of the benefits of breast cancer screening were consumer counselling in the Netherlands ($r=-0.18$, 95% CI$=-0.35$ to -0.01) and in Italy ($r=-0.17$, 95% CI$=-0.27$ to -0.07), and patient counselling ($r=-0.16$, 95% CI$=-0.26$ to -0.06) and self-help groups ($r=-0.12$, 95% CI$=-0.22$ to -0.02) in Italy alone.

The results for PSA screening confirmed the general conclusion that consultation of sources of medical information is not associated with knowledge of the benefits of screening. For men in Austria, Germany, the Netherlands, Russia, and Spain, there was no single source whose frequent use was associated with better understanding of benefits. Information from health insurances was associated with less overestimation in France ($r=-0.11$, 95% CI$=-0.20$ to -0.02), Poland ($r=-0.13$, 95% CI$=-0.25$ to -0.01), and Italy ($r=-0.18$, 95% CI$=-0.29$ to -0.08), and information from radio with less overestimation in the UK ($r=-0.11$, 95% CI$=-0.21$ to -0.01).

For both mammography and PSA screening, there was no single country in which frequent consulting of general practitioners and health pamphlets improved understanding of benefits. The overall effect across all nine countries was a slight positive correlation between overestimation and frequency of consultation for general practitioners ($r=0.07$, 95% CI$=0.05$–0.09) and health pamphlets ($r=0.06$, 95% CI$=0.04$–0.08).

Table 5.4 Percentage of participants reporting that they use specific sources of health information sometimes or frequently

Source	Mean[a]	Germany	France	Austria	Netherlands	Italy	UK	Spain	Poland	Russia
Family/friends	62	65	60	61	50	62	53	47	67	69[b]
General practitioner	59	68	69	68	50	79[b]	53	72	43	44
Pharmacist	54	56	62	59	54	70[b]	49	66	49	43
Television	43	45	57[b]	43	51	38	35	32	42	42
Popular magazines	26	36	39[b]	33	33	20	22	21	30	18
Daily newspaper	25	29	38[b]	38	30	19	25	24	25	20
Radio	23	20	36[b]	34	28	12	22	21	30	23
Leaflets and pamphlets by health organisations	21	41[b]	36	23	30	13	14	17	12	14
Reference books about health topics	20	20	23	23	27[b]	15	25	15	15	22
Health insurance company	17	19	27	20	44	3	9	54[b]	21	4
Internet (e.g. health portals)	15	17	21	17	42[b]	11	26	16	14	7
Consumer counselling	6	3	8	4	20[b]	4	3	9	4	6
Patient counselling	6	2	3	3	20[b]	6	5	8	9	5
Self-help organisations	4	3	5	2	8[b]	2	4	6	3	4

Response alternatives were never, rarely, sometimes, frequently, and don't know

[a] Mean across all nine countries was weighted by sample size

[b] Highest value for each source

5.3 Discussion and Conclusions

In this survey of more than 10,000 people in nine European countries, 92% of women and 89% of men overestimated the benefits of mammography and PSA screening, respectively, by an order of magnitude or more, or stated that they did not know what the benefits were. This percentage was the lowest in Russia, with 82% for women and 77% for men. Consulting general practitioners, health pamphlets, and other information sources generally did not increase accurate knowledge of benefits; the only major exception was information from health insurances about PSA screening.

Our use of a numerical response scale with particular categories (0, 1, 10, 50, 100, 200) may have influenced participants' estimates and may have contributed to the large amount of overestimation observed. However, we have indirect evidence that an open response format might not reduce the degree of overestimation. At the time of the study reported in this chapter (December 2006), we conducted an independent survey with a different polling institute (TNS Emnid) in Germany and with a new representative sample of 1,018 citizens, in which we included the question: "Early detection with mammography reduces the risk of dying from breast cancer by 25%. Assume that 1,000 women aged 40 and older participate regularly in screening. How many fewer would die of breast cancer?" No response categories were used. The proportion of correct answers was equally low, and overestimation was even larger, with a median estimate of 500 lives saved for every 1,000 women screened by mammography (Gigerenzer et al. 2007).

The study reported in this chapter did not assess perceived harms and economic costs, or whether the degree of overestimation of benefit translates into higher participation in screening. An association between overestimation and participation has been demonstrated in other studies, although this association was not observed for African American women (Miller and Champion 1997; Price et al. 1992). We also do not know whether the results are generalisable to other countries. Domenighetti et al. (2003) found similar overestimation of mammography in telephone interviews conducted with women in Switzerland and the USA and also reported overestimation for women in the UK and Italy, but we are not aware of any surveys of the perceived benefit of PSA tests that were conducted simultaneously in different countries. Nor are we aware of any representative nation-wide survey of the perceived quantitative benefit of mammography or PSA screening in the USA. A study with 145 American women with above-average education reported an average perceived breast cancer-specific mortality reduction of 60 in 1,000 (Black et al. 1995) and a study of 207 women attending general internal medicine clinics in Wisconsin reported that 76% overestimated the relative risk reduction (Haggstrom and Schapira 2006).

We do not know why women and men overestimate the benefits of screening, but the results in Table 5.4 may indicate potential reasons. After family and friends, whose information might actually derive from the other sources in Table 5.4, the most frequently mentioned sources were general practitioner and pharmacist.

Studies on physicians' lack of knowledge about the benefits of screening and conflicts of interest support the possibility that these professionals contribute to overestimation (Gigerenzer et al. 2007; Steurer et al. 2009; Welch 2004). The observation that health-specific sources rarely improve understanding of screening (except for health insurance in several countries) also implicates these sources as a further potential cause, a hypothesis that is consistent with the findings that few pamphlets, letters of invitation, and websites explain the size of the benefit. If they do, the explanation is almost always in terms of a relative risk reduction rather than in the more transparent form of an absolute risk reduction (Gigerenzer et al. 2007).

In conclusion, the study reported in this chapter documents that information about the benefits of mammography and PSA screening has not reached the general public in nine European countries, including the age group targeted by screening programmes. Knowing the benefit of a treatment is a necessary condition for informed consent and rational decision-making. At present, however, the available information sources are not designed to communicate benefits clearly. As a consequence, preconditions for informed decisions about participation in screening are largely non-existent in Europe.

References

Andriole, G. L., Grubb, R. L., Buys, S. S., Chia, D., Church, T. R., Fouad, M. N., et al. (2009). Mortality results from a randomized prostate-cancer screening trial. *The New England Journal of Medicine, 360*, 1310–1319.

Binkowska, M., & Debski, R. (2005). Screening mammography in Polish female population aged 45 to 54. *Ginekologia Polska, 76*, 871–878.

Black, W. C., Nease, R. F., & Tosteson, A. N. A. (1995). Perceptions of breast-cancer risk and screening effectiveness in women younger than 50 years of age. *Journal of the National Cancer Institute, 87*, 720–731.

Concato, J., Wells, C. K., Horwitz, R. I., Penson, D., Fincke, G., Berlowitz, D. R., et al. (2006). The effectiveness of screening for prostate cancer: A nested case-control study. *Archives of Internal Medicine, 166*, 38–43.

Domenighetti, G., D'Avanzo, B., Egger, M., Berrino, F., Perneger, T., Mosconi, P., et al. (2003). Women's perception of the benefits of mammography screening: Population-based survey in four countries. *International Journal of Epidemiology, 32*, 816–821.

Elmore, G., Barton, M. B., Moceri, V. M., Polk, S., Arena, P. J., & Fletcher, S. W. (1998). Ten-year risk of false positive screening mammograms and clinical breast examinations. *The New England Journal of Medicine, 338*, 1089–1096.

Frank, R. (2007). European consumer study—Gesundheit in Europa. Nuremberg: GfK e.V.

GfK-Nürnberg e.V., & Frank, R. (2007). *Health in Europe. European consumer study 2007*. Nuremberg: GFK.

Gigerenzer, G., Gaissmaier, W., Kurz-Milcke, E., Schwartz, L. M., & Woloshin, S. (2007). Helping doctors and patients to make sense of health statistics. *Psychological Science in the Public Interest, 8*, 53–96.

Gøtzsche, P. C., & Nielsen, M. (2006). Screening for breast cancer with mammography. *Cochrane Database of Systematic Reviews, 4*, CD001877.

Haggstrom, D. A., & Schapira, M. M. (2006). Black-white differences in risk perceptions of breast cancer survival and screening mammography benefit. *Journal of General Internal Medicine, 21*, 371–377.

Humphrey, L. L., Helfand, M., Chan, B. K. S., & Woolf, S. H. (2002). Breast cancer screening: A summary of the evidence for the US Preventive Services Task Force. *Annals of Internal Medicine, 137*, 347–360.

Miller, A. M., & Champion, V. L. (1997). Attitudes about breast cancer and mammography: Racial, income, and educational differences. *Women and Health, 26*, 41–63.

Nystrom, L., Andersson, I., Bjurstam, N., Frisell, J., Nordenskjold, B., & Rutqvist, L. E. (2002). Long-term effects of mammography screening: Updated overview of the Swedish randomised trials. *Lancet, 359*, 909–919.

Price, J. H., Desmond, S. H., Slenker, S., Smith, D. E., & Stewart, P. W. (1992). Urban black women's perceptions of breast cancer and mammography. *Journal of Community Health, 17*, 191–204.

Rozhkova, N. I., & Kochetova, G. P. (2005). Analysis of equipment of the Russian X-ray Mammological Service in 2003 and 2004. *Biomedical Engineering, 39*, 242–244.

Särndal, C. E., Swensson, B., & Wretman, J. (1992). *Model assisted survey sampling* (2nd ed.). New York: Springer.

Schroeder, F. H., Hugosson, J., Roobol, M. J., Tammela, T. L. J., Ciatto, S., Nelen, V., et al. (2009). Screening and prostate-cancer mortality in a randomized European study. *The New England Journal of Medicine, 360*, 1320–1328.

Schwartz, L. M., Woloshin, S., Fowler, F. J., & Welch, H. G. (2004). Enthusiasm for cancer screening in the United States. *Journal of the American Medical Association, 291*, 71–78.

Steurer, J., Held, U., Schmidt, M., Gigerenzer, G., Tag, B., & Bachmann, L. M. (2009). Legal concerns trigger PSA testing. *Journal of Evaluation in Clinical Practice, 15*, 390–392.

U.S. Preventive Services Task Force. (2002). Screening for prostate cancer: Recommendation and rationale. *Annals of Internal Medicine, 137*, 915–916.

Welch, H. G. (2004). *Should I be tested for cancer?* Berkeley: University of California Press.

World Health Organisation (2008). *World health statistics*. http://www.who.int/whosis/whostat/2008/en/index.html, accessed July 30, 2012.

Chapter 6
Symptom Recognition of Heart Attack and Stroke*

Jutta Mata, Ronald Frank, and Gerd Gigerenzer

Abstract Cardiovascular diseases are the number one cause of death and a source of chronic disability. In this chapter, we assess recognition of and reaction to symptoms of heart attack and stroke, and how recognition is related to the frequency of consulting physicians and other information sources. Participants (*N* = 10,228 persons) were representative samples from nine European countries, namely Austria, France, Germany, Italy, Netherlands, Poland, Russia, Spain, and UK, aged 14–98. Results show that the majority of citizens in these countries recognize few heart attack and stroke symptoms and many do not know how to react in case of a stroke. This low level of knowledge constitutes a major health risk, and likely leads to delay in treatment, contributing to the high mortality and morbidity from these diseases.

*In this chapter, we partially reproduced the article Mata, J., Frank, R., & Gigerenzer, G. (in press). Symptom recognition of heart attack and stroke in nine European countries: A representative survey. *Health Expectations*.

J. Mata, Ph.D. (✉)
University of Basel, Missionsstrasse 62a, Basel 4055, Switzerland
e-mail: jutta.mata@unibas.ch

R. Frank, M.Ed.
Gesellschaft für Konsumforschung Association,
Nordwestring 101, Nuremberg 90419, Germany
e-mail: ronald.frank@gfk-verein.org

G. Gigerenzer, Ph.D.
Harding Center for Risk Literacy, Center for Adaptive Behavior and Cognition,
Max Planck Institute for Human Development, Lentzeallee 94, Berlin 14195, Germany
e-mail: gigerenzer@mpib-berlin.mpg.de

R. Garcia-Retamero and M. Galesic (eds.), *Transparent Communication of Health Risks: Overcoming Cultural Differences*, DOI 10.1007/978-1-4614-4358-2_6,

6.1 Introduction and Background

Cardiovascular diseases are the number one cause of death worldwide and are the top two leading causes of death in Europe (World Health Organization 2011). Both heart attack and stroke are also a significant cause of chronic disability (Murray and Lopez 1997; World Health Organization 2008). Because many forms of therapy have to be applied within a few hours (Qureshi et al. 2005; Wardlaw et al. 2003), rapid access to treatment reduces deaths and disability. To avoid delay of treatment, people have to recognize the symptoms quickly *and* know what to do. Patients for whom an ambulance has been called are up to four times more likely to get to an emergency unit within 3 h of onset of symptoms than those brought by other modes of transportation (Kothari et al. 1999; Lacy et al. 2001). Thus, public knowledge about symptoms and best action appears to be a major potential factor for reducing morbidity and mortality from heart attack and stroke.

Many previous studies on the subject measured recall of symptoms rather than recognition. Yet, this may not be the best test, given that recognition, not recall, of symptoms is the relevant skill for detecting whether someone has had a heart attack or stroke. Memory research has found consistent differences between recall and recognition. For instance, one may be unable to recall a name yet easily recognize it (Anderson and Bower 1973; Postman 1963). Consequently, participants asked to recall symptoms name fewer correct symptoms. For example, one review reported that between 30 and 60% of individuals in the UK, the US, and Australia could not recall a single symptom of stroke in an open-ended question format (Nicol and Thrift 2005); however, they were able to recognize correctly between 10 and 95% of symptoms from a list. Some reviews did not differentiate between recall and recognition (e.g., Stroebele et al. 2011), making it difficult to compare knowledge of symptoms across studies and participants.

Most previous research on knowledge about heart attack and stroke was conducted in convenience samples of patients (e.g., people in the emergency unit, self-help groups) in the US, with a few studies in Australia, the UK, and Germany. In this chapter, we present the first European-wide survey on representative samples on heart attack and stroke to investigate symptom recognition, action knowledge, and information sources. Our survey was conducted in nine countries: eight countries of the European Union (which include about 75% of the total population of 500 million in the 27 European Union countries) and in the European part of Russia. Table 6.1 lists the countries in the order of health expenditure in % GDP and provides basic health variables relevant to heart attack and stroke. As can be seen in the table, health care expenditure is lowest in the Eastern European countries, namely Poland and Russia, and highest in Germany and France. Life expectancy at birth is comparable across the countries surveyed, with the exception of Poland and Russia, where life expectancy is lower. The number of deaths from ischemic heart and cerebrovascular disease are particularly high in Austria and Poland.

Table 6.1 Structural and health characteristics in the nine European countries

	Germany	France	Spain	Austria	Poland	Italy	Netherlands	UK	Russia
Health expenditure 2004 in % GDP (per capita in US$)	10.9 (3,052)	10.0 (3,016)	7.8 (1,908)	7.5 (2,365)	6.4 (810)	8.7 (2,424)	9.8 (3,056)	8.1 (2,531)	5.3 (571)
Life expectancy at birth[a,b,c]	78.6	80.3	80.5	79.3	74.6	79.7	78.8	78.5	65.6
Deaths from ischemic heart disease per 100,000 per year[d]	119.5	45.3	61.5	123.7	124.5	76.8	72.2	123.2	–
Deaths from cerebrovascular disease per 100,000 per year[d]	53.1	37.3	52.0	56.0	95.2	60.6	50.3	34.8	–
Internet access in 2006 in %[e]	67	41	39	52	36	40	80	63	–

[a] Statistisches Bundesamt (2006 a)
[b] Eurostat (2011 b)
[c] Statistisches Bundesamt (2006 b)
[d] Eurostat (2011 a)
[e] Eurostat (2009)

6.2 Study: Recognition of Symptoms in Nine European Countries

The main research questions behind the survey were: (1) What proportion of the general public in nine European countries recognizes the main symptoms for heart attack and stroke? And what differences in recognition levels exist between countries? (2) What proportion of citizens knows what to do in the event of a stroke? And (3) Do those who consult their doctors (or other sources of information) have better symptom recognition and action-relevant knowledge?

6.2.1 Method

The data analyzed were collected as part of the European Consumer Study 2007 conducted between September and December 2006 by the GfK-Group (Gesellschaft für Konsumforschung, "Society for Consumer Research"; Frank 2007). Wording of the questions was developed in collaboration with specialists in internal medicine. The questions were first formulated in German, then translated by professional translators into the languages of the other participating countries, and finally translated back into German to assure the accuracy and equivalence of the questions for participants in all countries. The questions and answer categories were field-tested to detect potential problems and then revised as needed. Participants were visited by interviewers in their home and questioned face-to-face in computer-assisted personal interviews, except in Russia, where interviewers used paper and pencil for security reasons. In general, the interviewer entered participants' responses into the computer, but if participants preferred, they could always enter the information themselves without the interviewer seeing their responses. The interviews were conducted in agreement with the ethical regulations of the GfK-Group and the Standards for Quality Assurance in Market and Social Research of ADM (Arbeitskreis Deutscher Markt- und Sozialforschungsinstitute "Research Group of German Market and Social Research Institutes," Frankfurt am Main, Germany). All participants were informed about the purpose of the survey and told that they could stop the survey at any time without negative consequences.

6.2.1.1 Participants

The total number of participants was 10,228: 2,054 from Germany and 2,019 from Russia (the countries with the largest populations); 1,005 from France, 1,042 from the UK, 1,007 from Italy, 1,019 from Poland, and 1,024 from Spain; as well as 501 from Austria and 557 from the Netherlands (the two countries with the smallest populations) see Chap. 5 for more details about the sample of participants). To obtain a representative sample of the population 14 years and older for each of the nine

European countries, a quota method was used, a systematic sampling method that determines the proportion of individuals to be sampled from different subcategories. The five subcategories used were region, size of household, gender, profession, and age, according to the official statistics in each country. The resulting samples are stratified and reflect the population structure in each country relative to these subcategories.

6.2.1.2 Stimuli and Procedure

The original questions used in this study are presented in Table 6.2. Briefly, participants were asked to indicate which of 7 conditions were possible symptoms of heart attack and which of 15 conditions possible symptoms of stroke. In both cases, multiple answers were possible and one of the symptoms offered was not an actual symptom. All symptoms were described in lay terms to ensure they were understandable to the general population. Participants were also given different options of what they would do if they saw a person suffering from short-term impaired vision, speech problems, numbness or a one-sided debility and again could choose multiple answers. Also, participants were asked whether they knew if their blood pressure was currently high, too low, or normal, and to report their height and current weight.

6.2.2 Results

Our research questions examined (1) mean differences between countries (i.e., comparing across the nine European countries surveyed the proportion of the general public that recognized symptoms of heart attack and stroke as well as the proportion that knew what to do in the event of a stroke) and (2) the association between knowledge and consulted information sources on heart attack and stroke. For mean differences (1), we calculated the mean number of symptoms recognized and the 95% confidence interval of this mean (95% CI) or the mean difference of a group comparison and its 95% confidence interval (95% CI_{diff}). For associations between knowledge and consulted information sources (2), we ran correlation analyses; r describes the strength of association (from 0 to 1). All correlations reported in this results section have a 95% confidence interval that does not include zero, that is, the strength of association is different from zero.

What proportion of the general public recognizes symptoms of heart attack? Chest pain was the only symptom of heart attack to be recognized by more than half of the Europeans interviewed. The two other symptoms recognized most often were shortage of breath and pain in arm and/or shoulder (Table 6.3). Germans identified the highest number of symptoms (M=3.15; 95% CI=3.08–3.22), followed by Austrians (M=2.91 symptoms; 95% CI=2.72–3.12). Participants in Italy, Spain, Poland, and Russia identified the lowest number. As many as 18% of participants (averaged across all countries) were not familiar with any symptom of heart attack except for chest pain, and 8% knew no single symptom.

Table 6.2 Original questions used in the study

Type of question	Questions and response options
Symptoms of a heart attack[a]	Which of the following conditions are possible symptoms of a heart attack? Multiple answers are possible *Options*: Chest pain, shortage of breath, feeling of anxiety, shoulder and/or arm pain, stomach pain, intense nausea and dizziness, headache
Symptoms of a stroke[b]	Which of the following conditions are possible symptoms of a stroke? Multiple answers are possible *Options*: Numbness, prickly feeling, paralysis, debility, slurred speech, spit running out of mouth, problems eating, frequent difficulty swallowing (particularly when drinking), lopsided face, runny eyes, dizziness, inclination to fall to one side (suddenly or increasingly more often), sudden one-sided blindness, sudden confusion/discomposure, earache
Information sources used	Please rate how often you consult this information source for health information on a four-point scale (never, rarely, sometimes, frequently) *Information sources*: General practitioner, pharmacist, health insurance company, family/friends, daily newspaper, popular magazines, leaflets and pamphlets by health organizations, radio, television, Internet (e.g., health portals), reference books about health topics, consumer counseling, patient counseling, and self-help organizations/groups
Reaction to a person suffering from stroke symptoms	What would you do if you saw a person suffering from short-term impaired vision, speech problems, numbness or a one-sided debility? Multiple answers are possible *Options*: Tell the sufferer to go to bed and wait, give the person a sip of fluid, advise her/him to see a doctor, call a doctor immediately, call an ambulance
Risk factors	Do you know whether your blood pressure is currently too high, too low, or normal? What is your height without shoes? What is your current weight without clothing?

[a]All conditions except headache are typical symptoms
[b]All conditions except earache are typical symptoms

Across all countries, the youngest age group recognized fewer heart attack symptoms than the two older age groups (young vs. middle: 2.20 vs. 2.47, 95% CI_{diff} of the mean difference −0.50 to −0.38; young vs. old: 2.20 vs. 2.43, 95% CI_{diff} = −0.49 to −0.33). More symptoms were identified by people with high level of education than by people with low (2.71 vs. 2.43, 95% CI_{diff} = 0.20–0.37) or medium level (2.71 vs. 2.60, 95% CI_{diff} = 0.17–0.34; except in Russia, where level of education was not assessed). Women recognized a higher number of symptoms than men did (2.47 vs. 2.19, 95% CI_{diff} = 0.32–0.22). The means for each country are shown in Table 6.4.

In addition, people at higher risk because of overweight (2.39 vs. 2.24, 95% CI_{diff} = 0.10–0.22) or obesity (2.50 vs. 2.24, 95% CI_{diff} = 0.18–0.34) identified more

Table 6.3 Percentage of participants who recognized a condition as a symptom of heart attack (all conditions except headache are typical symptoms). Mean across the nine countries was weighted by sample size. The highest recognition value for each symptom is bolded

	Nine countries	Germany	France	Spain	Austria	Poland	Italy	Netherlands	UK	Russia
Chest pain	79.9	85	84.5	65.3	84.2	83	66.5	87.5	**90.9**	79.1
Shortage of breath	49.3	62	42.2	33.4	60.4	52.1	26.8	42.2	**68.2**	50.7
Shoulder and/or arm pain	48.4	66.8	66.8	59.6	56.7	20.1	63.1	69.4	**72.4**	14.4
Feeling of anxiety	21.4	**51.2**	15.1	11.6	44.9	17.9	6.7	14.8	21.3	15.9
Intense nausea and dizziness	21.2	**40.7**	17.4	11.7	37.4	17.5	8.4	23.5	26.5	17.2
Headache	12	12	11.2	9.8	11.9	9.9	3.5	4.2	9.3	**19.1**
Stomach pain	7.5	9.5	5	5.2	8.1	3.7	**21.7**	4.1	6.2	3.9
I don't know	7.6	5.4	4.9	2.0	0.6	10.0	8.0	5.0	3.3	**11.5**
Mean of correct symptoms	2.3	**3.2**	2.3	1.9	2.9	1.9	1.9	2.4	2.9	1.8

Table 6.4 Mean numbers of correct heart attack symptoms recognized, separated by age, education, gender, blood pressure, and BMI. The highest average of recognized symptoms in each group is bolded

		Nine countries	Germany	France	Spain	Austria	Poland	Italy	Netherlands	UK	Russia
Age	14–35	2.2	2.6	2.3	1.8	**3.1**	1.8	1.8	2.3	2.8	1.5
	36–64	2.5	**3.4**	2.3	1.9	3.2	2.1	2.1	2.6	3.0	2.0
	65+	2.4	**3.3**	2.3	1.8	3.0	2.1	1.8	2.3	2.5	2.2
Education	Low	2.4	**3.1**	2.1	1.6	2.3	1.8	1.9	2.4	2.6	–
	Medium	2.6	3.2	2.3	1.8	**3.4**	2.1	2.0	2.5	3.1	–
	High	2.7	**3.3**	2.6	2.0	3.1	2.2	2.0	2.4	3.1	–
Sex	Male	2.2	**3.0**	2.2	1.8	2.8	1.9	1.8	2.2	2.7	1.6
	Female	2.5	**3.3**	2.4	1.9	3.1	2.0	2.0	2.6	3.0	2.0
Blood pressure	Normal	2.3	**3.2**	2.4	1.9	3.0	1.9	2.0	2.4	2.9	1.7
	High	2.4	**3.4**	2.3	2.0	2.9	2.3	1.9	2.7	2.8	2.2
BMI	Normal	2.2	**3.0**	2.3	1.9	2.9	2.0	2.0	2.4	2.8	1.7
	Overweight	2.4	**3.3**	2.4	1.8	3.1	2.0	1.8	2.5	2.9	1.9
	Obese	2.5	**3.5**	2.2	1.8	3.0	2.2	2.0	2.6	3.0	2.2

heart attack symptoms than did those with normal weight, but the effects are small. When testing countries separately, these effects hold only in Germany and Russia (Table 6.4).

What proportion of the general public recognizes symptoms of stroke? The stroke symptoms most frequently recognized were slurred speech, paralysis, and lopsided face. Yet none of the 14 stroke symptoms was recognized by more than 50% of the Europeans interviewed (Table 6.5). Once again, participants in Germany ($M=5.01$; 95% CI=4.85–5.17) and Austria ($M=4.94$; 95% CI=4.49–5.40) were familiar with more symptoms than were participants in other countries. As for heart attack symptoms, participants in Italy, Spain, Poland, and Russia recognized the lowest number of stroke symptoms. Nineteen percent of the Europeans interviewed did not recognize any stroke symptom at all.

The association between stroke symptom recognition and age was weakly positive ($r=0.08$) across all countries, mirroring the results for heart attack symptoms. When tested separately for each country, associations were strongest in Germany ($r=0.14$), Russia ($r=0.19$), and Poland ($r=0.08$), and weakest in France ($r=-0.08$; see Table 6.6 for means). The higher the level of education, the more stroke symptoms people identified (see Table 6.6), and women identified them more frequently than men did (3.62 vs. 3.01, 95% $CI_{diff}=0.72–0.49$).

Across all countries, people at higher risk for stroke owing to hypertension did not recognize more symptoms than did those with normal blood pressure (see Table 6.6 for means). People classified as overweight (3.55 vs. 3.25, 95% $CI_{diff}=0.17–0.43$) or obese (3.71 vs. 3.25, 95% $CI_{diff}=0.27–0.64$) identified more stroke symptoms than did those with normal weight. However, between countries, this difference holds only in Germany and Russia. Outside of these two countries, people at higher risk owing to hypertension or obesity were not better informed about stroke.

What proportion of the general public knows what to do in case of a stroke? Fifty-one percent of participants would take the most appropriate action and call an ambulance (Table 6.7). Surprisingly, in Germany and Austria—the two countries where people identified most symptoms of a stroke—only 33% and 34% would have called an ambulance immediately; instead, one of about three Germans and Austrians would advise the sufferer to go to bed or take a sip of water.

Across all countries, those participants who would call an ambulance or a doctor immediately recognized on average 3.6 symptoms, and those who would not do so recognized 3.1 (95% $CI_{diff}=0.32–0.55$). Spain was the only country where no difference was found.

Contribution of information source to symptom knowledge. Participants were asked how often they used 14 different sources of health information. Sixty-two percent said that they sometimes or frequently rely on friends and family for health information, followed by 59% stating their general practitioner and 54% their pharmacist as primary source. The next most frequently consulted sources were mass media (TV, 43%; popular magazines, 26%; daily newspaper, 25%; radio, 23%). Leaflets and pamphlets by health organizations were used by 21% and reference books about

Table 6.5 Percentage of participants who recognized a condition as a symptom for a stroke (all conditions except for earache are typical symptoms). Mean across the nine countries was weighted by sample size. The highest recognition value for each symptom is bolded

	Nine countries	Germany	France	Spain	Austria	Poland	Italy	Netherlands	UK	Russia
Slurred speech	44.0	53.2	41.6	27.4	49.7	36.2	36.2	64.7	**65.7**	38.6
Paralysis	43.0	74.4	43.3	34.9	**74.9**	40.2	31.3	49.5	38.5	31.4
Lopsided face	38.3	60.2	50.3	27.0	64.1	19.4	14.1	**74.1**	48.1	29.6
Dizziness	32.5	45.4	42.3	26.0	**47.3**	39.9	19.1	20.6	29.7	28.2
Inclination to fall to one side	29.8	**45.8**	44.9	21.8	39.7	17.4	16.9	35.1	38.0	20.6
Sudden confusion	26.2	41.5	41.7	20.8	**42.9**	15.0	24.4	31.3	34.5	11.2
Prickly feeling	24.7	26.9	19.5	3.0	20.4	15.2	20.5	3.2	25.1	**39.5**
Numbness	23.2	33.7	29.0	5.0	28.3	34.3	19.4	20.5	**52.5**	6.5
Debility	18.9	26.9	23.3	10.4	23.4	7.2	5.4	11.9	13.0	**27.0**
Sudden one-sided blindness	17.9	30.1	**31.9**	10.6	31.5	15.3	7.9	21.0	25.8	7.4
Spit running out of mouth	15.4	28.9	17.3	7.9	**32.3**	11.0	4.3	28.8	24.5	8.6
Problems eating	9.5	**19.0**	15.6	4.5	21.4	3.2	3.0	6.2	10.3	6.8
Earache	5.9	6.0	**10.9**	5.6	4.5	2.4	2.0	1.1	3.4	8.0
Frequent difficulties swallowing	5.6	10.4	**11.6**	4.7	11.3	4.0	1.2	3.4	5.4	3.0
Runny eyes	4.0	4.9	5.1	4.3	**7.1**	3.4	0.8	3.1	5.4	3.7
I don't know	19.1	9.8	14.3	16.2	2.8	27.6	**28.2**	7.1	14.3	26.0
Mean number of correct symptoms	3.3	**5.0**	4.2	2.1	4.9	2.6	2.0	3.7	4.2	2.6

Table 6.6 Number of correct stroke symptoms recognized, separated by age, education, gender, blood pressure, and BMI. The highest average of recognized symptoms in each group is bolded

		Nine countries	Germany	France	Spain	Austria	Poland	Italy	Netherlands	UK	Russia
Age	14–35	3.3	4.0	4.3	2.1	**6.3**	2.4	1.9	3.9	3.9	2.0
	36–64	3.9	5.5	4.4	2.1	**5.6**	2.8	2.2	4.0	4.6	3.0
	65+	3.5	**5.1**	3.5	2.0	4.9	2.7	1.9	3.1	3.3	3.2
Education	Low	3.4	**5.0**	3.4	1.7	4.9	2.2	2.0	3.1	3.5	–
	Medium	4.0	5.2	4.0	2.0	**5.6**	3.00	2.1	4.0	4.7	–
	High	4.4	5.2	5.4	2.5	**6.0**	3.4	2.3	4.1	5.0	–
Sex	Male	3.0	4.7	3.9	2.1	**4.9**	2.5	1.9	3.4	3.7	2.1
	Female	3.6	**5.3**	4.4	2.1	5.0	2.7	2.2	4.0	4.6	3.1
Blood pressure	Normal	3.6	5.1	4.3	2.1	**6.1**	2.6	2.1	3.7	4.2	2.5
	High	3.7	**5.6**	4.1	2.1	3.2	3.1	2.0	4.0	4.1	3.2
BMI	Normal	3.3	4.8	4.2	2.2	**5.4**	2.5	2.1	3.8	4.0	2.3
	Overweight	3.6	5.1	4.3	2.1	**5.4**	2.8	1.9	3.8	4.4	2.9
	Obese	3.7	**5.8**	3.6	1.7	**5.8**	3.0	2.5	4.0	4.2	3.4

Table 6.7 Percentage of participants who would take the following actions if they saw a person with stroke symptoms. The highest percentage for each action is bolded

Action	Nine countries	Germany	France	Spain	Austria	Poland	Italy	Netherlands	UK	Russia
Call an ambulance	51	33	43	42	34	**66**	49	41	58	64
Call doctor immediately	44	46	60	**61**	53	31	47	55	42	32
Recommend going to bed and waiting	16	12	23	13	13	6	5	1	3	**32**
Advise seeing a doctor	16	**35**	11	12	34	11	7	18	18	10
Give a sip of fluid	8	16	7	8	**17**	3	5	1	3	7

health topics by 20%. Health insurance companies were consulted by 17% and the Internet by only 15% of the population (when this survey was conducted in 2006, Internet was available to 49% of citizens in the 27 countries of the European Union; see Table 6.1 for availability per country; data for Russia are not available). Information from consumer counseling and patient counseling was sought by 6% for each, and from self-help organizations by 4% (for more details on use of information sources, see Chap. 5 and Gigerenzer et al. 2009).

Across all countries, the highest correlations between the frequency of consulting a source and the number of symptoms of heart attack known were found for leaflets and pamphlets by health organizations ($r=0.16$) and reference books on health topics ($r=0.15$). For individual countries, reference books on health topics were the source most frequently related to recognition of heart attack symptoms (Germany, $r=0.23$; France $r=0.14$; Austria, $r=0.19$; Italy, $r=0.18$; and Russia, $r=0.20$). Usage of the Internet for health information and recognition of heart attack symptoms was correlated in Germany ($r=0.08$), France ($r=0.09$), Italy ($r=0.09$), the UK ($r=0.06$), and Russia ($r=0.05$). The correlation between the frequency with which participants consult their general practitioner and the number of heart attack symptoms recognized was positive in Germany ($r=0.14$), Poland ($r=0.13$), Italy ($r=0.10$), and Russia ($r=0.13$); in all other countries there was no correlation (all 95% CIs include 0).

As for recognition of heart attack symptoms, those who most frequently consulted either leaflets and pamphlets by health organizations or reference books on health topics mentioned a higher number of correct stroke symptoms ($r=0.16$). In the different countries, reference books on health topics were again most frequently associated with symptom recognition (Germany, $r=0.20$; France, $r=0.18$; Spain, $r=0.16$; Italy, $r=0.20$; Poland, $r=0.16$; the Netherlands, $r=0.18$; Russia, $r=0.19$). The frequency of using the Internet for health information and recognition of stroke symptoms was correlated in seven of the nine countries (Germany, $r=0.08$; France, $r=0.13$; Spain, $r=0.13$; Italy, $r=0.11$; Netherlands, $r=0.16$; UK, $r=0.08$; Russia, $r=0.05$). Mirroring the results for heart attack, there was a relation between the frequency of consulting a general practitioner for health information and recognition of stroke symptoms in a few countries, namely in Germany ($r=0.10$), Poland ($r=0.14$), and Russia ($r=0.12$).

Use of information sources and reaction to stroke symptoms. Across all countries, people who would call an ambulance did not consult health information sources more frequently. A striking result is that in no country except the UK did people who sometimes or frequently consult their general practitioner say more often than others that they would call an ambulance or doctor if they saw a person suffering stroke symptoms (all $\chi^2<2.68$, all $p>0.12$; exception UK, $\chi^2=10.22$, $p=0.001$).

6.3 Discussion and Conclusions

To our knowledge, the study reported in this chapter is the first representative survey in nine European countries relating symptom recognition and action-relevant knowledge of heart attack and stroke with information sources consulted. We found that of six valid signs listed for heart attack, only chest pain was recognized by a majority of Europeans. Out of 14 symptoms for stroke, none was recognized by more than 50% of Europeans interviewed; one in five did not recognize any symptoms. Only about half of the 10,228 persons would call an ambulance immediately when witnessing someone suffering stroke symptoms. Interestingly, people at higher risk were generally not better informed about symptoms or what to do in case of stroke.

In all countries, women recognized more heart attack and stroke symptoms than men. Recognition of symptoms for both heart attack and stroke was highest in Germany and Austria, whereas only about half as many symptoms were recognized in Spain, Poland, Italy, and Russia. At the same time, Poland has the highest mortality rate from ischemic heart disease and cerebrovascular disease of all countries surveyed and among the highest mortality rates from cerebrovascular disease (numbers for Russia are not available). Ignorance about heart attack and stroke symptoms might well contribute to this high mortality rate and is thus especially worrisome.

The findings of our study differ from results from other studies. For instance, 92% of participants in a random US sample recognized chest pain or discomfort as heart attack symptoms; 31% of the participants recognized five symptoms (Fang et al. 2008). The numbers across the European countries we surveyed were substantially lower, with an average of 80% recognizing chest pain and 6% recognizing five or more symptoms. Also, recognition of stroke symptoms in our study, at up to 44% for slurred speech, was substantially lower than knowledge in previous studies in the US (Greenlund et al. 2003), Ireland (Parahoo et al. 2003), or Spain (Segura et al. 2003), where 88–95% of participants recognized symptoms. Only the study by Yoon et al. (2001) reported similarly low numbers for stroke symptom recognition: In a community sample in Australia, each of 11 listed symptoms was recognized by between 4 and 24% of participants. One possible explanation for the lower level of knowledge of heart attack and stroke symptoms in our European sample in comparison to earlier studies is that we used a representative sample and did not recruit participants through random digit dialing (Greenlund et al. 2003), random selection from a telephone directory (Yoon et al. 2001), or systematic random sampling (Parahoo et al. 2003). It was shown, for example, that participants randomly selected through random dialing were better educated than a sample representative for the population at large. When individuals are randomly called, well-educated individuals are more likely to participate (Wang et al. 2009), suggesting that studies using random procedures or community samples might actually overestimate knowledge in the population. However, a representative sample in Spain (Segura et al. 2003) also showed a higher proportion of participants that recognized symptoms than in our study.

Not only is recognizing symptoms important but also knowing what to do in the event of heart attack or stroke. When asked what they would do in the event of an acute stroke, 43% of participants in a Turkish community sample (Evci et al. 2007), 45% of a Spanish representative sample (Segura et al. 2003), 67% in an Australian community sample (Carroll et al. 2004), and 76% in a US community sample (Blades et al. 2005) said they would call an ambulance. However, when the same Australian community sample was presented with symptoms that are typical of a stroke (instead of the diagnosis "stroke"), the percentage that would call an ambulance ranged from only 1% if witnessing dizziness to 20% if witnessing weakness or paralysis (Carroll et al. 2004). These proportions approximately doubled if "going to the hospital casualty/emergency department" is also counted as a correct response (Yoon et al. 2001). Findings are analog for the US community sample (Blades et al. 2005): If symptoms were given instead of the diagnosis "stroke," the proportion of participants that would call an ambulance if witnessing weakness or paralysis dropped to 49%. Among patients in a UK hospital who had experienced a stroke within the last 48 h and recognized that they were experiencing a stroke, 25% had called an ambulance; of those patients who did not recognize that they were experiencing a stroke only 12.5% had called an ambulance (Carroll et al. 2004). In a Brazilian community sample presented with the scenario of a relative who is experiencing a number of symptoms typical for a stroke, such as difficulty speaking and walking, 51% would call an ambulance (Evci et al. 2007). Similarly, across all nine European countries surveyed in our study, 51% would call an ambulance if they saw a person experiencing symptoms typical of a stroke. This proportion is comparable to the results in community samples in Australia, Turkey, and Brazil described above, where participants were presented a description of a person suffering symptoms that are typical of a stroke but they were not told that this person was having a stroke. Therefore, the higher proportions of those who would call an ambulance found in other studies might be due to the presentation format of the question, that is, when participants are explicitly told that the person is suffering a stroke. As in the study among hospitalized UK stroke patients described above (Carroll et al. 2004), those who recognized that they were experiencing a stroke were more likely to call an ambulance. Increasing recognition of stroke symptoms and awareness of the most adequate response thus seems central to ensuring that more than half of the population knows what to do when they see someone experiencing a stroke.

Findings from previous studies also showed family and friends to be one of the most frequently consulted sources of health information knowledge (for a review, see Nicol and Thrift 2005). In contrast, participants in our survey more often asked their physician or pharmacist for advice. Other studies in the US and Australia had found that their participants relied on mass media more often than on physicians or hospital personnel, whom only 11–20% of participants consulted (Hesse et al. 2005; Nicol and Thrift 2005). We are not aware of other studies that related the frequency with which certain sources of health information were consulted to level of knowledge. Our study found very low correlations between level of knowledge and use of any information source. It should be noted that one source of medical knowledge that was not included in this survey is personal experience or witnessing others who have personal experience with a medical condition such as heart attack or stroke (for a review, see Stroebele et al. 2011). Nonetheless, even given personal experience with heart attack or stroke, participants likely consulted the information sources assessed in this survey to gather further information about their (or their loved ones') condition.

For the interpretation of our findings it should also be noted that some structural differences in the health care systems surveyed have elsewhere been suggested to affect how often and which health services are frequented. For example, nationalized publicly funded health systems as in the UK seem to be most effective at reducing inequalities in access to medical services (Gelormino et al. 2011), and might increase the number of times patients see their GP in these countries. In France, health insurance is also universal, but roughly 25% of the costs are covered by patients' co-payments, leading to a high frequency of supplementary health insurance. Patients with supplementary health insurance visit their GP significantly more often than those without it (Buchmueller et al. 2004); the importance of the GP as a source of health information might hence differ between those with and without supplementary insurance in France. However, empirical studies on factors that affect accessibility of health care in Europe are sparse and generally of poor quality (Gelormino et al. 2011). Another important difference is the availability of thrombolytic therapy in the countries surveyed. A pan-European survey showed that between 44% (Eastern Europe) and 73% (UK and Ireland) of patients with a heart attack received thrombolytic therapy (Fox et al. 2000). For people living in countries in which thrombolytic therapy is provided more often, arriving at the hospital within a few hours is even more important.

Another structural aspect related to heart attack and stroke knowledge and access to health-related information that was not considered in our survey is numeracy, or skills necessary to understand and manipulate different numerical expressions of probability about health (see Chap. 1), the ability to understand written information in situations that are encountered in daily life. Reading literacy differs between the countries (Chaps. 2 and 3; see also Galesic and Garcia-Retamero 2010). A further possible limitation is that the data reported in this chapter were collected in 2006 and reflect the state of heart attack and stroke symptoms in that year, without taking into account potential changes in relevant knowledge. Since then, for instance, public awareness campaigns as well as health care system reforms have been launched. This together with the structural differences between countries described above should be taken into consideration when interpreting the present study's findings on consultation of health information sources and knowledge about heart attack or stroke.

In spite of these limitations, the present survey of representative samples of nine European countries provides a major new contribution, making it possible to compare knowledge between countries and relate knowledge level of stroke and heart attack to characteristics of the health system. Altogether, awareness of warning signs of stroke and heart attack was found to be low among the European population, particularly among participants in Italy, Spain, Poland, and Russia. Although people at risk due to hypertension or obesity should be better informed than those who are not (compare e.g., Stroebele et al. 2011), we did not find that they were. In Germany and Austria, few were aware that calling an ambulance immediately is the most efficient action to save lives and avoid disability. This poor action-relevant knowledge in both countries is in stark contrast to their high level of symptom recognition and is in line with another German survey that also showed a large discrepancy between high symptom and poor action-relevant knowledge among a smaller, non-representative sample (Weltermann et al. 2000). These findings suggest that public health campaigns, particularly in Germany and Austria, should target action-relevant knowledge more strongly. Furthermore, the observation that, in all European countries, frequent consulting of a general practitioner contributes so little to people's understanding of the warning signals for stroke and heart disease deserves further investigation.

References

Anderson, J. R., & Bower, G. H. (1973). *Human associative memory*. Washington, DC: Winston.

Blades, L. L., Oser, C. S., Dietrich, D. W., Okon, N. J., Rodriguez, D. V., Burnett, A. M., et al. (2005). Rural community knowledge of stroke warning signs and risk factors. *Preventing Chronic Diseases, 2*, A14.

Buchmueller, T. C., Couffinhal, A., Grignon, M., & Perronnin, M. (2004). Access to physician services: Does supplemental insurance matter? Evidence from France. *Health Economics, 13*, 669–687.

Bundesamt, S. (2006a). *Europäische union*. Wiesbaden: Statistisches Bundesamt.

Bundesamt, S. (2006b). *Länderprofil Russische Föderation 2006*. Wiesbaden: Statistisches Bundesamt.

Carroll, C., Hobart, J., Fox, C., Teare, L., & Gibson, J. (2004). Stroke in Devon: Knowledge was good, but action was poor. *Journal of Neurology, Neurosurgery, and Psychiatry, 75*, 567–571.

Eurostat (2009). *Internet usage in 2009—Households and Individuals*. Luxembourg: Eurostat. http://gsmonline.pl/download/files/eurostat_broadband_internet_usage_in_2009.pdf, accessed July 30, 2012.

Eurostat (2011a). *Death due to ischaemic heart diseases, by gender—Standardised death rate by 100 000 inhabitants*. Luxembourg: Eurostat. http://epp.eurostat.ec.europa.eu/tgm/table.do?tab=table&init=1&plugin=1&language=en&pcode=tps00119, accessed July 30, 2012.

Eurostat (2011b). *Healthy life years and life expectancy at birth, by sex*. Luxembourg: Eurostat. http://epp.eurostat.ec.europa.eu/portal/page/portal/product_details/dataset?p_product_code=TSDPH100, accessed July 30, 2012.

Evci, E. D., Memis, S., Ergin, F., & Beser, E. (2007). A population-based study on awareness of stroke in Turkey. *European Journal of Neurology, 14*, 517–522.

Fang, J., Keenan, N., Dai, S., & Denny, C. (2008). Disparities in adult awareness of heart attack warning signs and symptoms—14 states, 2005. *Morbidity and Mortality Weekly Report, 57*, 175–179.

Fox, K. A. A., Cokkinos, D. V., Deckers, J., Keil, U., Maggioni, A., Steg, G., et al. (2000). The ENACT study: A pan-European survey of acute coronary syndromes. *European Heart Journal, 21*, 1440–1449.

Frank, R. (2007). *European consumer study—Gesundheit in Europa*. Nuremberg: GfK e.V.

Galesic, M., & Garcia-Retamero, R. (2010). Statistical numeracy for health: A cross-cultural comparison with probabilistic national samples. *Archives of Internal Medicine, 170*, 462–468.

Gelormino, E., Bambra, C., Spadea, T., Bellini, S., & Costa, G. (2011). The effects of health care reforms on health inequalities: A review and analysis of the European evidence base. *International Journal of Health Services, 41*, 209–230.

Gigerenzer, G., Mata, J., & Frank, R. (2009). Public knowledge of benefits of breast and prostate cancer screening in Europe. *Journal of the National Cancer Institute, 101*, 1216–1220.

Greenlund, K. J., Neff, L. J., Zheng, Z. J., Keenan, N. L., Giles, W. H., Ayala, C. A., et al. (2003). Low public recognition of major stroke symptoms. *American Journal of Preventive Medicine, 25*, 315–319.

Hesse, B. W., Nelson, D. E., Kreps, G. L., Croyle, R. T., Arora, N. K., Rimer, B. K., et al. (2005). Trust and sources of health information: The impact of the Internet and its implications for health care providers. Findings from the first Health Information National Trends Survey. *Archives of Internal Medicine, 165*, 2618–2624.

Kothari, R., Jauch, E., Broderick, J., Brott, T., Sauerbeck, L., Khoury, J., et al. (1999). Acute stroke: Delays to presentation and emergency department evaluation. *Annals of Emergency Medicine, 33*, 3–8.

Lacy, C. R., Suh, D. C., Bueno, M., & Kostis, J. B. (2001). Delay in presentation and evaluation for acute stroke: Stroke time registry for outcomes knowledge and epidemiology (S.T.R.O.K.E.). *Stroke, 32*, 63–69.

Murray, C. J., & Lopez, A. D. (1997). Mortality by cause for eight regions of the world: Global burden of disease study. *Lancet, 349*, 1269–1276.

Nicol, M. B., & Thrift, A. G. (2005). Knowledge of risk factors and warning signs of stroke. *Vascular Health and Risk Management, 1*, 137–147.

Parahoo, K., Thompson, K., Cooper, M., Stringer, M., Ennis, E., & McCollam, P. (2003). Stroke: Awareness of the signs, symptoms and risk factors—A population-based survey. *Cerebrovascular Diseases, 16*, 134–140.

Postman, L. (1963). One trial learning. In C. F. Cofer & B. S. Musgrave (Eds.), *Verbal behavior and learning* (pp. 295–332). New York: McGraw-Hill.

Qureshi, A. I., Kirmani, J. F., Sayed, M. A., Safdar, A., Ahmed, S., Ferguson, R., et al. (2005). Time to hospital arrival, use of thrombolytics, and in-hospital outcomes in ischemic stroke. *Neurology, 64*, 2115–2120.

Segura, T., Vega, G., Lopez, S., Rubio, F., Castillo, J., & Span, C. D. S. G. (2003). Public perception of stroke in Spain. *Cerebrovascular Diseases, 16*, 21–26.

Stroebele, N., Muller-Riemenschneider, F., Nolte, C. H., Muller-Nordhorn, J., Bockelbrink, A., & Willich, S. N. (2011). Knowledge of risk factors, and warning signs of stroke: A systematic review from a gender perspective. *International Journal of Stroke, 6*, 60–66.

Wang, P. P., Dicks, E., Gong, X., Buehler, S., Zhao, J., Squires, J., et al. (2009). Validity of random-digit-dialing in recruiting controls in a case-control study. *American Journal of Health Behavior, 33*, 513–520.

Wardlaw, J. M., Sandercock, P. A., & Berge, E. (2003). Thrombolytic therapy with recombinant tissue plasminogen activator for acute ischemic stroke: Where do we go from here? A cumulative meta-analysis. *Stroke, 34*, 1437–1442.

Weltermann, B. M., Rogalewski, A., Homann, J., Berger, K., Schulte, H., Assmann, G., et al. (2000). Knowledge about stroke among the German population. *Deutsche medizinische Wochenschrift, 125*, 416–420.

World Health Organization (2008). *Deaths from stroke. Cardiovascular disease atlas, 16*. http://www.who.int/cardiovascular_diseases/en/cvd_atlas_16_death_from_stroke.pdf, accessed July 30, 2012.

World Health Organization (2011). *The top 10 causes of death*. http://www.who.int/mediacentre/factsheets/fs310/en/index.html, accessed July 30, 2012.

Yoon, S. S., Heller, R. F., Levi, C., Wiggers, J., & Fitzgerald, P. E. (2001). Knowledge of stroke risk factors, warning symptoms, and treatment among an Australian urban population. *Stroke, 32*, 1926–1930.

Part II
Transparent Communication of Health-Related Risks Across Cultures

Chapter 7
Communicating Information About Preventive Medical Treatments and Screenings*

Mirta Galesic and Rocio Garcia-Retamero

Abstract Analogies are often used to explain health-related concepts in medical practice, but it is unclear whether they actually improve understanding and if so, why. Here, we studied these issues in experiments on probabilistic national samples in two countries, focusing on two questions. First, we investigated whether analogies are helpful in communicating medical information to people with different levels of numeracy and for tasks of different levels of difficulty. Second, following existing theories of analogies, we studied what characteristics of analogies improve their helpfulness. Our results revealed that for difficult medical problems, analogies were helpful to high-numeracy people but less so to low-numeracy people. For easy medical problems, the results were reversed. Different analogies were successful in different cultural contexts. Our results are in accord with our theoretical expectations and have practical implications for the design and use of analogies to communicate health-related information.

---

*In this chapter, we partially reproduced the article Galesic, M., & Garcia-Retamero, R. (2012). Using analogies to communicate information about health risks. *Applied Cognitive Psychology*. doi: 10.1002/acp.2866

M. Galesic, Ph.D. (✉)
Center for Adaptive Behavior and Cognition, Max Planck Institute for Human Development, Lentzeallee 94, Berlin 14195, Germany
e-mail: galesic@mpib-berlin.mpg.de

R. Garcia-Retamero, Ph.D.
Departamento de Psicología Experimental, Facultad de Psicología, University of Granada, Campus Universitario de Cartuja s/n, Granada 18071, Spain

Center for Adaptive Behavior and Cognition, Max Planck Institute for Human Development, Lentzeallee 94, Berlin 14195, Germany
e-mail: rretamer@ugr.es

R. Garcia-Retamero and M. Galesic (eds.), *Transparent Communication of Health Risks: Overcoming Cultural Differences*, DOI 10.1007/978-1-4614-4358-2_7,

7.1 Introduction and Background

Many patients have little understanding of basic statistical concepts—such as probabilities and the notion of a random toss—that are prerequisites for understanding information about the risks and benefits of health-related behaviors and medical treatments (see Chap. 2). As a consequence, they are at risk of making inadequate health-related choices, and in turn of suffering illness and having higher mortality (Reyna et al. 2009). Visual aids can improve understanding in patients with low numeracy who understand basic graphs (Gaissmaier et al. 2011; see also Chaps. 9–11). However, a significant portion of the general population-up to one third-lacks the basic skills required to understand both numerical and visual formats (see Chap. 4). Therefore it is crucial to explore alternative ways to communicate medical information to this particularly vulnerable group of people.

In this chapter we investigate a method that may improve understanding of complex medical information even in patients that lack basic numeracy and graph literacy: using analogous examples from everyday life (Sopory and Dillard, 2002; see also Chap. 8). Analogies, metaphors, and related figures of speech compare objects from different domains to illuminate some of their aspects (Holyoak et al. 2001). To illustrate, consider the following analogy that a doctor might use in medical practice: "Cancer screening is to cancer as a car alarm is to car theft." The analogy explains the relationship between cancer screening and cancer (the *target* of the analogy) by means of the relationship between car alarm and car theft, one that is well grounded in everyday experience (the *base* of the analogy). The relationship that holds in the car domain (i.e. the fact that a car alarm sometimes signals theft but sometimes gives false alarm or does not activate when it should) is applicable to the cancer domain, as well.

Analogies have long been used in science education to explain a wide range of concepts (Oppenheimer 1956). For instance, Mintz and Ostbye (1992) used analogies from legal practice to explain statistical concepts to medical professionals. Boyle et al. (2004) explained the complexities involved in a team approach to cancer treatment by comparing it to a rugby game. Newby et al. (1995) successfully used analogies to improve understanding and recall of advanced physiological concepts. Halpern et al. (1990) used the analogy of judges who make and dissolve marriages to explain the workings of enzymes in the body. Doctors have also been using analogies to explain medical concepts to patients since the dawn of medicine. As Edwards (2003) illustrated, one doctor used the following story to explain the limited sensitivity of some medical tests to patients: "Imagine you are a fire fighter called to a burning house. From inside, you hear screaming. You manage to rescue *x* of the *y* occupants, but despite your best efforts *z* perish. Should you be hailed as a hero or indicted for homicide?"

Although metaphoric language and analogies are used in medical practice (Sopory 2005), there is a lack of published research investigating whether they are helpful to patients—that is, whether they actually improve understanding of medical information. To the best of our knowledge, only few studies investigated this issue.

To illustrate, Edwards et al. (2006) conducted an experimental study with patients in the United Kingdom. These authors used familiar examples, such as the likelihood of a road accident, the chance of winning a lottery, and the success of treatments for common infections and hypertension, as analogies to explain the risks and benefits of different approaches to managing diabetes. The authors did not find a reliable effect of these analogies on patients' decisional conflict (i.e., their subjective uncertainty about which approach is best) or on their satisfaction with the information. The authors also used graphical displays to communicate the risks and benefits but found no effects of those aids, either. It is possible that the analogies and the graphs did not help because the task was relatively easy for these participants, for two reasons. First, the participants were well educated (68% had some form of higher education, compared to 31% of such people in the United Kingdom overall; Department for Innovation, Universities and Skills 2008). Second, participants were either diabetic patients or their caregivers and hence might already have had a vast amount of knowledge about diabetes treatments. For these participants, understanding information about risks and benefits of different approaches to managing diabetes might have been relatively easy even without aids. In sum, additional aids may not be helpful when there is no problem in understanding the risk information in the first place. However, Edwards et al. (2006) did not control for individual differences in risk understanding or for problem difficulty in their study.

Other studies (e.g., Dillard & Phau, 2002; Sopory & Dillard, 2002) showed that metaphors can be effective persuasion tools for risk communication. For example, Krieger et al. (2011) examined the influence of metaphors on behavioral intentions to participate in clinical trials among rural, low-income, older women. The authors showed that culturally derived metaphors (e.g., sex of a baby when a woman becomes pregnant) helped participants understand the concept of chance and randomization, and increased their intentions to participate in a clinical trial. However, the use of metaphors has also been found to have unintended effects-including failure to understand health messages and information about diagnosis (Chapman et al. 2003), and promoting uninformed decision making about medical treatments (Snowdon et al. 1997). These findings suggest that metaphoric language is not equally useful for everyone and that individual differences or task characteristics may play a role.

In the study reported in this chapter, we address two research questions. First, we investigate in what circumstances analogies can be helpful. Specifically, we investigate whether analogies help people with low and high numeracy skills, understand easy and difficult medical problems. Previous studies on the effect of individual differences on understanding of metaphors and analogies have produced mixed results. Trick and Katz (1986) found that participants with high rather than low analogical reasoning ability were better at recognizing successful metaphors. Whitney et al. (1996) found that people with a low reading memory span, but not those with a high span, were aided by metaphoric rather than literal summaries of complex texts. It is possible that individual abilities interact with problem difficulty: For people with high abilities, analogies may be helpful only when problems are relatively difficult; when problems are easy, their performance could already be so good that it can hardly be further improved. In contrast, people with low abilities may have such low understanding of some of the more difficult problems that analogies cannot help them because they do not understand what parts of the problems are explained by analogies. For easier problems they may have enough understanding to map the analogies to appropriate parts of the task and improve their performance.

We use participants' numeracy skills as a proxy for their abilities, as numeracy has been shown to affect people's understanding of medical information (see Chaps. 2, 3 and 8–11; see also Lipkus 2007; Peters et al. 2007; Reyna et al. 2009; Schwartz et al. 1997). More generally, numeracy enables greater depth of processing, decreases unintended effects of mood and framing on understanding of information, and improves decision making (Peters 2012). Our first hypothesis (H1) is that analogies are helpful to high-numeracy people for difficult problems and to low-numeracy people for easy problems.

Second, we investigate what makes an analogy helpful. In other words, how can we design a good analogy to communicate medical information? Numerous theoretical accounts of analogies and metaphors have been proposed (see Gentner 1983; Hummel and Holyoak 1997; Lakoff and Johnson 1980; Ortony et al. 1978; Tourangeau and Sternberg 1981). In this chapter we focus on those accounts that can help us discern which characteristics of analogies contribute most to successful communication of medical information to patients (Gentner 1983; Marschark et al. 1983; Tourangeau and Sternberg 1981, 1982; Trick and Katz 1986). Specifically, we investigate the role of (a) the similarity of the target and the base of the analogies, (b) the familiarity with the base of the analogies, and (c) the ease of visualization of the base of the analogies.

Similarity is often considered to be the foundation of metaphors and analogies: Their meaning depends on the common features of compared objects. However, more similarity is not necessarily better. As Aristotle (350 B.C.E) stated in his *Rhetoric*, "metaphors must not be far-fetched, or they will be difficult to grasp, nor obvious, or they will have no effect" (trans. W. R. Roberts, Book 3, Chapter 10). In their domains-interaction theory of metaphors, Tourangeau and Sternberg (1981, 1982) differentiated between two types of similarity: within-domain similarity and between-domain similarity. A metaphor is apt when the objects that are involved come from distant domains (i.e., when it has low between-domain similarity) but have similar positions within those domains (i.e., when it has high within-domain similarity). For instance, in the metaphor "the lion is the king among animals," the lion and the king come from distant domains (animals and humans) but occupy similar (i.e., dominating) positions within their domains.

In a similar vein, Gentner (1983) distinguished between the similarity of the *features* of the objects involved in the target and the base of an analogy, and the similarity of the *relationship* between the objects involved in the target to the *relationship* between the objects involved in the base. For example, in the analogy "A lion is among animals [target] as a king is among humans [base]," the lion and the king, as well as animals and humans, have relatively few features in common (i.e., the analogy has low similarity of features). However, the relationship between lions and animals (within the target) is similar to the relationship between kings and humans (within the base; the analogy has high similarity of relationships). Gentner showed that for a successful analogy, the similarity of the relationships is much more important than the similarity of the features. Based on this account, we hypothesized (H2a) that the helpfulness of an analogy in communicating health-related information would not be related to the similarity of the target and base features but would increase with the increasing similarity of the relationships.

Familiarity with the objects in the base of the analogies may be another important factor influencing helpfulness: It has been shown that familiarity increases comprehension of metaphors (Marschark et al. 1983). Analogies based on more familiar concepts are also likely to be better understood (Trick and Katz 1986). The linguists Lakoff and Johnson (1980) argued that everyday experiences are often used to form metaphors for more complex, unobservable concepts. For example, bodily sensations are used to form metaphoric expressions such as *important is big*, *more is up*, *knowing is seeing*, *understanding is grasping*, and *bad is stinky*. In these metaphors, bodily sensations provide a connection between direct experiences and the more abstract concepts. Inspired by this line of reasoning, we hypothesize (H2b) that analogies based on concepts that are part of people's everyday experiences are more helpful than analogies based on less familiar concepts. In addition, while Lakoff and Johnson (1980) remain mostly silent on the role of one's specific cultural experiences in formation of metaphors (but see Lakoff 1987), we find it plausible that differences between cultures in familiarity with certain concepts could partially explain why some analogies work better than others.

Finally, the ease of visualization of the objects in the base of analogies may also be important. Note that ease of visualization is not equivalent to familiarity. In the context of the present study, while many participants may be familiar with the notion of heart attack or cancer, they might have difficulties visualizing these concepts. When visualization is possible, imagery could help people recognize properties of the base that could be useful for explaining the target (Marschark et al. 1983). In addition, according to Paivio's dual-coding theory (Paivio 1969, 1986), imagery helps encoding of information and in turn enhances recall. Higher imaginability has been shown to enhance recall of numerical consequences of health-related behaviors (see Chap. 8; see also Garcia-Retamero et al. 2011). However, empirical evidence does not offer clear support of the importance of imaginability in metaphors and analogies. Marschark et al. (1983) found that imaginability of metaphoric vehicles (equivalent to the base of an analogy) was negatively related to degree of "metaphoricity." In a further study, they found no relationship between vehicle imaginability and recall (see also Marschark and Hunt 1986). Similarly, Honeck (1973) and Reichmann and Coste (1980) did not find a relationship between imagery and recall of proverbs. One reason for the mixed findings in the literature could be that heightened imaginability of an otherwise bad analogy does not help. If the relationship between the objects in the base of the analogy does not map well to the relationship between the objects of the target of the analogy, then increasing the ease of visualization of the objects in the base could deter performance because it may foster using an inappropriate analogy. Therefore, we hypothesize (H2c) that ease of visualization of the objects in the base of the analogy would improve helpfulness only when the analogy is otherwise successful (e.g., when people are familiar with the base of the analogy).

7.2 Studies: Using Analogies to Communicate Medical Information to People with High and Low Numeracy

In two experiments, we sought to answer two main research questions: whether analogies are helpful, and what makes an analogy helpful. To answer these questions, we designed several analogies for communicating benefits of medical treatments and screenings and tested them using probabilistic national samples of low- and high-numeracy people in two different countries, the United States and Germany. These countries differ in several aspects that could affect helpfulness of a particular analogy, such as language, cultural traditions, and various aspects of everyday life (see Chap. 1). We operationalized helpfulness of analogies as the increase in the percentage of participants who gave correct answers when analogies were present versus absent. We measured helpfulness immediately-upon reading the analogy-and after a delay of 3 weeks. The rationale is that an analogy that helps once but whose effect is lost in the next similar situation would not be very helpful in the context of health, where similar decisions often need to be made repeatedly (e.g., whether to go to mammography screenings, or take aspirin to reduce the risk of stroke).

7.2.1 Method

7.2.1.1 Participants

The experiments were conducted on probabilistic national samples in the USA and Germany as part of the project "Helping people with low numeracy understand medical information," funded by the Foundation for Informed Medical Decision Making. The project involved a survey that gathered data for a number of studies related to understanding and communicating risks, conducted in two waves (see also Chaps. 2, 4, 8–11, and 13). In the first wave, large national samples of participants ($n=1{,}009$ in the USA and $n=1{,}001$ in Germany) completed a numeracy scale consisting of nine items selected from Schwartz et al. (1997) and Lipkus et al. (2001; see Chap. 15). Participants with numeracy scores in the top and bottom third of the whole sample ($n=507$ in the USA, and $n=533$ in Germany) were invited to the second wave 3 weeks later.

Approximately half of the participants in the first wave of the overarching project ($n=517$ in the USA, and $n=499$ in Germany) participated in this study. In the first wave, they answered questions about medical treatments and screenings presented with or without analogies. In the second wave, approximately half of the participants who participated in the first wave answered the same questions again ($n=274$ in the USA, and $n=267$ in Germany). Their answers were used to test hypothesis H1. In addition, some participants in the second wave who did *not* answer the questions about medical treatments and screenings in the first wave ($n=233$ in the USA, and $n=266$ in Germany) were asked in the second wave to evaluate the

Table 7.1 Structure of the sample of participants in terms of numeracy, gender, age, and education

	USA		Germany	
	Low numeracy	High numeracy	Low numeracy	High numeracy
First-wave participants in Experiments 1 and 2				
N	277	240	251	248
Mean numeracy (max.=9)	3.8	8.0	4.2	8.1
% Female	56	47	60	39
Mean age (years)	47.0	43.0	47.8	45.5
% High school only[a]	57	28	83	65
Second-wave participants in Experiments 1 and 2				
N	124	150	134	133
Mean numeracy (max.=9)	3.3	8.1	3.4	8.6
% Female	58	47	60	39
Mean age (years)	46.0	42.0	49.2	43.8
% High school only[a]	49	31	87	61
Second-wave participants who evaluated analogies				
N	97	136	126	140
Mean numeracy (max.=9)	3.1	8.1	3.3	8.6
% Female	59	47	60	40
Mean age (years)	44.7	45.2	49.9	43.3
% High school only[a]	55	28	91	59

[a]For comparison, the percentage of the general population with only a high school education (in Germany this means no Abitur) is 47% in the USA and 73% in Germany

characteristics of analogies that were used in the study. Their evaluations were used to test hypotheses H2a–c. The structure of each of these groups of participants, by low and high numeracy, is described in Table 7.1 (see Chap. 2 for more details about the methodology of the survey). This sample enables us to generalize results to low- and high-numeracy people within each country and to compare these groups between countries. In our analyses, we split the participants into two groups according to the median numeracy score for the total sample (i.e., 6; see Peters et al. 2006 for a similar procedure). The average numeracy scores in each of the resulting groups in each country are shown in Table 7.1.

7.2.1.2 Stimuli and Procedure

The questionnaire was administered through the Web and the participants completed it on their home computers. The materials for the English and German versions were carefully developed to be comparable (see Chap. 2 for more details about the translation of the materials and the programmed questionnaire). The Ethics Committee of the Max Planck Institute for Human Development approved the methodology, and all participants consented to participation through an online consent form at the beginning of the survey.

Participants completed two experiments in a randomized order: In Experiment 1 they had to solve two difficult medical problems, and in Experiment 2, two easy medical problems. Difficulty of problems was determined in a pretest with 400 participants in the USA and 400 participants in Germany, drawn from volunteer Web-access panels maintained by the company Survey Sampling International. Difficult problems were solved correctly by, on average, 34% of participants with low numeracy and 45% of those with high numeracy skills (chance level was 33%), whereas easy problems were solved correctly by 54 and 70% of participants with low and high numeracy skills, respectively (chance level was 40%). For each problem, we developed four analogies that could help people find the correct answer. The analogies that worked best were selected and refined in a pretest in our lab at the Max Planck Institute, involving 60 students and 60 older adults. In the pretest, we also checked whether all questions and measures were understandable to participants with different levels of numeracy.

Experiment 1: Difficult medical problems. In these problems, participants were asked about the effectiveness of preventive medical treatments to reduce the risk of a disease. The problems were adapted from the Medical Data Interpretation Test by Schwartz et al. (2005). One problem described a fictitious medical drug—Gritagrel—that reduced the risk of stroke. The other problem described a fictitious toothpaste—Zendil—that promised reduction of the frequency of gum inflammation (see Appendix available online for full text)[1]. Each problem included a question with six possible response options in a randomized order and participants had to select only one option. To illustrate, in the problem describing the fictitious drug Gritagrel, participants received the following information:

> Imagine that you see the following advertisement for a new drug: Gritagrel—50% reduction of strokes. Gritagrel is a new pill meant to prevent strokes. People taking Gritagrel had half as many strokes as people taking a placebo (i.e., a sugar pill). Which one of the following pieces of information would best help you determine how much a person could benefit from Gritagrel?

Response options were: (1) the risk of stroke for people who do not take Gritagrel, (2) the risk of stroke for people who take a different drug for the same purpose, (3) how many people there were in the group taking a placebo (sugar pill), (4) how old the people who participated in the study were, (5) how much a weekly dose of Gritagrel costs, (6) whether Gritagrel has been recommended by a doctors' association for this use (1 is the correct answer).

In the first wave, participants were assigned randomly to one of five groups differing in the introduction that preceded the two problems. One group (namely, the control group) received a general introduction without analogies; the rest of the groups (namely, the analogies groups) received the same introduction and one of four different analogies (listed in the Appendix available online)[1]. To illustrate, participants in the control group received the following introduction:

> Please read the following information carefully. It will help you answer the questions that follow. We often hear in the media that a certain medicine will reduce the chance of getting

[1]Appendix is available at https://sites.google.com/site/mirtagalesic/home/Galesic_Garcia Retamero_Analogies_Appendix.pdf

> some disease by, for example, 50%. To understand how useful this drug could be, it would be good to know how high the risk of getting this disease is in the first place.

Participants in one of the analogies groups received the same introduction as in the control group, and in addition they were told:

> Similarly, to determine how useful taking aspirin is for reducing the risk of a heart attack, it would be good to know how high the risk of having a heart attack is in the first place.

This analogy related taking the new drug that promised to reduce the risk of stroke to taking aspirin to reduce the risk of a heart attack. In the second wave, half of the participants in the first wave read the same problems and answered the two questions again, but without any introduction. The order of the two problems and the response options was randomized in both waves.

Experiment 2: Easy medical problems. In these problems, participants were asked about medical screenings. One of the problems was about using mammography to detect breast cancer, while the other was about the prostate-specific antigen (PSA) test to detect prostate cancer (see Appendix available online for full text)[1]. Each problem included a question with five possible response options in a randomized order and participants had to select only one option. To illustrate, in the problem describing mammography to detect breast cancer, participants received the following information:

> Mammography screening is an X-ray of breasts that can help discover breast cancer. A positive result on the mammography screening does not always mean that a woman has breast cancer. Which one of the following questions would best help you determine how much a woman can profit from mammography screening?

Response options were: (1) how many women who have breast cancer get a positive mammogram? (2) how many women who get a positive mammogram actually have breast cancer? (3) what percentage of women go to mammography screening? (4) how much does mammography screening cost? (5) is mammography screening recommended by doctors' associations? (2 is the correct answer).

As for the difficult problems, participants in the first wave were randomly assigned to one of five groups—determined independently of their group in the difficult problems. One group of participants (namely, the control group) received a general introduction without analogies; the rest of the groups (namely, the analogies groups) received the same introduction and one of four analogies (see Appendix available online for full text)[1]. To illustrate, participants in the control group received the following introduction:

> Please read the following information carefully. It will help you answer the questions that follow. One often hears that medical screenings can help in the early detection of diseases. However, getting a positive result from a screening test does not always mean you have the disease.

Participants in one of the analogies groups received the same introduction as in the control group, and in addition they were said:

> Similarly, not all activated car alarms mean that somebody is trying to steal that car.

This analogy related the use of mammography to detect breast cancer to the use of a car alarm to detect car theft. In the second wave, half of the participants read the same problems and answered the two questions again but did not receive any introduction. The order of the two problems and the response options was randomized in both waves.

Evaluations of analogies. To evaluate the properties of the analogies that we used, we asked six different subgroups of participants to evaluate these analogies in the second wave of the study. These participants did not participate in Experiments 1 and 2. They rated the analogies in terms of (a1) the similarity of the corresponding objects in the base and the target (e.g., for the analogy relating mammography to a car alarm, participants were asked: "How similar would you say that mammography is to a car alarm?" and "how similar would you say that breast cancer is to having a car stolen?"); (a2) the similarity of the relationship between the objects involved in the base to the relationship between the objects involved in the target (e.g., for the same analogy, a group of participants was asked: "How similar is using mammography screenings to detect cancer to using a car alarm to detect that somebody is trying to steal a car?"); (b) the familiarity with the base (e.g., "How familiar does each of the following activities seem to you?" which included, among others, "the use of a car alarm to detect that somebody is trying to steal a car"); and (c) the ease of visualization of the base of the analogies (e.g., "How easy it is for you to visualize each of the following activities?" which included, among others, "the use of a car alarm to detect that somebody is trying to steal a car"). Each participant evaluated one of these properties for all the analogies used in the difficult medical problems and a different property for all the analogies used in the easy medical problems. For each of the questions about similarity (a1 and a2), ratings for Gritagrel and Zendil were collected separately and then averaged for the purpose of analysis. We followed the same procedure in the questions about similarity for mammography and the PSA test. Each property was evaluated on a scale ranging from 1 (*not at all*) to 7 (*a lot*) by a different subgroup of, on average, 39 participants in the USA and 44 participants in Germany.

In sum, one group of participants answered questions about difficult and easy medical problems, with or without the addition of analogies. We analyzed whether analogies helped them answer the questions correctly and whether the analogies were similarly helpful to participants with high and low numeracy skills. A separate group of participants evaluated the analogies we used regarding several properties that have been suggested to improve the helpfulness of analogies. We used these evaluations to investigate what makes an analogy helpful for understanding medical problems. In what follows, we present the results of these analyses.

7.2.2 Results

While analogies were helpful on average, not all analogies worked equally well for all participants in both countries. Table 7.1 shows percentage of participants answering at least one of two tasks correctly in each Experiment, by analogy, country, and

Table 7.2 Percentage of participants answering at least 1 of 2 tasks in each Experiment correctly

	United States				Germany			
	Low numeracy		High numeracy		Low numeracy		High numeracy	
	Wave 1	Wave 2	Wave 1	Wave 2	Wave 1	Wave 2	Wave 1	Wave 2
Experiment 1: Preventive treatment to disease is like …								
Aspirin to heart attack	49	13	58	22	39	38	59	69
Flu vaccine to flu	40	10	76	70	44	42	66	61
Fire insurance to bankruptcy	43	25	49	78	32	53	54	40
Broccoli to cancer	49	28	90	72	35	47	54	60
Control (no analogy)	51	32	58	48	24	36	45	56
Experiment 2: Screening test to disease is like …								
Cough to pneumonia	81	50	71	66	64	73	70	58
Stomach pain to ulcer	72	64	61	85	40	33	67	81
Car alarm to theft	51	21	82	88	64	70	84	75
Metal detector to weapon	75	23	77	83	72	74	69	83
Control (no analogy)	52	38	84	71	59	49	86	79

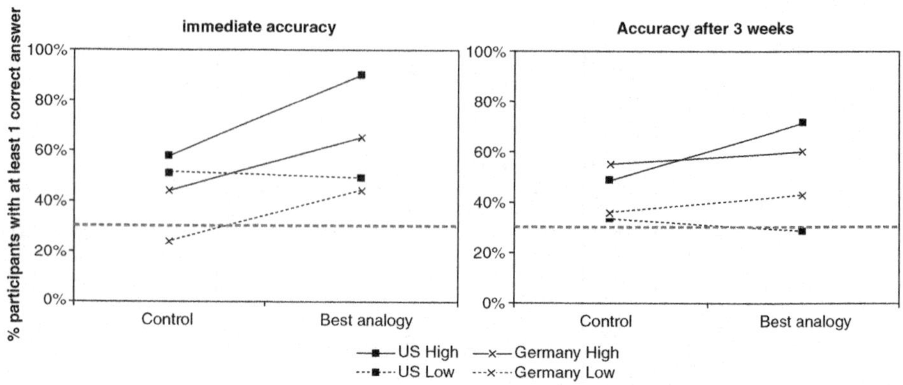

Fig. 7.1 Percentage of participants with high and low numeracy, in each country, correctly answering at least one of the *difficult* problems (Experiment 1), without analogies (control) and with the analogy that most improved immediate accuracy and accuracy after 3 weeks. *Horizontal dotted line* indicates chance level of performance (33%)

numeracy group. For difficult problems, the most helpful analogy in the United States for both low- and high-numeracy participants was "Gritagrel is to stroke/Zendil is to gum inflammation as broccoli is to cancer." In contrast, the most helpful analogy for both low- and high-numeracy people for difficult problems in Germany was "Gritagrel is to stroke/Zendil is to gum inflammation as flu vaccine is to flu" (note that the actual text of the analogies was longer and more elaborated—see the Appendix available online[1]). For easy problems, the most helpful analogy for low-numeracy participants in the United States was "PSA test is to prostate cancer/mammography screening is to breast cancer as cough is to pneumonia," while for low-numeracy people in Germany the most helpful analogy was "PSA test is to prostate cancer/mammography screening is to breast cancer as metal detector is to a weapon." Finally, the most helpful analogy for high-numeracy people in easy problems and in both countries was "PSA test is to prostate cancer/mammography screening is to breast cancer as car alarm is to car theft."

Are Analogies Helpful? Fig. 7.1 shows the percent of participants correctly answering at least one of the two difficult medical problems in Experiment 1 without analogies (control group) and with the analogy that worked best in each numeracy group and country. The figure shows immediate accuracy and accuracy 3 weeks after reading the analogy that worked best. Fig. 7.2 shows the same results for the easy problems in Experiment 2.

In line with the pretest results, the tasks in Experiment 1 were more difficult than those in Experiment 2. Without analogies, on average 37% of low-numeracy and 53% of high-numeracy participants in the first wave answered correctly at least one of the two difficult problems. In contrast, 56% of low-numeracy and 85% of high-numeracy participants answered at least one of the two easy problems correctly. Chance performance was 33% and 40% for difficult and easy problems, respectively.

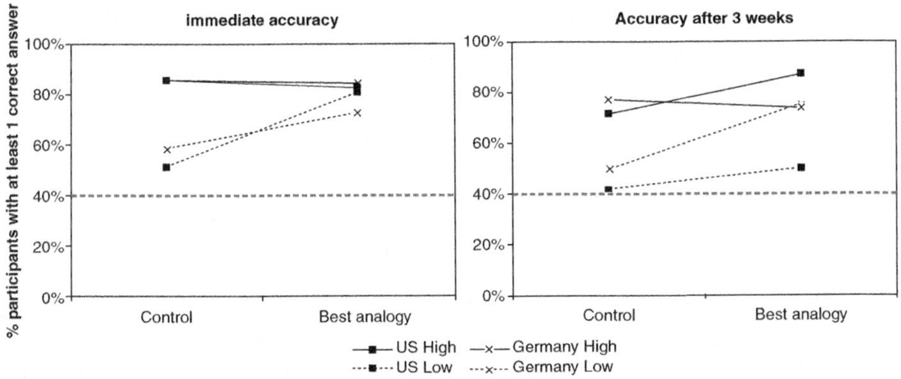

Fig. 7.2 Percentage of participants with high and low numeracy, in each country, correctly answering at least one of the *easy* problems (Experiment 2), without analogies (control) and with the analogy that most improved immediate accuracy and accuracy after 3 weeks. *Horizontal dotted line* indicates chance level of performance (40%)

As the figures show, there was an interaction between problem difficulty and numeracy when accuracy was measured immediately. When the problems were *difficult* (Fig. 7.1, left panel), analogies reliably improved the performance of *high-numeracy* participants in both countries. Compared to the control group, there was an increase of 32 percentage points among high-numeracy participants in the USA and an increase of 21 percentage points among those in Germany. The improvement in participants with low numeracy was smaller: In Germany, it was 20 percentage points over the control group, and in the USA we actually observed an unreliable decrease of 2 percentage points. An analysis of variance (ANOVA) with presence of analogies (yes vs. no), numeracy (high vs. low), and country (USA vs. Germany) as independent variables and percentage of participants correctly answering at least one problem as the dependent variable showed comparable results:[2] The main effect of analogies, $F_{1,341}=13.37$, $p=0.001$, was qualified by an interaction between analogies, numeracy, and country, $F_{1,341}=4.53$, $p=0.034$.

After 3 weeks, the overall performance on difficult problems decreased (Fig. 7.1, right panel). The improvement due to analogies was still present but was only of 23 and 5 percentage points for high-numeracy Americans and Germans, respectively. The improvement was 7 percentage points among low-numeracy Germans. The performance of low-numeracy Americans again decreased slightly with analogies—5 percentage points compared to the control group. An ANOVA equivalent to that reported above indicated no reliable effect of analogies, $F_{1,194}=1.37$, $p=0.244$, and no reliable interactions with numeracy and country in accuracy after 3 weeks.

[2] In this analysis we followed Lunney (1970; see also Cleary and Angel 1984), who showed that ANOVA can be used to obtain conservative results for large samples of a dichotomous dependent variable.

Table 7.3 Results of the regression of the percentage of participants answering at least one of two questions correctly on properties of the analogies

	Immediate accuracy		Accuracy after 3 weeks	
	Beta	*p*	Beta	*p*
Similarity of objects	–0.60	0.03	–0.80	0.02
Similarity of relationships	0.77	0.04	0.79	0.08
Familiarity	0.64	0.05	0.08	0.82
Ease of visualization	−1.13	0.00	–0.83	0.03
Country (0 = USA, 1 = Germany)	–0.06	0.80	0.57	0.08
Adjusted R^2	0.58		0.57	

For the *easy problems*, analogies improved immediate understanding but only for participants with *low numeracy*—29 percentage points in the USA and 14 in Germany (Fig. 7.2, left panel). The performance of high-numeracy participants was approximately the same with and without analogies. As hypothesized, it is possible that this latter group had already reached their ceiling performance and could not be helped more. An ANOVA equivalent to the one conducted before echoed these findings: The main effect of analogies, $F_{1,308}=4.17$, $p=0.042$, was qualified by an interaction between analogies and numeracy, $F_{1,308}=7.72$, $p=0.006$. In contrast to difficult problems, the overall positive effects of analogies in easy problems remained after 3 weeks (Fig. 7.2, right panel), $F_{1,161}=4.539$, $p=0.035$. As the performance of the high-numeracy control groups decreased somewhat, the main effect of analogies was now also positive for high-numeracy people in the USA (i.e., there were no reliable interactions between analogies and numeracy). In sum, in accord with Hypothesis H1, analogies were more helpful to high-numeracy participants for difficult problems and to low-numeracy participants for easy problems. (see Appendix available online for full text)[1]

What Makes an Analogy Helpful? For each type of problem (difficult and easy), four groups of participants received different analogies. What properties of the analogies made some of them more helpful than others? As explained in Sect. 7.2.1.2, a group of participants in the second wave of the study rated four characteristics of each analogy: (a1) the similarity of corresponding objects in the base and the target, (a2) the similarity of the relationship between the objects involved in the base to the relationship between the objects involved in the target, (b) the familiarity with the base, and (c) the ease of visualization of the base. To investigate independent contributions of each of the four factors to the helpfulness of analogies, we regressed the average ratings for each of the eight analogies, calculated separately for each country (i.e., a total of 16 observations) on the percentage of people correctly answering at least one of the problems after reading the analogy. The results are shown in Table 7.3. We have also conducted a simpler analysis by calculating the partial correlations of each characteristic with accuracy, after controlling for the other three characteristics. The pattern of the results remained the same.

As Table 7.3 shows, helpfulness of analogies is explained well by combining the four properties of the analogies and the country. In fact, the combination explains 58% of the variance in immediate accuracy and 57% in accuracy after 3 weeks.

The pattern of regression coefficients is the same at both time points. As predicted by Hypothesis H2a, the higher the similarity of the *relationship* between the objects in the base to the *relationship* between objects in the target of the analogy (a2), the more successful the analogy was. In contrast, higher similarity of the objects in the base and the target of an analogy (a1) made the analogy less successful. Independently of similarity, familiarity with the base of the analogies (b) positively affected their success, in line with Hypothesis H2b. Finally, ease of visualization (c) had an overall negative effect. Further analysis showed that its negative influence was most pronounced when analogies were otherwise not helpful—low in similarity of the relationships and in familiarity. The accuracy achieved with helpful analogies (high in similarity of the relationships and/or familiarity) *increased* from 59% when the analogies were relatively difficult to visualize to 67% when they were easy to visualize, in line with Hypothesis H2c. However, when analogies were not helpful (low in similarity of the relationships and/or familiarity), then ease of visualization further *decreased* performance, from 64% for analogies that were difficult to visualize to 51% for those that were easy to visualize.

7.3 Discussion and Conclusions

To the best of our knowledge, the experiments described in this chapter are the first to investigate whether analogies help communicate medical information to low- and high-numeracy people, for difficult and easy medical problems, and in different countries using probabilistic national samples.

We found that helpfulness critically depended on both problem difficulty and people's numeracy skills. In difficult medical problems, analogies worked for high-numeracy participants but less so for low-numeracy participants. In contrast, in easy medical problems, analogies did not bring further improvement to high-numeracy participants but did enhance understanding of the low-numeracy participants. How can we explain this pattern of results? It is possible that in the difficult problems, low-numeracy participants lacked even a basic understanding of the medical information. Therefore, these participants could not parse the critical information in the target of the analogy that should be compared with the information in the base. To illustrate, one of the analogies used in the difficult problems was "the flu vaccine is to flu as Gritagrel (a stroke-prevention drug) is to stroke." To provide a correct answer in our study, participants had to understand not only that helpfulness of a flu vaccine depends on the base rate of flu, but also which of the response options corresponds to the base rate of stroke. The concept of base rate may have been so novel to low-numeracy people (in particular those in the USA; see Chap. 2) that they could not have profited from the analogies. In contrast, their basic understanding of the easy problems may have been sufficient to discern the relevant information in the target that should be compared to the base.

The interaction between people's numeracy skills and problem difficulty may explain why Edwards et al. (2006) did not find analogies particularly useful. Their participants were highly educated and had good knowledge about their disease. For these participants the task could have been relatively easy even without analogies. Our results highlight the need to tailor the analogies to patients' abilities and knowledge (see also Dillard and Phau 2002; Krieger et al. 2011 for a similar conclusion). If everything is clear, as it might have been for most of our high numeracy participants in Experiment 2, analogies are not needed. In fact they might even be bothersome, as in Edwards et al study. On the other hand, when a patient finds a task so difficult and unclear that she cannot even map the analogies to appropriate parts of the task, then analogies will not improve her performance.

We found that the helpfulness of specific analogies varied across numeracy groups and across countries. Although some analogies performed consistently well across different groups of participants, there was a lot of variability in the success of different analogies in different groups. We tested theory-driven hypotheses about what makes analogies more or less successful for different people. We showed that the most helpful analogies have relatively high similarity of the relationships between objects in the base and objects in the target, but relatively low similarity of the corresponding objects in the base and the target. For example, the analogy "mammography screening is to breast cancer as a metal detector is to a weapon" was quite successful across countries and numeracy groups: The average percentage of participants correctly answering at least one question with the help of this analogy was 74%. In accord with theoretical explanations, it had relatively high similarity of the relationships (3.6) compared to the similarity of objects (2.1 on average across countries). In contrast, the analogy "mammography screening is to breast cancer as stomach pain is to an ulcer," which had somewhat lower similarity of relationships (3.1) and higher similarity of objects (2.9), was much less successful: Across countries and numeracy groups, the average percentage of participants correctly answering at least one question with the help of this analogy was 60%. Higher familiarity with the base of an analogy also contributes to its helpfulness, while easy visualization of the base can backfire when the analogy is otherwise bad. Obviously, factors that influence helpfulness of analogies (e.g., similarity and familiarity) are to a large extent subjective and depend on people's personal experiences. An implication of this finding is that analogies would be most helpful when doctors know their patients reasonably well and can choose an analogy that is related to their patients' everyday experiences.

Our results are in line with recent research on health literacy and medical decision making, which shows that in many countries doctors and their patients have severe problems grasping a host of numerical concepts that are prerequisites for understanding health-relevant risk information (see Chaps. 8–11; see also Ancker and Kaufman 2007; Fagerlin et al. 2007; Fuller et al. 2002; Lipkus and Peters 2009). With results consistent with our findings, this research shows that these problems do not simply occur because of cognitive biases that prevent good decision making (Gigerenzer et al. 2007). In contrast, errors occur because inappropriate information formats complicate and mislead adaptive decision makers. Using *ecologically rational formats* that benefit from the way information is represented in the human mind (Gigerenzer and Edwards 2003; Gigerenzer and Gray 2011) might enhance risk comprehension, communication, and recall, and might help both doctors and their patients to make better decisions about health. Examples of these formats are the use of natural frequencies to improve people's risk understanding (Gigerenzer and Hoffrage 1995), and the use of visual aids to enhance risk understanding and risk communication (Ancker et al. 2006; Lipkus and Hollands 1999; Waters et al. 2007; Zikmund-Fisher et al. 2010; see also Chap. 9), or to eliminate biases (Peters et al. 2009, see also Chap. 10) and errors induced by framed messages (see Chap. 11). Other examples include making consequences of risky behaviors more tangible to enhance risk communication (see Chap. 8), and using evolutionarily plausible group sizes to improve risk understanding and recall (Garcia-Retamero & Galesic, 2011). In sum, ecological information formats are powerful tools that can facilitate the communication and comprehension of information about health.

A limitation of our experiments is that we used only two types of medical problems, which investigated understanding of the importance of base rate for evaluating preventive medical treatments, and understanding the importance of positive predictive value for evaluating medical screenings. Both types of problems are relatively complex and represent only a small portion of the medical problems that patients can face. Future research might investigate whether analogies are helpful to understanding equally essential, but simpler concepts such as relative and absolute risk reduction, conditional probabilities, and single event probabilities. In line with our results, we hypothesize that in these easier problems analogies will be especially useful for patients with low numeracy. A further limitation is that in this study we could not observe the real interaction between patients and doctors. In particular, doctors may differ in their willingness to use analogies. Some particularly disadvantaged groups of patients—for instance, older adults with low numeracy skills—may have problems understanding analogies. This is certainly an important avenue for further research. A final unanswered question is whether analogies would be helpful to people who not only have low numeracy but also have low graph literacy skills, preventing them from profiting from visual aids (see Chap. 4).

In sum, analogies can improve understanding of information about medical treatments and screenings. They can be a useful tool to improve communication with patients in everyday medical practice. If they are well designed and tailored to abilities and circumstances of different patients, they could help both low- and high-numeracy people make better decisions about their health.

References

Ancker, J. S., & Kaufman, D. (2007). Rethinking health numeracy: A multidisciplinary literature review. *Journal of the American Medical Informatics Association, 14*, 713–721.

Ancker, J. S., Senathirajah, Y., Kukafka, R., & Starren, J. B. (2006). Design features of graphs in health risk communication: A systematic review. *Journal of the American Medical Informatics Association, 13*, 608–618.

Aristotle (350 B.C.E.). *Rhetoric* (book 3, chapter 10). (W. R. Roberts, Trans.). http://classics.mit.edu/Aristotle/rhetoric.3.iii.html, accessed July 30, 2012.

Boyle, F., Robinson, E., Heinrich, P., & Dunn, S. (2004). Cancer: Communicating in the team game. *ANZ Journal of Surgery, 74*, 477–481.

Chapman, K., Abraham, C., Jenkins, V., & Fallowfield, L. (2003). Lay understanding of terms used in cancer consultations. *Psycho-Oncology, 12*, 557–566.

Cleary, P. D., Angel, R. (1984). The analysis of relationships involving dichotomous dependent-variables. *Journal of Health and Social Behavior, 25*, 334–348.

Department for Innovation, Universities and Skills (2008). *The level of highest qualification held by adults: England 2007* (rev.). London, UK: Author. http://www.education.gov.uk/rsgateway/DB/SFR/s000798/dsfr05-2008.pdf, accessed July 30, 2012.

Edwards, A. (2003). Communicating risks through analogies. *British Medical Journal, 327*, 749.

Edwards, A., Elwyn, G., & Mulley, A. (2002). Explaining risks: Turning numerical data into meaningful pictures. *British Medical Journal, 324*, 827–830.

Edwards, A., Thomas, R., Williams, R., Ellner, A. L., Brown, P., & Elwyn, G. (2006). Presenting risk information to people with diabetes: Evaluating effects and preferences for different formats by a web-based randomised controlled trial. *Patient Education and Counselling, 63*, 336–349.

Fagerlin, A., Ubel, P. A., Smith, D. M., & Zikmund-Fisher, B. J. (2007). Making numbers matter: Present and future research in risk communication. *American Journal of Health Behavior, 31*, 47–56.

Fagerlin, A., Wang, C., & Ubel, P. A. (2005). Reducing the influence of anecdotal reasoning on people's health care decisions: Is a picture worth a thousand statistics? *Medical Decision Making, 25*, 398–405.

Fuller, R., Dudley, N., & Blacktop, J. (2002). How informed is consent? Understanding of pictorial and verbal probability information by medical inpatients. *Postgraduate Medical Journal, 78*, 543–544.

Galesic, M., Garcia-Retamero, R., & Gigerenzer, G. (2009a). Using icon arrays to communicate medical risks: Overcoming low numeracy. *Health Psychology, 28*, 210–216.

Galesic, M., Gigerenzer, G., & Straubinger, N. (2009b). Natural frequencies facilitate accurate judgments about medical screenings for elderly and people with lower numeracy skills. *Medical Decision Making, 29*, 368–371.

Garcia-Retamero, R., & Galesic, M. (2011). Using plausible group sizes to communicate information about medical risks. *Patient Education and Counseling, 84*, 245–250.

Garcia-Retamero, R., Galesic, M., & Gigerenzer, G. (2010). Do icon arrays help reduce denominator neglect? *Medical Decision Making, 30*, 672–684.

Garcia-Retamero, R., Galesic, M., & Gigerenzer, G. (2011). Enhancing understanding and recall of quantitative information about medical risks: A cross-cultural comparison between Germany and Spain. *Spanish Journal of Psychology, 14*, 213–221.

Gentner, D. (1983). Structure-mapping: A theoretical framework for analogy. *Cognitive Science, 7*, 155–170.

Gigerenzer, G., & Edwards, A. (2003). Simple tools for understanding risks: From innumeracy to insight. *British Medical Journal, 327*, 741–744.

Gigerenzer, G., Gaissmaier, W., Kurz-Milcke, E., Schwartz, L. M., & Woloshin, S. (2007). Helping doctors and patients make sense of health statistics. *Psychological Science in the Public Interest, 8*, 53–96.

Gigerenzer, G., & Gray, J. A. M. (2011). Launching the century of the patient. In G. Gigerenzer & J. A. Muir Gray (Eds.), *Better doctors, better patients, better decisions: Envisioning health care in 2020. Strüngemann Forum Report* (pp. 3–28). Cambridge, MA: MIT Press.

Gigerenzer, G., & Hoffrage, U. (1995). How to improve Bayesian reasoning without instruction: Frequency formats. *Psychological Review, 102*, 684–704.

Halpern, D. F., Hansen, C., & Riefer, D. (1990). Analogies as an aid to understanding and memory. *Journal of Educational Psychology, 82*, 298–305.

Holyoak, K., Gentner, D., & Kokinov, B. (2001). The place of analogy in cognition. In K. Holyoak, D. Gentner, & B. Kokinov (Eds.), *The analogical mind: Perspectives from cognitive science* (pp. 1–19). Cambridge, MA: MIT Press.

Honeck, R. P. (1973). Interpretive versus structural effects on semantic memory. *Journal of Verbal Learning and Verbal Behavior, 12*, 448–455.

Hummel, J. E., & Holyoak, K. J. (1997). Distributed representations of structure: A theory of analogical access and mapping. *Psychological Bulletin, 104*, 427–466.
Krieger, J. L., Parrot, R. L., & Nussbaum, J. F. (2011). Metaphor use and health literacy: A pilot study of strategies to explain randomization in cancer clinical trials. *Journal of Health Communication, 16*, 3–16.
Lakoff, G. (1987). *Women, fire, and dangerous things: What categories reveal about the mind.* Chicago, IL: University of Chicago Press.
Lakoff, G., & Johnson, M. (1980). *Metaphors we live by*. Chicago, IL: University of Chicago Press.
Lipkus, I. M. (2007). Numeric, verbal, and visual formats of conveying health risks: Suggested best practices and future recommendations. *Medical Decision Making, 27*, 696–713.
Lipkus, I. M., & Hollands, J. G. (1999). The visual communication of risk. *Journal of the National Cancer Institute Monographs, 25*, 149–163.
Lipkus, I. M., & Peters, E. (2009). Framework and practical insights understanding the role of numeracy in health: Proposed theoretical insights. *Health Education and Behavior, 36*, 1065–1081.
Lipkus, I. M., Samsa, G., & Rimer, B. K. (2001). General performance on a numeracy scale among highly educated samples. *Medical Decision Making, 21*, 37–44.
Marschark, M., & Hunt, R. R. (1986). On memory for metaphor. *Memory and Cognition, 13*, 412–424.
Marschark, M., Katz, A. N., & Paivio, A. (1983). Dimensions of metaphor. *Journal of Psycholinguistic Research, 12*, 17–40.
Mintz, E., & Ostbye, T. (1992). Teaching statistics to health professionals: The legal analogy. *Medical Teacher, 14*, 371–374.
Newby, T. J., Ertmer, P. A., & Stepich, D. A. (1995). Instructional analogies and the learning of concepts. *Educational Technology Research and Development, 43*, 5–18.
Oppenheimer, R. (1956). Analogy in science. *American Psychologist, 11*, 127–135.
Ortony, A., Reynolds, R. E., & Arter, J. A. (1978). Metaphor: Theoretical and empirical research. *Psychological Bulletin, 85*, 919–943.
Paivio, A. (1969). Mental imagery in associative learning and memory. *Psychological Review, 76*, 241–263.
Paivio, A. (1986). *Mental representations: A dual coding approach.* New York, NY: Oxford University Press.
Peters, E. (2012). Beyond comprehension: The role of numeracy in judgments and decisions. *Current Directions in Psychological Science, 21*, 31–35.
Peters, E., Dieckmann, N. F., Västfjäll, D., Mertz, C. K., Slovic, P., & Hibbard, J. (2009). Bringing meaning to numbers: The impact of evaluative categories on decisions. *Journal of Experimental Psychology: Applied, 15*, 213–227.
Peters, E., Hibbard, J. H., Slovic, P., & Dieckmann, N. F. (2007). Numeracy skill and the communication, comprehension, and use of risk and benefit information. *Health Affairs, 26*, 741–748.
Peters, E., Västfjäll, D., Slovic, P., Mertz, C. K., Mazzocco, K., & Dickert, S. (2006). Numeracy and decision making. *Psychological Science, 17*, 407–413.
Reichmann, P., & Coste, E. (1980). Mental imagery and the comprehension of figurative language: Is there a relationship? In R. P. Honeck & R. Hoffman (Eds.), *Cognition and figurative language* (pp. 183–200). Hillsdale, NJ: Erlbaum.
Reyna, V. R., Nelson, W. L., Han, P., & Dieckmann, N. F. (2009). How numeracy influences risk comprehension and medical decision making. *Psychological Bulletin, 135*, 943–973.
Schwartz, L. M., Woloshin, S., Black, W. C., & Welch, H. G. (1997). The role of numeracy in understanding the benefit of screening mammography. *Annals of Internal Medicine, 127*, 966–972.
Schwartz, L. M., Woloshin, S., & Welch, G. (2005). Can patients interpret health information? An assessment of the medical data interpretation test. *Medical Decision Making, 25*, 290–300.

Snowdon, C., Garcia, J., & Elbourne, D. (1997). Making sense of randomization: Responses of parents of critically ill babies to random allocation of treatment in a clinical trial. *Social Science and Medicine, 45*, 1337–1355.

Sopory, P. (2005). Metaphor in formative evaluation and message design: An application to relationships and alcohol use. *Health Communication, 17*, 149–172.

Sopory, P., & Dillard, J. (2002). The persuasive effects of metaphor: A meta-analysis. *Human Communication Research, 28*, 382–419.

Tourangeau, R., & Sternberg, R. (1981). Aptness in metaphor. *Cognitive Psychology, 13*, 27–55.

Tourangeau, R., & Sternberg, R. (1982). Understanding and appreciating metaphors. *Cognition, 11*, 203–244.

Trick, L., & Katz, A. (1986). The domain interaction approach to metaphor processing: Relating individual differences and metaphor characteristics. *Metaphor and Symbolic Activity, 1*, 185–213.

Waters, E. A., Weinstein, N. D., Colditz, G. A., & Emmons, K. M. (2007). Reducing aversion to side effects in preventive medical treatment decisions. *Journal of Experimental Psychology. Applied, 13*, 11–21.

Whitney, P., Budd, D., & Mio, J. S. (1996). Individual differences in metaphoric facilitation of comprehension. In J. S. Mio & A. N. Katz (Eds.), *Metaphor: Implications and applications* (pp. 203–214). Mahwah, NJ: Erlbaum.

Zikmund-Fisher, B. J., Fagerlin, A., & Ubel, P. A. (2010). A demonstration of "less can be more" in risk graphics. *Medical Decision Making, 30*, 661–671.

Chapter 8
Helping People Memorize Consequences of Risky Behaviors

Mirta Galesic and Rocio Garcia-Retamero

Abstract In this chapter, we investigated whether presenting consequences of health-related behaviors in terms of life expectancy, rather than risk of disease, improves recall and, if yes, through which underlying mechanisms. We also investigated whether these effects hold for both low- and high-numeracy people and in two countries with different cultural environments and medical systems. The study was conducted within a computerized survey on probabilistic national samples in the USA and Germany. Results showed that recall was better when consequences of health-related behaviors were presented in terms of changes in life expectancy than when they were presented in terms of risks of a disease both after 10 min and after 3 weeks. This was so for participants of both high and low numeracy and in both countries. The improved recall seems to be due to better imaginability of changes in life expectancy. When communicating with patients about medical risks, we recommend using concepts that they can readily relate to their own everyday experiences.

---

* In this chapter, we partially reproduced the article Galesic, M., & Garcia-Retamero, R. (2011). Communicating consequences of risky behaviors: Life expectancy versus risk of disease. *Patient Education and Counseling, 82*, 30–35.

M. Galesic, Ph.D. (✉)
Center for Adaptive Behavior and Cognition, Max Planck Institute for Human Development, Lentzeallee 94, Berlin 14195, Germany
e-mail: galesic@mpib-berlin.mpg.de

R. Garcia-Retamero, Ph.D.
Departamento de Psicología Experimental, Facultad de Psicología, University of Granada, Campus Universitario de Cartuja s/n, Granada 18071, Spain

Center for Adaptive Behavior and Cognition, Max Planck Institute for Human Development, Lentzeallee 94, Berlin 14195, Germany
e-mail: rretamer@ugr.es

R. Garcia-Retamero and M. Galesic (eds.), *Transparent Communication of Health Risks: Overcoming Cultural Differences*, DOI 10.1007/978-1-4614-4358-2_8,

8.1 Introduction and Background

Doctors and health authorities frequently communicate consequences of unhealthy behaviors in terms of risks of different diseases. For example, the Centers for Disease Control and Prevention, on their web page dedicated to educating general public about smoking (http://www.cdc.gov/tobacco/), include the following information: "The risk of dying from lung cancer is more than 23 times higher among men who smoke cigarettes, and about 13 times higher among women who smoke cigarettes compared with never smokers." For some people, understanding and memorizing such messages can be difficult for two reasons. First, people who have low numeracy often have problems with correct interpretation of statistical expressions such as percentages and odds (see Chap. 2). Second, people may have problems mapping abstract concept of risk to practical consequences for their everyday life. As a result, such messages may fail to guide their health-related behavior.

In this chapter, we explore whether relating consequences of health-related behaviors to people's everyday experiences improves their understanding and recall. Studies of human memory suggest that consequences expressed in ways that are easier to connect with everyday experiences may facilitate encoding, leading to a richer memory trace and enhanced subsequent recall (Baddeley 1997). For example, consequences of unhealthy behaviors could be communicated in terms of *changes in life expectancy*. This concept is naturally familiar to all people, as everybody is exposed to the experience of getting older and watching others grow old and die. In addition, life expectancy is expressed in terms of simple integers (years or months), therefore requiring less quantitative sophistication than probabilities and percentages, which are ratios.

How could communicating in terms of life expectancy instead of in terms of risk of diseases facilitate encoding? There are two possible mechanisms: one primarily cognitive and the other primarily emotional. The first one is based on the imaginability of consequences. Following Paivio's dual-coding theory (Paivio 1969, 1971, 1986), concrete words more readily invoke mental images than abstract words, and therefore enable both verbal and visual encoding in memory. This in turn enhances subsequent recall of the concrete compared to the more abstract words. In a similar vein, Gollwitzer and others have shown that imagining a task that needs to be done is a successful way of improving prospective memory for that task (Chasteen et al. 2001; Gollwitzer 1999; Liu and Park 2004). In the present study, it could be that the concept of life expectancy is more concrete and easier to imagine than the concept of risk of a disease, and that it will therefore be easier to encode and later recall. The second mechanism is based on emotions evoked by different consequences of risk behaviors. Emotions—in particular negative emotions—have been shown to increase the distinctiveness of an event in memory and subsequently improve its recall (Brown and Kulik 1977; Christianson 1992; Ochsner 2000). In the context of this study, if consequences of unhealthy behaviors are perceived to be less desirable when using one of the information formats than the other (either increased risk of disease or reduction in life expectancy), they could invoke a stronger negative affect and therefore be encoded and later recalled better.

8.2 Study: Communicating Consequences of Risky Behaviors

In this study, we investigate four questions. First, we test whether different ways of describing consequences of risky behaviors—in terms of life expectancy versus in terms of risk of a disease—affect their recall. Second, we analyze the mechanisms that might underlie the potential improvements—namely, imaginability and undesirability of consequences. Third, we study whether these effects hold in two distinct population groups: people with low- and high-numeracy skills. The former group is particularly vulnerable to misunderstanding of health-related information (Estrada et al. 2004; Galesic et al. 2009; Nelson et al. 2008; Peters et al. 2006; Schwartz et al. 1997; Woloshin et al. 2001), and our hope is to find ways to raise their understanding to the level of high-numeracy people. Fourth, we investigate whether the effects of different descriptions hold in two countries with different cultural environments and medical systems: the USA and Germany. As we mentioned in Chap. 1, in the USA, but not in Germany, patient-centered advertising of prescription drugs is allowed, exposing US patients to concepts such as risks of diseases and efficiency of treatments. Also, many US patients need to make health decisions on their own because of insufficient medical insurance (see Chap. 2; see also Galesic and Garcia-Retamero 2010). It is therefore possible that their understanding and recall of abstract risk reductions will be better than that of their German counterparts. Consequently, the life expectancy format could lead to smaller improvements over the risk reduction format in the USA compared to Germany.

8.2.1 *Method*

8.2.1.1 Participants

The study was conducted on probabilistic national samples in the USA and Germany as part of the project "Helping people with low numeracy understand medical information," funded by the Foundation for Informed Medical Decision Making. The project involved a survey that gathered data for a number of studies related to understanding and communicating risks, conducted in two waves (see Chaps. 2, 4, 7, 9–11, and 13). In the first wave, large national samples of participants ($n = 1{,}009$ in the USA and $n = 1{,}001$ in Germany) completed a numeracy scale consisting of nine items selected from Schwartz et al. (1997) and Lipkus et al. (2001; see Chap 15). Participants with numeracy scores in the top and bottom third of the whole sample were invited to the second wave 3 weeks later. A sample of 1,047 participants of the overarching project completed the two waves of this study (513 participants from the USA and 534 from Germany). The structure of the resulting sample is presented in Table 8.1 (see Chap. 2 for more details about the methodology of the survey). This sample enables us to compare people with low- and high-numeracy scores within each country, as well as each of those groups between countries. In our analyses,

Table 8.1 Structure of the sample of participants in the study in terms of numeracy, gender, age, and education

	USA		Germany	
	Low numeracy	High numeracy	Low numeracy	High numeracy
Total	255	258	261	273
Mean numeracy[a]	35	90	38	95
Gender				
Male	41	54	40	60
Female	59	46	60	40
Age				
25–39	37	37	21	41
40–54	31	44	41	37
55–69	32	19	38	32
Education				
High school or less	52	29	89	60
Some college or more[b]	48	71	11	40
Income[c]				
Lower third	41	20	43	20
Middle third	36	28	40	48
Upper third	23	52	17	32

[a]Numeracy scores are transformed to a 0–100-point scale
[b]In Germany, this category includes people with Abitur
[c]Thirds are based on the distribution of household income in the general population of the USA (Germany). Lower third includes participants with household income up to \$30,000 (18,000€), middle third those with household income from \$30,000 to \$60,000 (18,000€–36,000€), and upper third those with household income of \$60,000 (36,000€) or more

we split the participants into two groups according to the median numeracy score for the total sample (i.e., 6; see Peters et al. 2006 for a similar procedure). The average numeracy scores in each of the resulting groups in each country are shown in Table 8.1.

8.2.1.2 Stimuli and Procedure

In the first step, besides completing the numeracy scale, a random half of participants completed two tasks on consequences of risky behaviors, described in the next section. The other half of the participants completed only unrelated questions about health risks. In the second step 3 weeks later, all participants who completed the two tasks in the first step ($n=274$ in the USA and $n=274$ in Germany) were asked to recall the information presented in these tasks. The other half ($n=239$ in the USA and $n=260$ in Germany) were asked to evaluate the scenarios in the two tasks in terms of their imaginability and undesirability.

We used two tasks involving realistic risks related to obesity and physical inactivity. The information was taken from published studies (Fontaine et al. 2003; Franco et al. 2005; Kenchaiah et al. 2002; Miller et al. 1997). Half of the participants got the information in terms of expected risk of heart failure. Specifically, they were told: "People who are overweight have a 36% risk of heart failure—18% higher than an average person" and "people who exercise regularly have a 27% risk of cardiovascular disease—13% lower than an average person." The other half got the information in terms of life expectancy: "People who are overweight have life expectancy of 73 years—60 months shorter than an average person" and "people who exercise regularly have life expectancy of 81 years—36 months longer than an average person." We took care to make the two presentation formats as comparable as possible in terms of complexity—as much as we could while keeping the information truthful. Both formats used two sets of two-digit numbers (i.e., months rather than years to express life expectancy), and the number of words and the sentence structure were similar. The only difference was that the numbers in the risk of disease scenario represented percentages, and in the life expectancy scenario months of life. Participants were *not* specifically instructed to memorize this information. On 7-point scales, they were only asked to evaluate how important it was for them (1) not to be overweight and (2) to exercise regularly.

After completing unrelated questions about health risks, which took approximately 10 min, participants were asked to recall the information presented in these two tasks. Specifically, participants who got the information in terms of expected risk of heart failure answered the question "How much higher is the risk of heart failure for people who are overweight, compared to an average person?" on a scale ranging from 9 to 54%, marked with intervals of 9% points, and the question "How much lower is the risk of cardiovascular disease for people who exercise regularly, compared to an average person?" on a scale ranging from 3 to 23%, marked with intervals of 5 percentage points. Participants who got the information in terms of life expectancy answered the question "How much shorter is life expectancy for people who are overweight, compared to an average person?" on a scale ranging from 20 to 100 months, marked with intervals of 20 months, and the question "How much longer is life expectancy for people who exercise regularly, compared to an average person?" on a scale ranging from 18 to 90 months, marked with intervals of 18 months. The same procedure was repeated in the second step, conducted after 3 weeks.

As mentioned in the previous section, a random half of participants did not get these tasks but were instead asked to evaluate all four of the scenarios described above for their imaginability and undesirability. This enabled us to test two theoretically plausible explanations for improvements in recall. Specifically, these participants answered the question "How easy is it for you to imagine yourself in each of the following scenarios?" on 7-point scales ranging from 1 (*very easy*) to 7 (*very difficult*), and the question "How desirable or undesirable is each of the following scenarios for you?" on 7-point scales ranging from 1 (*very desirable*) to 7 (*very undesirable*).

The materials for the English and German versions were carefully developed to be comparable (see Chap. 2 for more details about the translation of the materials and the programmed questionnaire). The Ethics Committee of the Max Planck Institute for Human Development approved the methodology of the study, and all participants consented to participation through an online consent form at the beginning of the survey.

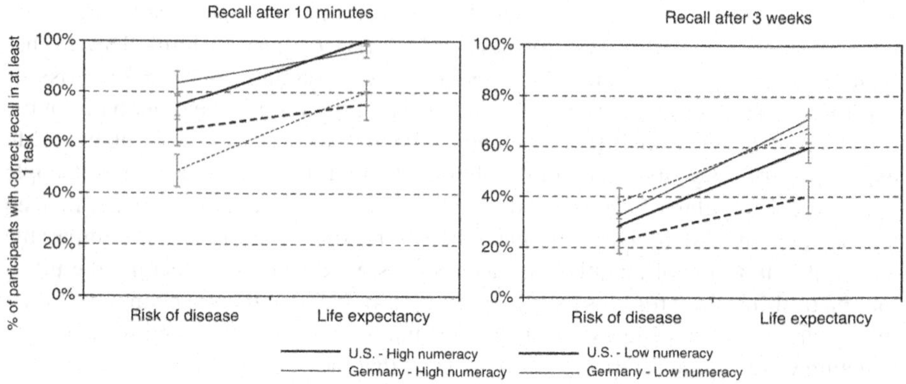

Fig. 8.1 Recall of information about consequences of risky behaviors at two time points (after 10 min and 3 weeks), by presentation format, country, and numeracy skills. Error bars represent ±1 SE

In sum, there were two experimental groups: One received information about the consequences of being overweight and exercising in terms of risk of heart disease, and the other in terms of life expectancy. Two separate groups of participants, who did not participate in the experiment but were part of the same sample, evaluated the imaginability and undesirability of each scenario. The main dependent variable is the percentage of participants in each experimental group who recalled the information after 10 min and after 3 weeks. To test the effects of format, numeracy, and country, on percentage of participants who recalled the information correctly in each time period, we used analysis of variance (ANOVA). In this we followed Lunney (1970; see also Cleary and Angel 1984), who showed that ANOVA can be used to obtain conservative results for large samples of a dichotomous-dependent variable.

8.2.2 Results

Do different ways of describing consequences of risky behaviors affect recall? Does performance improve for both low and high-numeracy participants and in both countries? As Fig. 8.1 shows, when the information about consequences of risky behaviors was presented as months of life lost or gained, recall was better than when it was presented in terms of risks of a disease. The recall was better both after 10 min, Cohen's $h=0.51$, $F_{1,543}=34.12$, $p=0.001$, and after 3 weeks, $h=0.62$, $F_{1,543}=48.98$, $p=0.001$. This was so for participants of both high and low numeracy, and in both countries. There was no interaction between numeracy or country and the presentation format. Recall of high-numeracy participants was considerably better than that of low-numeracy persons after 10 min, $h=0.52$, $F_{1,543}=35.09$, $p=0.001$, but after 3 weeks the recall of high- and low-numeracy groups was similar, $h=0.11$, $F_{1,543}=1.76$, $p=0.185$. These results remained unchanged even after

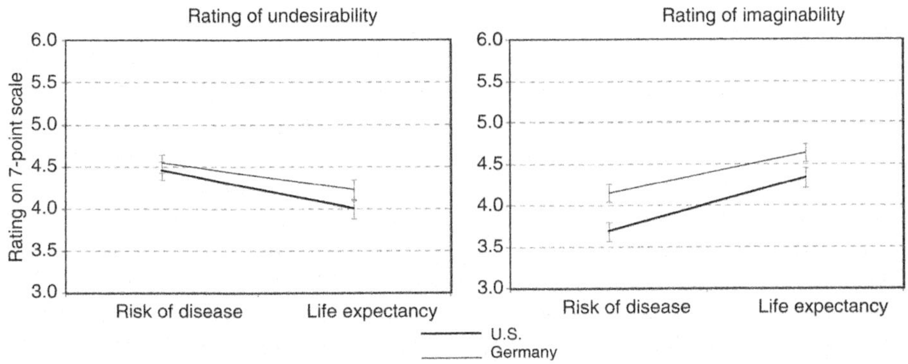

Fig. 8.2 Ratings of undesirability and imaginability of different consequences of risky behaviors, by country. Error bars represent ±1 SE

controlling for sex, age, and income of different numeracy groups. Furthermore, the presentation format did not affect ratings of importance of maintaining healthy weight and exercising within any numeracy group in either country.

What mechanisms underlie differences in recall? As outlined before, we tested for two possible mechanisms: one based on imaginability and the other on undesirability of consequences. The more imaginable and the less desirable the consequences, the better they should be encoded and subsequently recalled. We collected ratings of imaginability and undesirability from separate groups of participants who were not involved in the main experiment but were part of the same sample. As Fig. 8.2 shows, the two types of consequences differed both in undesirability and imaginability. Decrease in life expectancy was rated as more undesirable than increase in risk of disease: in the USA, $d=0.31$, $t_{99}=3.08$, $p=0.003$; in Germany, $d=0.18$, $t_{130}=2.04$, $p=0.044$. At the same time, changes in life expectancy were easier to imagine than changes in risk of disease: in the USA, $d=0.49$, $t_{138}=5.71$, $p=0.001$; in Germany, $d=0.37$, $t_{128}=4.22$, $p=0.001$. Importantly, only the differences in imaginability of the consequences correspond to the results presented in Fig. 8.1. This supports the hypothesis that encoding and recall are enhanced when information is easier to imagine.

8.3 Discussion and Conclusions

We found much better recall for consequences of health-related behaviors when they were expressed as changes in life expectancy rather than in terms of risk of getting a disease. The improvements in the recall persisted as long as 3 weeks. At the same time, the life expectancy format did not bias perceptions of risk. Rated importance of maintaining healthy weight and exercising was the same for both presentation formats. This result is promising for public health campaigns aimed at improving people's awareness about unhealthy consequences of risky lifestyles such as smoking, obesity, and physical inactivity.

These effects seem to be mediated by a primarily cognitive mechanism that acts through enhanced imaginability of the information, enabling better encoding and a richer memory trace. The other, primarily emotional mechanism acting through lower desirability of risk of disease might have played a role, but any effect of that factor was probably overpowered by the effect of imaginability. These results are in line with the dual-coding theory of Paivio (1969, 1971, 1986), who proposed that words higher in imaginability enable both verbal and visual encoding, thus enhancing subsequent recall. Studies on implementation of intentions (Chasteen et al. 2001; Gollwitzer 1999; Liu and Park 2004) in which patients who imagine a task (e.g., taking their prescription medication) are subsequently more likely to remember to do the task are also in accord with our findings.

Our results are consistent with previous findings that low-numeracy people have problems understanding statistical information about risks (Estrada et al. 2004; Galesic et al. 2009; Garcia-Retamero and Galesic 2009; Nelson et al. 2008; Peters et al. 2006; Schwartz et al. 1997; Woloshin et al. 2001). However, their performance was improved to the level of high-numeracy people when the consequences of risky behaviors were presented in terms of life expectancy, in both the USA and Germany. As low-numeracy people are often of lower socioeconomic status (see Table 8.1), and correspondingly more likely to lack health insurance (see Chap. 2; see also Galesic and Garcia-Retamero 2010) and have unhealthy lifestyles (Schoen et al. 2005), simple framing manipulations such as these are an important tool for improving this population's informed decision making about health.

This chapter makes several contributions to the existing literature on risk communication. First, to the best of our knowledge, no study so far has compared recall of health-related information expressed in terms of life expectancy versus risk reduction, although this is a very important aspect for developers and distributors of health information. If one of these formats produces superior recall without biasing risk perception, then this format should be preferred when planning public health campaigns. Second, we suggest and test two theoretical rationales about the mechanisms underlying improvements in recall, one primarily cognitive (imaginability) and the other primarily emotional (undesirability). Third, by using probabilistic national samples of low- and high-numeracy people in two countries, we test the generalizability of our findings to different patient groups.

Our findings have significant implications for medical practice. When it is desired that patients memorize certain information about medical risks, it is preferable to choose representations that patients can readily connect to their everyday experiences. Representing consequences of risky behaviors in terms of loss or gain in life duration uses the fact that we all experience the passage of years of our and others' lives, and that most people have thought about how long they might live. Therefore, this representation is easier to imagine than increase or reduction of risk of a disease—a concept that might be less intuitive for most people, in particular those with lower numeracy skills (Galesic and Garcia-Retamero 2010).

Framing information about risks using formats that enhance recall is justifiable to achieve the greatest public health gain (Edwards et al. 2002). Several studies have shown that the way risks and benefits are framed affects patients' readiness to accept medical screenings and treatments (see Chap. 11; see also Edwards et al. 2001, 2002; Rothman and Salovey 1997; Rothman et al. 1999; Salovey and Williams-Piehota 2004). For example, framing benefits of medical screenings in terms of potential losses enhances screening uptake more than "gain" framing (Banks et al. 1995; Kalichman and Coley 1995; Lauver and Rubin 1990; Lerman et al. 1992; Meyerowitz and Chaiken 1987; Myers et al. 1991; Rothman et al. 1993; Schneider et al. 2001). In line with these results, the present chapter shows that describing consequences of risky behaviors in terms of life years enhances recall of these consequences. Further research could investigate other ways to connect abstract medical information to everyday life, for example, by using analogies and metaphors (see Chap. 7; see also Edwards 2003).

A limitation of the study described in this chapter is that it focuses on just one of the many factors that affect what patients consider to be relevant risks and what determines whether they take actions to reduce or avoid them. Within this probabilistic national survey it was also not possible to observe and record actions that the participants would actually take. All of these limitations could be addressed in future research.

In conclusion, recall of consequences of health-related behaviors is better when the information is presented in terms of life years lost or gained, rather than in terms of increase or decrease of risk of diseases. These effects are persistent over the course of several weeks and are due to better imaginability of life years compared to risk of disease. When communicating with patients about medical risks, we recommend using concepts that they can readily connect to their everyday experiences. In our study, gain or loss in life duration—naturally experienced by all people—was easier to imagine than reduction or increase in risk of a disease, and has enhanced recall. This finding can be particularly useful when trying to improve patient's awareness about drawbacks of risky lifestyles such as smoking, obesity, and physical inactivity.

References

Baddeley, A. (1997). *Human memory: Theory and practice*. East Sussex: Psychology Press.

Banks, S. M., Salovey, P., Greener, S., Rothman, A. J., Moyer, A., Beauvais, J., et al. (1995). The effects of message framing on mammography utilization. *Health Psychology, 14*, 178–184.

Brown, R., & Kulik, J. (1977). Flashbulb memories. *Cognition, 5*, 73–99.

Chasteen, A. L., Park, D. C., & Schwarz, N. (2001). Implementation intentions and facilitation of prospective memory. *Psychological Science, 12*, 457–461.

Christianson, S. A. (1992). Emotional stress and eyewitness testimony: A critical review. *Psychological Bulletin, 112*, 284–309.

Cleary, P. D., & Angel, R. (1984). The analysis of relationships involving dichotomous dependent-variables. *Journal of Health and Social Behavior, 25*, 334–348.

Edwards, A. (2003). Communicating risks through analogies. *British Medical Journal, 327*, 749.

Edwards, A., Elwyn, G., Covey, J., Matthews, E., & Pill, R. (2001). Presenting risk information—A review of the effects of "framing" and other manipulations on patient outcomes. *Journal of Health Communication, 6*, 61–82.

Edwards, A., Elwyn, G., & Mulley, A. (2002). Explaining risks: Turning numerical data into meaningful pictures. *British Medical Journal, 324*, 827–830.

Estrada, C. A., Martin-Hryniewicz, M., Peek, B. T., Collins, C., & Byrd, J. C. (2004). Literacy and numeracy skills and anticoagulation control. *The American Journal of the Medical Sciences, 328*, 88–93.

Fontaine, K. R., Redden, D. T., Wang, C. X., Westfall, A. O., & Allison, D. B. (2003). Years of life lost due to obesity. *Journal of the American Medical Association, 289*, 187–193.

Franco, O. H., de Laet, C., Peeters, A., Jonker, J., Mackenbach, J., & Nusselder, W. (2005). Effects of physical activity on life expectancy with cardiovascular disease. *Archives of Internal Medicine, 165*, 2355–2360.

Galesic, M., & Garcia-Retamero, R. (2010). Statistical numeracy for health: A cross-cultural comparison with probabilistic national samples. *Archives of Internal Medicine, 170*, 462–468.

Galesic, M., Garcia-Retamero, R., & Gigerenzer, G. (2009). Using icon arrays to communicate medical risks: Overcoming low numeracy. *Health Psychology, 28*, 210–216.

Garcia-Retamero, R., & Galesic, M. (2009). Communicating treatment risk reduction to people with low numeracy skills: A cross-cultural comparison. *American Journal of Public Health, 99*, 2196–2202.

Gollwitzer, P. M. (1999). Implementation intentions—Strong effects of simple plans. *American Psychologist, 54*, 493–503.

Kalichman, S. C., & Coley, B. (1995). Context framing to enhance HIV-antibody-testing messages targeted to African-American women. *Health Psychology, 14*, 247–254.

Kenchaiah, S., Evans, J. C., Levy, D., Wilson, P. W. F., Benjamin, E. J., Larson, M. G., et al. (2002). Obesity and the risk of heart failure. *The New England Journal of Medicine, 347*, 305–313.

Lauver, D., & Rubin, M. (1990). Message framing, dispositional optimism, and follow-up for abnormal Papanicolaou tests. *Research in Nursing and Health, 13*, 199–207.

Lerman, C., Ross, E., Boyce, A., Gorchov, P. M., McLaughlin, R., Rimer, B., et al. (1992). The impact of mailing psychoeducational materials to women with abnormal mammograms. *American Journal of Public Health, 82*, 729–730.

Lipkus, I. M., Samsa, G., & Rimer, B. K. (2001). General performance on a numeracy scale among highly educated samples. *Medical Decision Making, 21*, 37–44.

Liu, L. L., & Park, D. C. (2004). Aging and medical adherence: The use of automatic processes to achieve effortful things. *Psychology and Aging, 19*, 318–325.

Lunney, G. H. (1970). Using analysis of variance with a dichotomous dependent variable—Empirical study. *Journal of Educational Measurement, 7*, 263–269.

Meyerowitz, B. E., & Chaiken, S. (1987). The effect of message framing on breast self-examination attitudes, intentions, and behavior. *Journal of Personality and Social Psychology, 52*, 500–510.

Miller, T. D., Balady, G. J., & Fletcher, G. F. (1997). Exercise and its role in the prevention and rehabilitation of cardiovascular disease. *Annals of Behavioral Medicine, 19*, 220–229.

Myers, R. E., Ross, E. A., Wolf, T. A., Balshem, A., Jepson, C., & Millner, L. (1991). Behavioral interventions to increase adherence in colorectal-cancer screening. *Medical Care, 29*, 1039–1050.

Nelson, W., Reyna, V. F., Fagerlin, A., Lipkus, I., & Peters, E. (2008). Clinical implications of numeracy: Theory and practice. *Annals of Behavioral Medicine, 35*, 261–274.

Ochsner, K. N. (2000). Are affective events richly recollected or simply familiar? The experience and process of recognizing feelings past. *Journal of Experimental Psychology: General, 129*, 242–261.

Paivio, A. (1969). Mental imagery in associative learning and memory. *Psychological Review, 76*, 241–263.

Paivio, A. (1971). *Imagery and verbal processes*. New York: Holt, Rinehart, & Winston.
Paivio, A. (1986). *Mental representations: A dual coding approach*. New York: Oxford University Press.
Peters, E., Vastfjall, D., Slovic, P., Mertz, C. K., Mazzocco, K., & Dickert, S. (2006). Numeracy and decision making. *Psychological Science, 17*, 407–413.
Rothman, A. J., Martino, S. C., Bedell, B. T., Detweiler, J. B., & Salovey, P. (1999). The systematic influence of gain- and loss-framed messages on interest in and use of different types of health behavior. *Personality and Social Psychology Bulletin, 25*, 1355–1369.
Rothman, A. J., & Salovey, P. (1997). Shaping perceptions to motivate healthy behavior: The role of message framing. *Psychological Bulletin, 121*, 3–19.
Rothman, A. J., Salovey, P., Antone, C., Keough, K., & Martin, C. (1993). The influence of message framing on health behavior. *Journal of Experimental Social Psychology, 29*, 408–433.
Salovey, P., & Williams-Piehota, P. (2004). Field experiments in social psychology—Message framing and the promotion of health protective behaviors. *American Behavioral Scientist, 47*, 488–505.
Schneider, T. R., Salovey, P., Apanovitch, A. M., Pizarro, J., McCarthy, D., Zullo, J., et al. (2001). The effects of message framing and ethnic targeting on mammography use among low-income women. *Health Psychology, 20*, 256–266.
Schoen, C., Doty, M. M., Collins, S. R., & Holmgren, A. L. (2005). Insured but not protected: How many adults are underinsured? *Health Affairs*, W5-289–W5-302.
Schwartz, L. M., Woloshin, S., Black, W. C., & Welch, H. G. (1997). The role of numeracy in understanding the benefit of screening mammography. *Annals of Internal Medicine, 127*, 966–972.
Woloshin, S., Schwartz, L. M., Moncur, M., Gabriel, S., & Tosteson, A. N. A. (2001). Assessing values for health: Numeracy matters. *Medical Decision Making, 21*, 382–390.

Chapter 9
Improving the Understanding of Treatment Risk Reduction*

Rocio Garcia-Retamero and Mirta Galesic

Abstract Visual aids have been proposed as a promising method for enhancing comprehension about medical risks. In this chapter, we describe a survey of probabilistic national samples in the USA and Germany, comparing the effectiveness of adding different types of visual aids (icon arrays and bar graphs representing either affected individuals only or the entire population at risk) to numerical information in either an absolute or a relative risk reduction format. We also analyzed whether people's numeracy and graph literacy skills affected the efficacy of the visual aids. Our results showed large improvements in accuracy both when icon arrays and when bar graphs were added to numerical information. Highest increases were achieved when the visual aids depicted the entire population at risk. Importantly, visual aids were most useful for the participants who had low-numeracy but relatively high-graph literacy skills. We conclude that visual aids help to modify incorrect expectations about treatment risk reduction.

---

*In this chapter, we partially reproduced the article Garcia-Retamero, R., & Galesic, M. (2010). Who profits from visual aids: Overcoming challenges in people's understanding of risks. *Social Science and Medicine, 70*, 1019–1025.

R. Garcia-Retamero, Ph.D. (✉)
Departamento de Psicología Experimental, Facultad de Psicología, University of Granada, Campus Universitario de Cartuja s/n, Granada 18071, Spain

Center for Adaptive Behavior and Cognition, Max Planck Institute for Human Development, Lentzeallee 94, 14195 Berlin, Germany
e-mail: rretamer@ugr.es

M. Galesic, Ph.D.
Center for Adaptive Behavior and Cognition,
Max Planck Institute for Human Development,
Lentzeallee 94, Berlin 14195, Germany
e-mail: galesic@mpib-berlin.mpg.de

R. Garcia-Retamero and M. Galesic (eds.), *Transparent Communication of Health Risks: Overcoming Cultural Differences*, DOI 10.1007/978-1-4614-4358-2_9,

9.1 Introduction and Background

Increased emphasis on patient-centered decision making has shifted responsibility to patients, who now more than ever need to understand numerical information to actively participate in making decisions about their health (Barry 1999; Hanson 2008). Informed consent laws, for instance, mandate that patients must be informed about risks before any treatment can be implemented (Garcia-Retamero and Galesic 2009b). Understanding a treatment risk reduction implies taking into account the number of treated and nontreated people who die or survive out of those who do and do not receive the treatment (i.e., the entire population at risk; Gigerenzer and Edwards 2003). However, a growing literature attests that many patients, especially those with low numeracy skills, have difficulties with understanding these and other health-relevant numerical concepts (see Chaps. 2 and 3; see also Baker et al. 2008; Kutner et al. 2006; Lipkus et al. 2001; Peters et al. 2006).

Visual aids have been proposed as a potentially promising method for efficiently communicating treatment risk reductions (see Chap. 4; see also Edwards et al. 2002). They can also improve understanding of risks and benefits associated with different treatments, screenings, and life-styles (Ancker et al. 2006; Galesic et al. 2009; Lipkus 2007; Lipkus and Hollands 1999; Paling 2003), and promote consideration of beneficial treatments that have side effects (Waters et al. 2007). Visual aids are also effective in eliminating errors induced by anecdotal narratives (Fagerlin et al. 2005), biases (see Chap. 10; see also Garcia-Retamero and Dhami 2011; Garcia-Retamero and Galesic 2009a; Garcia-Retamero et al. 2010; Peters et al. 2009), and framed messages (see Chap. 11; see also Garcia-Retamero and Cokely 2011; Garcia-Retamero and Galesic 2010). In addition, risk information presented via visual aids is perceived as easier to understand (Goodyear-Smith et al. 2008), and has been shown to increase risk avoidance substantially (Schirillo and Stone 2005). Yet our understanding of the effectiveness of visual aids in improving perceptions of treatment risk reduction remains incomplete.

First, most of the studies on the topic focus on the impact of a single type of visual aids (e.g., icon arrays or bar charts; Fagerlin et al. 2005; Rudski and Volksdorf 2002; Waters et al. 2006; Zikmund-Fisher et al. 2008), and only a few compare the efficacy of different displays (Brundage et al. 2005; Feldman-Stewart et al. 2000; Hawley et al. 2008; Schapira et al. 2001). Second, there is no research on whether the visual aids should reflect the number of affected individuals or the entire population at risk (Ancker et al. 2006; Stone et al. 2003) to improve perceptions of treatment risk reduction. Third, most studies on visual aids represent numerical information about risk using a single format (e.g., either absolute or relative risk reduction (RRR); Brundage et al. 2005; Fagerlin et al. 2005; Feldman-Stewart et al. 2000; Rudski and Volksdorf 2002; Schapira et al. 2001; Waters et al. 2006; Zikmund-Fisher et al. 2008). In contrast to previous research, we compare the effectiveness of different visual aids, representing either affected individuals only or the entire population at risk. In addition, we tested visual aids when the numerical information was presented in both absolute and RRR formats.

Fourth, to the best of our knowledge, all previous studies on the effectiveness of visual aids were conducted on convenient samples of specific groups of participants (e.g., patients with particular diseases or students). These studies provide valuable information about how these participants understand risks. However, as Lipkus (2007) pointed out, due to nonprobabilistic sampling methods, the results cannot be generalized to a wider population. This is problematic because it could prevent conclusions about the effects of different, important characteristics (e.g., people's numeracy) on the impact of using visual aids to improve risk understanding. In this study, therefore, we examined the accuracy of perceptions of treatment risk reduction in probabilistic national samples.

Fifth, people might differ in the extent to which they profit from visual displays when estimating risk reductions. For instance, icon arrays are especially useful for individuals who are more vulnerable to having difficulties when making decisions about health (e.g., the elderly or people with low numeracy skills; Galesic et al. 2009; Garcia-Retamero and Galesic 2009a; Garcia-Retamero et al. 2010). Adding icon arrays to numerical information about treatment risk reduction helps these people to make more accurate assessments. Those with fewer difficulties with numerical concepts, in contrast, often make accurate estimates even if icon arrays are not provided. Recently, research by Galesic and Garcia-Retamero (2011) revealed that people, regardless of their numeracy skills, differ substantially in their ability to understand graphically presented quantitative information about health. As Fagerlin et al. (2007) pointed out, it is still an open question whether people's numeracy and graph literacy skills affect the efficacy of different visual aids. Accordingly, we studied which visual aids, if any, were more convenient for people with high and low numeracy and graph literacy skills, and how these skills interacted with the type of numerical format, namely absolute vs. RRR.

Last but not least, there is no research on the effectiveness of visual aids in countries with different health systems such as the USA and Germany (Statistisches Bundesamt Deutschland 2007; World Health Organization 2012). As we mentioned in Chap. 1, most health expenditure in the USA is private-based (55%; World Health Organization 2012), and direct-to-consumer advertising of prescription drugs is allowed. Consequently, US citizens might be more often required to determine whether and which medical treatment they need than the citizens of Germany where only 23% of health expenditure is private-based, and most people have health insurance (99.7% compared to 85% in the USA; Schoen et al. 2005, 2011; Statistisches Bundesamt Deutschland 2007; U.S. Census Bureau 2007). In this chapter, we investigated whether visual aids can help US and German residents make appropriate decisions about their medical treatments.

9.2 Study: Who Profits from Visual Aids?

In a survey, we compared the effectiveness of adding different types of visual aids (icon arrays and bar graphs representing either affected individuals only or the entire population at risk) to the numerical information in either an absolute or a RRR format. We also analyzed whether people's numeracy and graph literacy skills affected the efficacy of the visual aids.

9.2.1 *Method*

9.2.1.1 Participants

The study was conducted on probabilistic national samples in the USA and Germany as part of the project "Helping people with low numeracy understand medical information" funded by the Foundation for Informed Medical Decision Making. The project involved a survey that gathered data for a number of studies related to understanding and communicating risks (see also Chaps. 2, 4, 7, 8, 10, 11, and 13). In particular, we selected large national samples of participants ($n=1,009$ in the USA and $n=1,001$ in Germany) for the overarching project. Randomly selected groups of 492 participants in the USA and of 495 in Germany were asked to answer the questions presented in this chapter. The sample structure is shown in Table 4.1 in Chap. 4 (see Chap. 2 for more details about the methodology of the survey).

9.2.1.2 Stimuli and Procedure

All participants completed a computerized questionnaire that was developed in English and translated into German (see Chap. 2 for more details about the translation of the materials and the programmed questionnaire). The Ethics Committee of the Max Planck Institute for Human Development approved the methodology of the study. At the beginning of the survey, all participants consented to participation through an online consent form and completed a numeracy and a graph literacy scale.

Measurement of numeracy: The numeracy scale consisted of nine items developed by Schwartz et al. (1997) and by Lipkus et al. (2001; see Chaps. 2 and 15). The items were selected based on their correlation with the total score, other items, and their difficulty, as found in a pilot study conducted on samples drawn from opt-in web panels in the USA ($n=414$) and Germany ($n=461$). In the analyses that follow, we split the participants into two groups according to their group's median numeracy scores. The low-numeracy group includes participants with six or fewer correct answers, while the high-numeracy group includes those with seven or more correct answers (see Peters et al. 2006 for a similar procedure).

Measurement of graph literacy: The graph literacy scale consists of 13 items developed by Galesic and Garcia-Retamero (2011; see Chap. 15). It measures three abilities of graph comprehension (Friel et al. 2001): (1) the ability to *read the data*, that is, to find specific information in the graph (for instance, the ability to read off the height of a particular bar within a bar chart); (2) the ability to *read between the data*, that is, to find relationships in the data as shown on the graph (for instance, the ability to read off the difference between two bars or sets of icons); and (3) the ability to *read beyond the data*, or make inferences and predictions from the data (for example, the ability to project a future trend from a line chart). For examples of items measuring each of the three abilities, see Fig. 4.1.

The scale is designed to cover four frequently used graph types—line plots, bar charts, pies, and icon arrays, and includes items dealing with the communication of medical risks, treatment efficiency, and prevalence of diseases. The complexity of the items was varied by changing the number of data series displayed on the same graph (one, two, or three). The scale has promising psychometric properties and is suitable for use in most clinical and research circumstances (see Chap. 4). In the analyses that follow, we split the participants into two groups according to their group's median graph literacy scores (i.e., 9). US and German participants were evenly distributed in both the numeracy and graph literacy groups.

After completing the scales, participants were presented with two medical scenarios of the usefulness of Vitarilen, a hypothetical new drug for reducing the risk of stroke (scenario 1) and heart attack (scenario 2) for patients with symptoms of arterial disease. In each scenario, participants were provided with the results of two randomly selected groups of 100 patients who took a placebo and Vitarilen, respectively. The order of the two scenarios was randomized.

Three independent variables were manipulated in the study. First, the drug's RRR was set at either 25% (scenario 1) or 75% (scenario 2). Second, half of the participants received the information about risk reduction in the form of absolute risk reduction (ARR) and the other half in the form of RRR. In scenario 1, participants got the following information in the ARR condition: "Of the patients who took a placebo, 20 had a stroke. Compared to the group that took a placebo, five fewer patients had a stroke in the group that took Vitarilen." Those in the RRR condition were told: "Compared to the group that took a placebo, the relative reduction in risk of having a stroke in the group that took Vitarilen was 25%." In scenario 2, 15 fewer patients had a heart attack (ARR) and the RRR of having a heart attack was 75% (RRR).

Finally, the provision of visual aids, in addition to the numerical information about risk reduction, was manipulated between-subjects with five conditions. In one condition (icons-sick), participants received two icon arrays using black circles to represent the number of patients who had a stroke (heart attack) when the drug was and was not taken, respectively. In a second condition (icons-overall), the number of healthy patients who did and did not take the drug, represented as white circles, was added to the information presented in the first condition. In this condition, therefore, icon arrays visually represented the entire population at risk (see Fig. 9.1). We used circles to represent patients because previous research did not find differences in effects of arrays with faces compared to more abstract symbols (Stone et al. 1997).

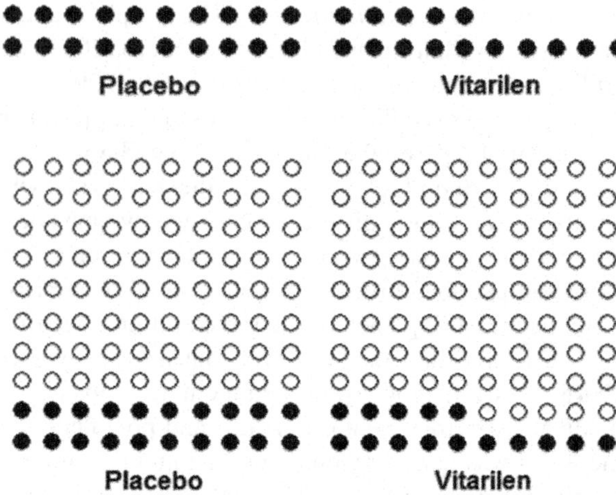

Fig. 9.1 Icon arrays presented in addition to numerical information about risk reduction in icon-sick (*top*) and icon-overall (*bottom*) conditions (Original material was in either English or German)

In a third condition (bars-sick), participants received a two-bar graph presenting the number of patients who had a stroke (heart attack) when the drug was and was not taken, respectively. The *y*-axis of the graph ranged from 0 to 25 to reflect only the number of patients with the disease. In a fourth condition (bars-overall), the same two-bar graph was presented but the *y*-axis ranged from 0 to 100 to reflect the overall number of patients who did and did not take the drug (see Fig. 9.2). Participants in the final condition (numerical) did not receive visual aids in addition to the numerical information.

As a dependent variable, we measured accuracy of risk understanding after reading the information about each medical scenario. First, following the procedure used by Schwartz et al. (1997), participants were asked how many of 1,000 patients with symptoms of arterial disease might have a stroke (heart attack) if they *do not* take the drug. Second, they were asked how many of 1,000 patients with symptoms of arterial disease might have a stroke (heart attack) if they *do* take the drug. By deducting the second from the first answer and dividing it by the first, we calculated the estimated RRR. Participants were classified depending on whether their estimates were correct in the two scenarios. Estimates were considered to be correct when there were exactly right.

To assess the effect of numerical format and visual aids, and their interaction with numeracy, graph literacy, and country on estimates of treatment risk reduction, we conducted mixed analyses of variance (ANOVAs), following Lunney (1970) and Cleary and Angel (1984). Tukey's HSD (honest significant difference) test was used for post hoc analyses.

9.2.2 Results

Which visual aids lead to the most accurate perceptions of risk reduction? Does depicting the overall population at risk improve accuracy? When information about

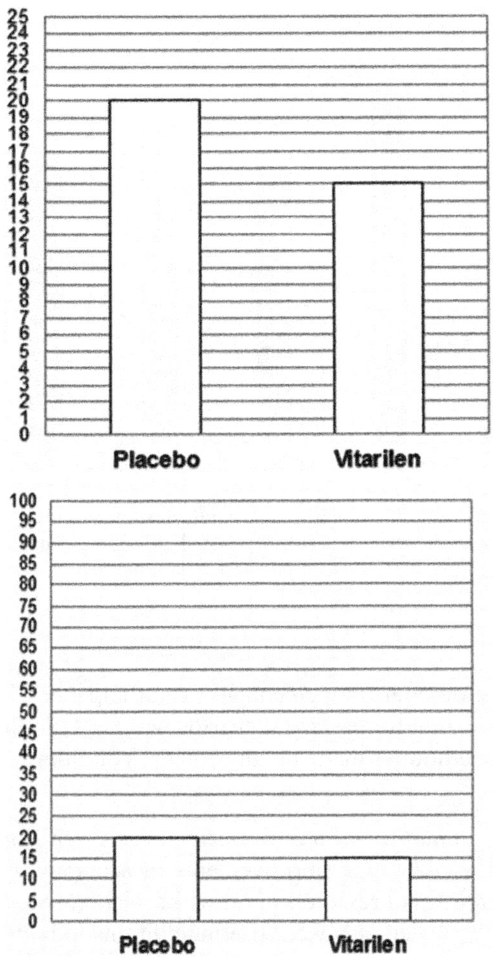

Fig. 9.2 Bar graphs presented in addition to numerical information about risk reduction in bar-sick (*top*) and bar-overall (*bottom*) conditions (Original material was in either English or German)

the drug was provided numerically, 35% (*SE*=3.3) of the participants provided correct estimates of risk reduction for the two scenarios. When visual aids were added to the numerical information, this percentage increased substantially, especially when they represented the overall number of patients who did and did not take the drug (i.e., in the icons-overall and bars-overall conditions). We observed similar increases with icon arrays and bar graphs: 62% (*SE*=3.3) and 64% (*SE*=3.6) of the participants, respectively, provided correct estimates of risk reduction for the two scenarios when icon arrays and bar graphs depicted the overall population at risk, whereas 48% (*SE*=3.3) and 48% (*SE*=3.8) gave correct answers when only sick individuals were shown. Consistent with this result, the ANOVA with visual aids as a between-subjects factor shows a main effect of visual aids, $F_{4,993}=11.99$, $p=0.001$.

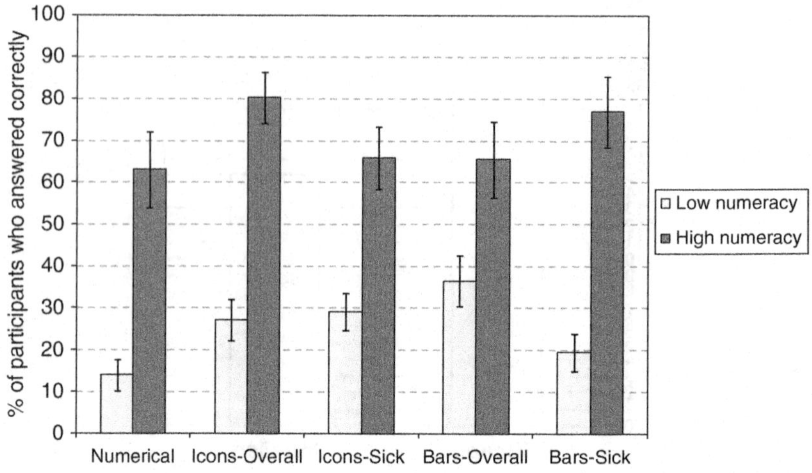

Fig. 9.3 Percentage of participants with *low graph literacy* and high or low numeracy who gave correct estimates for the two scenarios, by visual aids condition. Error bars represent one standard error

Post hoc analyses show that the percentage of participants who provided correct estimates of risk reduction for the two scenarios was larger in the icons-overall and the bars-overall conditions than in the other conditions ($p<0.004$ for all comparisons).

Do visual aids lead to additional improvements even when transparent numerical representations are used? Large improvements in accuracy were achieved when numerical information was presented in terms of ARR (56%; $SE=2.2$) instead of RRR (47%; $SE=2.2$). Visual aids were useful additions to both types of numerical representations: The percentage of participants who provide accurate estimates increased from 36 ($SE=4.7$) to 61% ($SE=6.5$) when visual aids were added to numerical information presented as ARRs, and from 33% ($SE=4.8$) to 50% ($SE=5.5$) when presented as RRRs. In line with these results, an ANOVA with numerical format and visual aids as between-subjects factors showed a main effect of numerical format, $F_{1,994}=4.39$, $p=0.036$. The interaction between the two factors was not significant.

Do participants differ in the extent to which they profit from visual aids when estimating risk reductions? For whom are visual aids most useful? When information about the drug was provided numerically, the percentage of participants with high numeracy who provided correct estimates for the two scenarios was higher than that of low-numeracy participants. Within each numeracy group, the percentage of participants with high graph literacy who provided correct estimates was similar to that of participants with low graph literacy (see Figs. 9.3 and 9.4 for participants with high and low graph literacy, respectively).

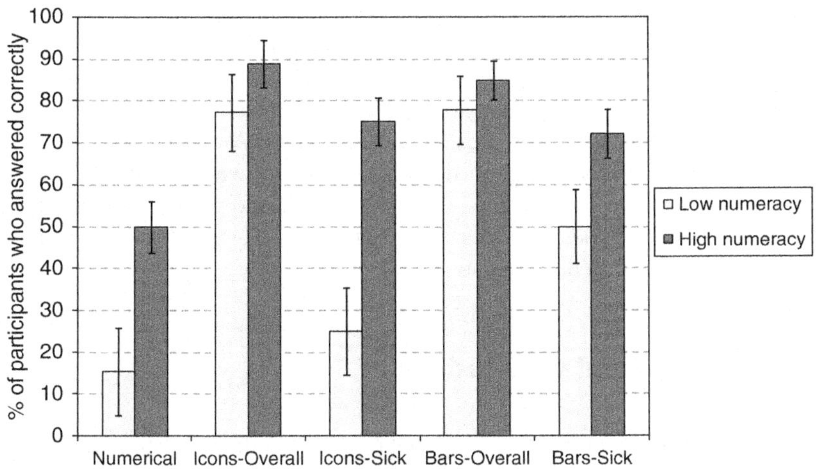

Fig. 9.4 Percentage of participants with *high graph literacy* and high or low numeracy who gave correct estimates for the two scenarios, by visual aids condition. Error bars represent one standard error

Visual aids were useful additions in particular for participants with low numeracy whose graph literacy skills were high compared to the average. The percentage of participants with low numeracy and high graph literacy who provided correct estimates especially increased when icon arrays and bar graphs represented the overall population at risk (i.e., in the icons-overall and bars-overall conditions). In contrast, there was only a minor increase in the percentage of participants with both high numeracy and high graph literacy who provided accurate estimates in these conditions, and almost no increase in those with low graph literacy even if they had high numeracy. Consistently, the ANOVA with visual aids, numeracy, and graph literacy as between-participants factors showed a significant main effect of numeracy, $F_{1,978}=112.45$, $p=0.001$, and graph literacy, $F_{1,978}=14.79$, $p=0.001$, and an interaction between visual aids, numeracy, and graph literacy, $F_{4,978}=3.24$, $p=0.007$. These results were not influenced by the format in which the numerical information was presented (i.e., all conclusions remained unchanged when numerical format was included in the analyses).

Do participants from the USA and Germany differ in the accuracy of their estimates? Do they differ in the extent to which they benefit from visual aids? Understanding medical information was more difficult for US than German participants—especially when the numerical information was presented in terms of RRR (40% correct, $SE=3.3$ in the USA vs. 49% correct, $SE=3.1$ in Germany) as opposed to ARR (57% correct, $SE=3.2$ in the USA vs. 52% correct, $SE=3.1$ in Germany). US participants, therefore, were less often correct when less transparent numerical representations were used. Similarly, a lower percentage of participants in the USA than in Germany provided accurate estimates when information about the drug was provided only numerically (29% correct, $SE=4.7$ in the USA vs. 40% correct, $SE=4.7$ in Germany). When visual aids were added to the numerical information, however, percentages were similar in the two countries (58%, $SE=2.4$ in the USA vs. 54%, $SE=2.6$ in Germany). Visual aids, therefore, were especially useful for the US participants. Consistent with these results, an ANOVA with country, visual aids, and numerical format as between-participants factors showed an interaction between country and numerical format, $F_{1,978}=5.9$, $p=0.015$, and country and visual aids, $F_{4,978}=5.56$, $p=0.001$. These results remained unchanged when numeracy and graph literacy were included in the analyses.

9.3 Discussion and Conclusions

Building on previous research showing that problems with understanding numerical information often do not reside in people's minds but in the representation of the problem (Gigerenzer et al. 2007; Gigerenzer and Hoffrage 1995), our results show that visual aids help to modify incorrect expectations about treatment risk reduction and have important implications for medical practice.

First, our findings showed large improvements in accuracy when either icon arrays or bar graphs were added to numerical information presented as either absolute or RRRs. Whether visual aids reflect the overall population at risk has a significant impact on people's perceptions: The highest increases in accuracy were achieved when the icon arrays and bar graphs represented visually the number of patients who did and did not take the treatment in addition to the number of treated and nontreated patients who suffered a disease. A plausible explanation for this result could be that presenting numerical information regarding the entire population at risk in imaginable and identifiable formats could help participants pay attention to part-to-whole relationships (Ancker et al. 2006) and represent superordinate classes (i.e., overall numbers of treated and nontreated patients; Reyna and Brainerd 2008). This explanation is compatible with previous results in marketing research by Stone and colleagues, who showed that numerically presented risks are perceived as more serious than equivalent risks presented visually only when visual aids reflect the overall population at risk (Stone et al. 1997, 2003). Our research, however, is unique in its efforts to study perceptions of part-to-whole relationships in problems involving risk reduction in a medical context. Furthermore, in contrast to research by Stone et al. (1997, 2003), which focused on people's willingness to pay for a product and risk aversion, our study focuses on accuracy of estimates (i.e., quantitative reasoning; Ancker et al. 2006).

Second, our results suggest suitable ways to communicate quantitative medical data to people who are especially vulnerable to having difficulty when making decisions about health: providing visual aids in addition to numerical information helps people with low numeracy make more accurate assessments of risk reduction. These results support our own and others' previous findings (Fagerlin et al. 2007; Galesic et al. 2009; Garcia-Retamero and Galesic 2009a; Garcia-Retamero et al. 2010). They also extend the literature, revealing a significant group of patients with low numeracy for whom graphically presented information is very useful, namely those who have high graph literacy skills. Because of their low numeracy skills, these people have particular difficulties grasping numerical concepts. However, they can be especially aided by using visual displays designed to enhance comprehension. People with both low numeracy and low graph literacy may require specially designed information formats undemanding in terms of both skills (e.g., analogies; see Chap. 7; see also Galesic and Garcia-Retamero 2012) and/or additional training in the use of graphs (Galesic and Garcia-Retamero 2011).

Last but not least, we found interesting cross-cultural differences between participants from the USA and Germany. In line with results in national studies investigating numerical skills (Kutner et al. 2006; Programme for International Student Assessment 2003; Rinderman 2007; Tuijnman 2000), US participants were particularly vulnerable to having difficulty when estimating treatment risk reduction. This result can be due to the differences in the educational systems between the USA and Germany (see Chap. 1). In fact, the stronger emphasis on math and science education in early grades in Germany compared to the USA (Stigler et al. 1999) is one of the reasons why German students score higher than US students on measures of quantitative literacy (Kutner et al. 2006; Programme for International Student Assessment 2003; Tuijnman 2000). These differences might also affect people's ability to reason about numerical concepts, including risks, in adulthood. This hypothesis is supported by the fact that residents in Germany also have higher scores on numeracy than those in the USA (see Chap. 2; see also Galesic and Garcia-Retamero 2010). Our findings are also compatible with research showing that residents in USA show more risk aversion than those in Germany (Renn and Rohrmann 2000; Weber and Hsee 1998). It is possible that these cultural differences in orientation towards risk and uncertainty could have made Americans particularly vulnerable to errors when estimating treatment risk reduction. Interestingly, our results show that these patients can be especially aided by using visual displays designed to enhance risk comprehension.

In sum, our study reveals a way to improve patients' medical decision making, namely by using visual aids that do not require high levels of numeracy and that represent the entire population of patients at risk, especially with those who possess high graph literacy skills. Further research is needed on suitable strategies for people with low numeracy and poor ability to understand graphically presented quantitative information about health.

References

Ancker, J. S., Senathirajah, Y., Kukafka, R., & Starren, J. B. (2006). Design features of graphs in health risk communication: A systematic review. *Journal of the American Medical Informatics Association, 13*, 608–618.

Baker, D. W., Wolf, M. S., Feinglass, J., Thompson, J. A., Gazmararian, J. A., & Huang, J. (2008). Health literacy and mortality among elderly persons. *Archives of Internal Medicine, 167*, 1503–1509.

Barry, M. D. (1999). Involving patients in medical decisions. *Journal of the American Medical Association, 282*, 2356–2357.

Brundage, M., Feldman-Stewart, D., Leis, A., Bezjak, A., Degner, L., Velji, K., et al. (2005). Communicating quality of life information to cancer patients: A study of six presentation formats. *Journal of Clinical Oncology, 23*, 6949–6956.

Cleary, P. D., & Angel, R. (1984). The analysis of relationships involving dichotomous dependent-variables. *Journal of Health and Social Behavior, 25*, 334–348.

Edwards, A., Elwyn, G., & Mulley, A. (2002). Explaining risks: Turning numerical data into meaningful pictures. *British Medical Journal, 324*, 827–830.

Fagerlin, A., Ubel, P. A., Smith, D. M., & Zikmund-Fisher, B. J. (2007). Making numbers matter: Present and future research in risk communication. *American Journal of Health Behavior, 31*, 47–56.

Fagerlin, A., Wang, C., & Ubel, P. A. (2005). Reducing the influence of anecdotal reasoning on people's health care decisions: Is a picture worth a thousand statistics? *Medical Decision Making, 25*, 398–405.

Feldman-Stewart, D., Kocovski, N., McConnell, B. A., Brundage, M. D., & Mackillop, W. J. (2000). Perception of quantitative information for treatment decisions. *Medical Decision Making, 20*, 228–238.

Friel, S. N., Curcio, F. R., & Bright, G. W. (2001). Making sense of graphs: Critical factors influencing comprehension and instructional implications. *Journal for Research in Mathematics Education, 32*, 124–158.

Galesic, M., & Garcia-Retamero, R. (2010). Statistical numeracy for health: A cross-cultural comparison with probabilistic national samples. *Archives of Internal Medicine, 170*, 462–468.

Galesic, M., & Garcia-Retamero, R. (2011). Graph literacy: A cross-cultural comparison. *Medical Decision Making, 31*, 444–457.

Galesic, M. & Garcia-Retamero, R. (2012). Using analogies to communicate information about health risks. Applied Cognitive Psychology. doi: 10.1002/acp.2866

Galesic, M., Garcia-Retamero, R., & Gigerenzer, G. (2009). Using icon arrays to communicate medical risks: Overcoming low numeracy. *Health Psychology, 28*, 210–216.

Garcia-Retamero, R., & Cokely, E. T. (2011). Effective communication of risks to young adults: Using message framing and visual aids to increase condom use and STD screening. *Journal of Experimental Psychology: Applied, 17*, 270–287.

Garcia-Retamero, R., & Dhami, M. K. (2011). Pictures speak louder than numbers: On communicating medical risks to immigrants with limited non-native language proficiency. *Health Expectations, 14*, 46–57.

Garcia-Retamero, R., & Galesic, M. (2009a). Do icon arrays help reduce denominator neglect? *American Journal of Public Health, 99*, 2196–2202.

Garcia-Retamero, R., & Galesic, M. (2009b). Trust in healthcare. In M. W. Kattan (Ed.), *The encyclopedia of medical decision making* (pp. 1153–1155). Thousand Oaks: SAGE.

Garcia-Retamero, R., & Galesic, M. (2010). How to reduce the effect of framing on messages about health. *Journal of General Internal Medicine, 25*, 1323–1329.

Garcia-Retamero, R., Galesic, M., & Gigerenzer, G. (2010). Do icon arrays help reduce denominator neglect? *Medical Decision Making, 30*, 672–684.

Gigerenzer, G., & Edwards, A. (2003). Simple tools for understanding risks: From innumeracy to insight. *British Medical Journal, 327*, 741–744.

Gigerenzer, G., Gaissmaier, W., Kurz-Milcke, E., Schwartz, L. M., & Woloshin, S. (2007). Helping doctors and patients make sense of health statistics. *Psychological Science in the Public Interest, 8*, 53–96.

Gigerenzer, G., & Hoffrage, U. (1995). How to improve Bayesian reasoning without instruction: Frequency formats. *Psychological Review, 102*, 684–704.

Goodyear-Smith, F., Arroll, B., Chan, L., Jackson, R., Wells, S., & Kenealy, T. (2008). Patients prefer pictures to numbers to express cardiovascular benefit from treatment. *Annals of Family Medicine, 6*, 213–217.

Hanson, J. L. (2008). Shared decision making: Have we missed the obvious? *Archives of Internal Medicine, 168*, 1368–1370.

Hawley, S. T., Zikmund-Fisher, B., Ubel, P., Jancovic, A., Lucas, T., & Fagerlin, A. (2008). The impact of the format of graphical presentation on health-related knowledge and treatment choices. *Patient Education and Counseling, 73*, 448–455.

Kutner, M., Greenberg, E., Jin, Y., & Paulsen, C. (2006). *The health literacy of America's adults: Results from the 2003 National Assessment of Adult Literacy (NCES 2006–483)*. Washington, DC: National Center for Education Statistics.

Lipkus, I. M. (2007). Numeric, verbal, and visual formats of conveying health risks: Suggested best practices and future recommendations. *Medical Decision Making, 27*, 696–713.

Lipkus, I. M., & Hollands, J. G. (1999). The visual communication of risk. *Journal of the National Cancer Institute Monographs, 25*, 149–163.

Lipkus, I. M., Samsa, G., & Rimer, B. K. (2001). General performance on a numeracy scale among highly educated samples. *Medical Decision Making, 21*, 37–44.

Lunney, G. H. (1970). Using analysis of variance with a dichotomous dependent variable—Empirical study. *Journal of Educational Measurement, 7*, 263–269.

Paling, J. (2003). Strategies to help patients understand risks. *British Medical Journal, 327*, 745–748.

Peters, E., Dieckmann, N. F., Västfjäll, D., Mertz, C. K., Slovic, P., & Hibbard, J. (2009). Bringing meaning to numbers: The impact of evaluative categories on decisions. *Journal of Experimental Psychology: Applied, 15*, 213–227.

Peters, E., Vastfjall, D., Slovic, P., Mertz, C. K., Mozzocco, K., & Dickert, S. (2006). Numeracy and decision making. *Psychological Science, 17*, 406–413.

Programme for International Student Assessment (PISA). (2003). *The PISA 2003 assessment framework—mathematics, reading, science, and problem solving knowledge and skills.* Paris: OEDC.

Renn, O., & Rohrmann, B. (2000). Cross-cultural risk perception: State and challenges. In O. Renn & B. Rohrmann (Eds.), *Cross-cultural risk perception: A survey of empirical studies* (pp. 211–233). Dordrecht: Kluwer.

Reyna, V. F., & Brainerd, C. J. (2008). Numeracy, ratio bias, and denominator neglect in judgments of risk and probability. *Learning and Individual Differences, 18*, 89–107.

Rinderman, H. (2007). The g-factor of international cognitive ability comparisons: The homogeneity of results in PISA, TIMSS, PIRLS and IQ-tests across nations. *European Journal of Personality, 21*, 667–706.

Rudski, J. M., & Volksdorf, J. (2002). Pictorial versus textual information and the ratio-bias effect. *Perceptual and Motor Skills, 95*, 547–554.

Schapira, M. M., Nattinger, A. B., & McHorney, C. A. (2001). Frequency or probability? A qualitative study of risk communication formats used in health care. *Medical Decision Making, 21*, 459–467.

Schirillo, J. A., & Stone, E. R. (2005). The greater ability of graphical versus numerical displays to increase risk avoidance involves a common mechanism. *Risk Analysis, 25*, 555–566.

Schoen, C., Doty, M. M., Collins, S. R., & Holmgren, A. L. (2005). Insured but not protected: How many adults are underinsured? *Health Affairs, 10*, W5-289–W5-302.

Schoen, C., Osborn, R., Doty, M. M., Bishop, M., Peugh, J., & Murukutla, N. (2007). Toward higher-performance health systems: Adults' health care experiences in seven countries, 2007. *Health Affairs, 26*, W717–W734.

Schwartz, L. M., Woloshin, S., Black, W. C., & Welch, H. G. (1997). The role of numeracy in understanding the benefit of screening mammography. *Annals of Internal Medicine, 127*, 966–972.

Statistisches Bundesamt Deutschland, Microcensus (2007). http://www-genesis.destatis.de/genesis/online/online?operation=abruftabellenVerzeichnis, accessed July 30, 2012.

Stigler, J. W., Gonzales, P., Kawanaka, T., Knoll, S., & Serrano, A. (1999). *The TIMSS videotape classroom study: Methods and findings from an exploratory research project on eighth-grade mathematics instruction in Germany, Japan, and the United States*. Washington, DC: U.S. Department of Education, National Center for Education Statistics.

Stone, E. R., Sieck, W. R., Bull, B. E., Yates, J. F., Parks, S. C., & Rush, C. J. (2003). Foreground: Background salience: Explaining the effects of graphical displays on risk avoidance. *Organizational Behavior and Human Decision Processes, 90*, 19–36.
Stone, E. R., Yates, J. F., & Parker, A. M. (1997). Effects of numerical and graphical displays on professed risk-taking behavior. *Journal of Experimental Psychology: Applied, 3*, 243–256.
Tuijnman, A. (2000). *Benchmarking adult literacy in America: An international comparative study (International Adult Literacy Survey)*. Washington, DC: Department of Education, OVAE.
U.S. Census Bureau (2011). *Number of uninsured and uninsured rate: 1987 to 2007*. http://www.census.gov/hhes/www/hlthins/data/incpovhlth/2007/fig06.pdf.
Waters, E. A., Weinstein, N. D., Colditz, G. A., & Emmons, K. (2006). Formats for improving risk communication in medical tradeoff decisions. *Journal of Health Communication, 11*, 167–182.
Waters, E. A., Weinstein, N. D., Colditz, G. A., & Emmons, K. M. (2007). Reducing aversion to side effects in preventive medical treatment decisions. *Journal of Experimental Psychology: Applied, 13*, 11–21.
Weber, E. U., & Hsee, C. K. (1998). Cross-cultural differences in risk perception, but cross-cultural similarities in attitude towards perceived risk. *Management Science, 44*, 1205–1217.
World Health Organization (2012). World Health Statistics 2012. http://www.who.int/gho/publications/world_health_statistics/2012/en/, accessed July 30, 2012.
Zikmund-Fisher, B. J., Ubel, P. A., Smith, D. M., Derry, H. A., McClure, J. B., Stark, A., et al. (2008). Communicating side effect risks in a tamoxifen prophylaxis decision aid: The debiasing influence of pictographs. *Patient Education and Counseling, 73*, 209–214.

Chapter 10
Reducing Denominator Neglect*

Rocio Garcia-Retamero, Mirta Galesic, and Mandeep K. Dhami

Abstract A prominent example of the difficulties that patients experience to understand health-relevant numerical concepts is *denominator neglect*, or the focus on the number of times a target event has happened (numerators), without consideration of the overall number of opportunities for it to happen (denominators). In this chapter, we describe two studies involving probabilistic national US and German samples (Study 1) and a large immigrant sample of Polish people living in the UK (Study 2) addressing the effect of denominator neglect in problems involving treatment risk reduction. We also analyzed whether people's comprehension can be aided with icon arrays. Results showed that participants—in particular those disadvantaged by their lack of numerical and language skills—showed substantial denominator neglect in their perceptions of treatment risk reduction. We further showed that

---

*In this chapter, we partially reproduced the articles Garcia-Retamero, R., & Galesic, M. (2009). Communicating treatment risk reduction to people with low numeracy skills: A cross-cultural comparison. *American Journal of Public Health, 99*, 2196–2202, and Garcia-Retamero, R., & Dhami, M. K. (2011). Pictures speak louder than numbers: On communicating medical risks to immigrants with limited non-native language proficiency. *Health Expectations, 14*, 46–57.

R. Garcia-Retamero, Ph.D. (✉)
Departamento de Psicología Experimental, Facultad de Psicología, University of Granada, Campus Universitario de Cartuja s/n, Granada 18071, Spain

Center for Adaptive Behavior and Cognition, Max Planck Institute for Human Development, Lentzeallee 94, Berlin 14195, Germany
e-mail: rretamer@ugr.es

M. Galesic, Ph.D.
Center for Adaptive Behavior and Cognition, Max Planck Institute for Human Development, Lentzeallee 94, Berlin 14195, Germany
e-mail: galesic@mpib-berlin.mpg.de

M.K. Dhami, Ph.D.
School of Psychology, University of Surrey, AD Building, Guildford, Surrey, GU2 7XH, UK
e-mail: m.dhami@surrey.ac.uk

R. Garcia-Retamero and M. Galesic (eds.), *Transparent Communication of Health Risks: Overcoming Cultural Differences*, DOI 10.1007/978-1-4614-4358-2_10,

the use of icon arrays was an effective method for eliminating denominator neglect. We concluded that problems with understanding health-related numerical information often reside not in people's mind but in their representation of the problem.

10.1 Introduction and Background

Ratio concepts—of which risks and probabilities are examples—are particularly challenging and prone to biases that undermine good judgment and decision making (Cuite et al. 2008; Garcia-Retamero and Galesic 2011; Garcia-Retamero et al. 2012). A prominent example of people's difficulties with ratio concepts is *denominator neglect* (Reyna 2004; Reyna and Brainerd 2008). That is, people often pay too much attention to the number of times a target event has happened (numerators) and insufficient attention to the overall number of opportunities for it to happen (denominators; Reyna and Brainerd 2008). The denominator neglect effect has been studied both in medical and non-medical contexts (Lloyd and Reyna 2001; Lloyd et al. 2001; Pacini and Epstein 1999a; Stanovich and West 2008). In an experiment by Yamagishi (1997), for instance, participants were presented with estimates of the number of deaths in the population due to 11 causes (e.g., cancer) and had to assess the risk of dying of such causes. Using a within-subjects design, these estimates were presented both as numbers of deaths out of 10,000 and of 100. Participants rated the likelihood of a cancer killing 1,286 out of 10,000 people (i.e., 12.86%) as higher than 24.14 out of 100 people (i.e., 24.14%). The degree of perceived riskiness, therefore, varied according to the number of deaths presented (numerators), irrespective of the total possible number of deaths (denominators).

Denominator neglect could have important consequences when estimating treatment risk reduction. In medical practice, for example, the overall number of patients who receive a certain treatment is often smaller than those who do not (Grossarth-Maticek and Ziegler 2008; Walitza et al. 2007). Therefore, patients and their doctors might be able to think of more people who did not have a particular screening or take a novel drug than those who did. If individuals disregard the overall number of treated and non-treated patients (e.g., 100 and 800, respectively), they might perceive the treatment to be more effective than it actually is. Thus, they might underestimate the number of patients who died after receiving the treatment, while overestimating the number of those who died and did not receive the treatment (e.g., 5 out of 100 and 80 out of 800 for a treatment risk reduction of 50%; see Fig. 10.1). However, most of the past research on people's perceptions of treatment risk reductions has employed samples of treated and non-treated patients of the same size (see Chap. 9; see also Fagerlin et al. 2007; Galesic et al. 2009), and even experts in medical decision making recommend doing so (Ancker et al. 2006; International Patient Decision Aids Standards 2005; Paling 2003). As an exception, Garcia-Retamero et al. (2010) conducted a study with unequal samples of (hypothetical) treated and non-treated patients, and showed that participants overestimated risk reduction

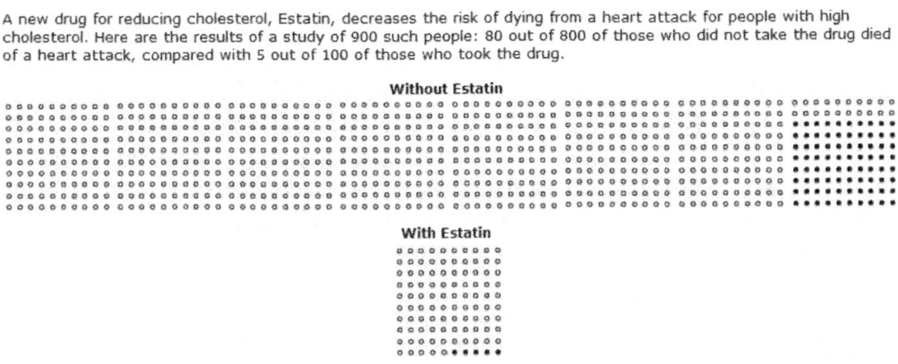

Fig. 10.1 Numerical information about relative risk reduction and additional visual information (icon array)

when the overall number of treated patients was lower than the number of patients who did not receive the treatment.

In this chapter, we report two studies in which we sought to address the effect of denominator neglect in problems involving treatment risk reduction. Study 1 involved probabilistic national US and German samples of participants with different levels of numeracy (see Garcia-Retamero and Galesic 2009). Study 2 involved a large sample of immigrants (i.e., Polish people living in the UK) with limited non-native language proficiency (Garcia-Retamero and Dhami 2011).

10.2 Study 1: On Communicating Treatment Risk Reduction in People with High and Low Numeracy

In the following study, we investigated whether people with low numeracy skills show more denominator neglect than those with high-numeracy skills. As Fagerlin et al. (2007) point out, low-numeracy patients might have more need for consistent denominators than would high-numeracy patients because their lack of numerical ability puts them at a disadvantage. In this study, we investigated this suggestion experimentally.

More importantly, there is a dearth of published research on whether people with low-numeracy skills can be aided when making decisions about their health by using displays designed to enhance comprehension (Ancker et al. 2006; Montori and Rothman 2005). As Reyna and Brainerd (2008) point out, visual displays can help people represent superordinate classes such as the overall number of patients who did and did not receive a treatment, thus reducing denominator neglect (Lloyd and Reyna 2001). Icon arrays have been shown to be a promising method for communicating medical risk reduction (see Chaps. 9 and 11; see also Fagerlin et al. 2005; Galesic et al. 2009; Zikmund-Fisher et al. 2008), and might then help draw people's attention to the overall number of unaffected patients, reducing denominator neglect. This might be especially the case in people with low-numeracy skills.

Finally, all of the studies on denominator neglect conducted so far (see Reyna and Brainerd 2008, for a review) have used relatively limited laboratory samples of participants. Although these studies provide valuable information about the accuracy of understanding of these participants, because of the non-probabilistic sampling methods employed, the results cannot be generalized to any wider population. We conducted a study on probabilistic national samples in two countries with very different medical systems—the USA and Germany (see Chap. 1)—to test the generalizability of denominator neglect and the effect of icon arrays on a wider population.

10.2.1 Method

10.2.1.1 Participants

The study was conducted on probabilistic national samples in the USA and Germany as part of the project "Helping people with low numeracy understand medical information," funded by the Foundation for Informed Medical Decision Making. The project involved a survey that gathered data for a number of studies related to understanding and communicating risks, conducted in two waves (see Chaps. 2, 4, 7–9, and 13). In the first wave, large national samples of participants ($n=1{,}009$ in the USA and $n=1{,}001$ in Germany) completed a numeracy scale consisting of nine items selected from Schwartz et al. (1997) and Lipkus et al. (2001; see Chap. 15). The scale does not contain any item that measures denominator neglect. Participants with numeracy scores in the top and bottom third of the whole sample were invited to participate in this study, resulting in a sample of 513 from the USA and 534 participants from Germany. The structure of the resulting sample is presented in Table 8.1 in Chap. 8 (see Chap. 2 for more details about the methodology of the survey). This sample enabled us to compare low- and high-numeracy people within each country, as well as each of those groups between countries. In our analyses, we split the participants into two groups according to the median numeracy score for the total sample (i.e., 6; see Peters et al. 2006 for a similar procedure). The average numeracy scores in each of the resulting groups in each country are shown in Table 8.1 in Chap. 8.

10.2.1.2 Stimuli and Procedure

All participants completed a computerized questionnaire, which was developed in English and translated into German (see Chap. 2 for more details about the translation of the materials and the programmed questionnaire). The Ethics Committee of the Max Planck Institute for Human Development approved the methodology, and all participants consented to participate through an online consent form at the beginning of the survey.

We presented participants with a medical scenario of the usefulness of "Estatin"—a hypothetical drug for reducing cholesterol that also decreases the risk of dying from a heart attack with a relative risk reduction of 50%. In one condition, for

Table 10.1 Number of treated and non-treated patients who died from a heart attack used in fictitious medical scenarios with different denominator sizes

Sizes of denominators[a]	Treated patients		Non-treated patients	
	Dead patients	Population size	Dead patients	Population size
800–800	40	800	80	800
100–800	5	100	80	800
800–100	40	800	10	100
100–100	5	100	10	100

Note: Treatment risk reduction is 50% in all conditions
[a]Treated and untreated people, respectively

instance, participants received the following information: "A new drug for reducing cholesterol, Estatin, decreases the risk of dying from a heart attack for patients with high cholesterol. Here are the results of a study of 900 such patients: 80 out of 800 of those who did not take the drug died of a heart attack, compared with 5 out of 100 of those who took the drug."

Two independent variables were manipulated between groups. Participants were randomly assigned to the conditions representing these variables. First, the overall numbers of treated and non-treated patients (i.e., the sizes of the denominators) were manipulated to be 800 and 800, 100 and 800, 800 and 100, or 100 and 100, where the first and second quantity reflect the overall number of patients who did and did not take the drug, respectively (Table 10.1). To achieve a relative risk reduction of 50%, the sizes of the numerators (i.e., the number of treated and non-treated patients who died) varied within conditions depending on the sizes of the denominators.

Independently of these manipulations, half of the participants received—in addition to the numerical information about risk reduction—two icon arrays presenting the risk of dying of a heart attack when the drug was and was not taken, respectively. All icon arrays contained either 800 or 100 circles depending on the overall number of patients who did and did not take the drug. Deceased patients were shown as black circles at the end of the array. An example of the condition involving icon arrays is shown in Fig. 10.1.

As a dependent variable, we measured participants' estimates of treatment risk reduction. First, following the procedure used by Schwartz et al. (1997), participants were asked how many of 1,000 patients with high cholesterol might die of a heart attack if they do not take the drug. Second, they were asked how many of 1,000 patients with high cholesterol might die of a heart attack if they do take the drug. By deducting the second from the first answer and dividing it by the first, we calculated the estimated relative risk reduction. Participants were classified depending on whether their estimates were accurate, lower, or higher than the exact value (i.e., 50%). Estimates were considered to be accurate only when they were exactly correct.

In sum, the design of the study had four between-subjects factors: the sizes of the denominators, icon arrays, numeracy, and nationality. To assess the effect of these factors on estimates of treatment risk reduction, we conducted analyses of variance (ANOVAs; see Cleary and Angel 1984; Lunney 1970).We conducted Tukey's honest significant difference test in post hoc analyses.

10.2.2 Results

Do participants show denominator neglect in their estimates of risk reduction? And, do participants with low numeracy show more denominator neglect than those with high numeracy? Figs. 10.2a, b shows the percentage of low- and high-numeracy participants, respectively, whose estimates of risk reduction were accurate, lower, or higher than the exact value. When information about the drug was provided numerically (no icon arrays) and the sizes of the denominators were different, many participants provided inaccurate estimates. This result held especially for participants with low numeracy. An ANOVA with numeracy and sizes of the denominators as between-subjects factors on the percentage of participants whose estimates of risk reduction were inaccurate showed a main effect of numeracy, $F_{1,593}=162.44$; $p=0.001$, and sizes of the denominator, $F_{3,593}=16.502$; $p=0.001$, when information about the drug was provided numerically.

As Fig. 10.2a, b shows, 71% of the participants with low numeracy *overestimated* risk reduction when the number of treated patients was lower than the number of those who did not receive the treatment (i.e., in the 100 and 800 denominator condition), whereas only 25% of the participants with high numeracy provided a lower estimate than the exact value in that condition ($p=0.001$). Note that in such a case, the number of patients who received the treatment and died ($n=5$) is much lower than the number of patients who did not receive the treatment and died ($n=80$; Table 10.1). Possibly, many participants—especially those with low numeracy—did not take proportions into account but only absolute numbers in the numerators, which might have led them to believe that the treatment had a *larger* effect than it actually did.

In contrast, 67% of the participants with low numeracy *underestimated* risk reduction when the number of treated patients was higher than the number of patients who did not receive treatment (i.e., in the 800 and 100 denominator condition), whereas only 19% of the participants with high numeracy provided a higher estimate than the exact value in that condition ($p=0.001$). In such a case, the number of patients who received the treatment and died ($n=40$) is higher than the number of patients who did not receive the treatment and died ($n=10$; see Table 10.1). This might have led participants—especially those with low numeracy—to believe that the treatment had a smaller effect than it actually did.

Finally, when the sizes of the denominators were equal, estimated risk reduction was inaccurate in only 6 and 56% of the participants with high and low numeracy, respectively ($p=0.001$). In these conditions, participants did not necessarily have to take proportions into account to make accurate estimates but could rely on only the absolute numbers in the numerators.

Do icon arrays help reduce denominator neglect? And, are icon arrays especially helpful for participants with low numeracy? As Fig. 10.2a, b shows, when icon arrays were added to the numerical information, the denominator neglect effectively disappeared. Interestingly, this was particularly the case in those participants who were less skilled in using numerical information. An ANOVA with numeracy,

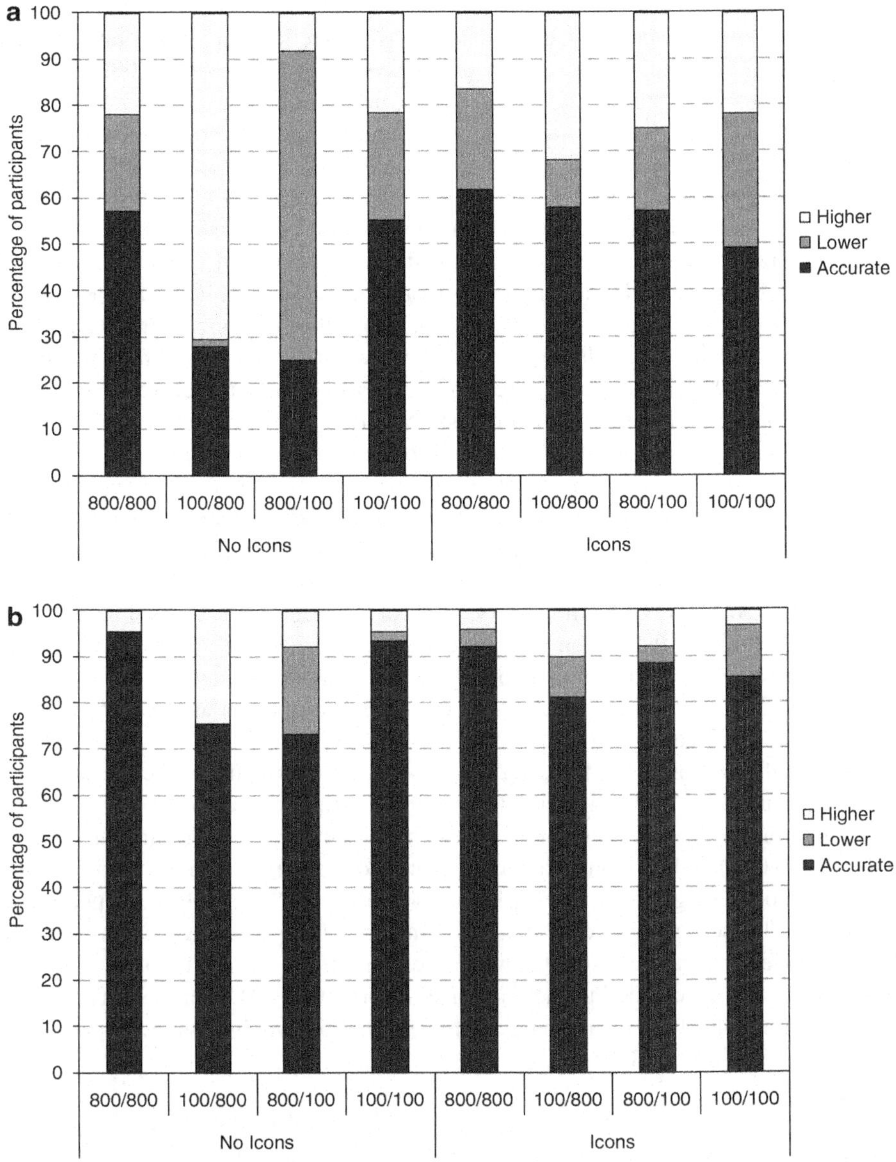

Fig. 10.2 Estimates of treatment risk reduction in Study 1: (**a**) Percentage of participants with *low* numeracy whose estimates of risk reduction were either accurate or lower or higher than the exact value as a function of the sizes of the denominators and icon arrays. (**b**) Percentage of participants with *high* numeracy whose estimates of risk reduction were either accurate or lower or higher than the exact value as a function of the sizes of the denominators and icon arrays

sizes of the denominators, and icon arrays as between-subjects factors on the percentage of participants whose estimates of risk reduction were inaccurate showed an interaction between numeracy and icon arrays, $F_{1,1100}=6.96$; $p=0.008$, and sizes of denominators and icon arrays, $F_{3,1100}=7.25$; $p=0.001$.

When the sizes of the denominators were different and icon arrays were added to the numerical information, the percentage of low-numeracy participants who estimated the treatment risk reduction incorrectly decreased from 74 to 42% ($p=0.001$), and from 26 to 15% in participants with high numeracy ($p=0.038$). The percentages when the sizes of the denominators were different (i.e., 42 and 15%) are similar to those when the sizes of the denominators were equal (i.e., for high numeracy, 45%, $p=0.744$; and for low numeracy, 22%, $p=0.343$). Thus, the percentages of participants who estimated risk reduction correctly were not influenced by the sizes of the denominators when icon arrays were provided. Participants, therefore, disregarded denominators when information about risk reduction was provided numerically but did not do so when icon arrays were added to the numerical information.

Which country shows more denominator neglect? And, do icon arrays improve accuracy of estimates of treatment risk reduction in both countries? Understanding medical information presented numerically was more difficult for US participants than for German participants. In addition, icon arrays were especially useful for US participants. An ANOVA with country, sizes of the denominators, and icon arrays as between-subjects factors on the percentage of participants whose estimates of risk reduction were inaccurate showed an interaction among the three factors ($F_{3,1100}=3.124$; $p=0.025$). The interaction remained significant after controlling for participants' numeracy.

When information about the drug was provided numerically, higher percentages of US participants (66%) provided inaccurate estimates when the sizes of the denominators were different compared with percentages of German participants (40%; $p=0.005$). When icon arrays were added to the numerical information, however, these percentages were similar in the two countries (31 and 36%, respectively; $p=0.473$). These percentages were also similar to the percentage of participants who provided inaccurate estimates when the sizes of the denominators were equal and icon arrays were added to the numerical information (30% for US participants, $p=0.976$; and 24% for German participants, $p=0.696$). We discuss the implications of these results in Sect. 10.4.

10.3 Study 2: On Communicating Treatment Risk Reduction in Immigrants with Limited Non-native Language Proficiency

Communication of treatment risk reduction has been infrequently studied in vulnerable populations, for example, those with difficulties in comprehension of health-related information. These populations include—but are not limited to—immigrant groups with low literacy or limited non-native language proficiency (Huerta and

Macario 1999), which might reduce their access to, and understanding of, medical risks (Fry et al. 2007; Shaw and Hurst 2009) thus mitigating the effectiveness of public health strategies (Andrulis et al. 2007; James et al. 2007; Taylor-Clark et al. 2007). To illustrate, since 2005, the UK has experienced an influx of immigrants from Eastern Europe, particularly Poland, whose first language is not English (BBC News 2009; Burrell 2009). Public sector bodies in the UK including medical centers and the criminal justice system have responded to communication problems by producing information in the immigrants' native language (e.g., Polish) and recruiting translators who speak these languages (Eurostat 2009). Due to limitations in non-native language proficiency, denominator neglect might undermine estimates of treatment risk reductions in immigrant populations—especially when the risk information is not provided in their native language. Testing this hypothesis was the first aim of this study.

There is also a dearth of published research on whether patients who are disadvantaged by their lack of non-native language skills can be aided when making decisions about their health (Andrulis et al. 2007; James et al. 2007; Larkey and Gonzalez 2007). In line with the results of the previous study, we hypothesized that icon arrays might reduce denominator neglect when assessing treatment risk reduction, especially when the risk information is not provided in people's native language. Testing this hypothesis was the second aim of the study. To test the two hypotheses, we conducted a study involving participants who were all Polish immigrants to the UK.

10.3.1 Method

10.3.1.1 Participants

Ninety-six Polish immigrants to the UK volunteered to participate in the study. Forty-nine percent were male. The average age of the sample was 27 years (range 19–44; SD=5.2). The majority (65%) had at most a secondary school education (i.e., up to age 16), and 34% had a university degree. Participants were recruited by a Polish research assistant from public places such as restaurants and gyms in the city of Cambridge (UK).

10.3.1.2 Stimuli and Procedure

The stimuli and procedure in this study were similar to those in Study 1. We employed a mixed design with three independent variables. The sizes of the denominators were manipulated within-subjects and had four levels (see Table 10.1). Icon arrays were manipulated between-subjects and had two levels: Icons in addition to the numerical information about risk reduction (see Fig. 10.1) and no icon arrays (i.e., numerical information only). Finally, language was a between-subjects factor and had two levels: Information about treatment risk reduction was provided either in participants' native language, Polish, or a non-native language, English. Participants were assigned randomly to one of four equally sized groups depending on icon arrays and language.

All materials were developed in English, translated into Polish by a skilled translator, and then back-translated into English by another translator. Thus, the two language versions were comparable. The Ethics Committee of the University of Granada approved the methodology, and all participants consented to participation through a consent form at the beginning of the study.

There were three dependent measures. We measured estimates of treatment risk reduction as in Study 1. We further measured confidence on estimates and perceptions of treatment effectiveness. In particular, participants were asked how confident they were in their answers to the above two questions on a 15-point scale from 1 (*not confident at all*) to 15 (*very confident*). Participants also evaluated the effectiveness of the treatment in preventing deaths by heart attack for patients with high cholesterol on a 15-point scale from 1 (*not at all effective*) to 15 (*very effective*).[1]

In sum, the design of the study had three variables, the sizes of the denominators, icon arrays, and language. To assess the effect of these factors on estimates of treatment risk reduction, confidence on estimates, and perceptions of treatment effectiveness, we conducted ANOVAs. Degrees of freedom for the analyses containing repeated-measures factors were corrected by using the Greenhouse and Geisser (1959) technique. Tukey's honest significant difference test was used for post hoc analyses.

10.3.2 Results

Do participants show denominator neglect in their estimates of risk reduction? And, is denominator neglect more pronounced when information about risk reduction is not in participants' native language? Figs. 10.3a, b shows the percentage of participants whose estimates of risk reduction were accurate, lower, or higher than the exact value when information about risk reduction was provided in English and Polish, respectively. As in Study 1, when information about the drug was provided numerically and the sizes of the denominators were different, many participants provided inaccurate estimates. This effect was particularly pronounced when the information was given in the participants' non-native language, English, rather than in their native language, Polish, and holds for all three dependent measures. The ANOVAs with sizes of denominators as a within-subjects factor and language as a

[1] In this study, we controlled for participants' numeracy skills. We measured numeracy using 12 items taken from Schwartz et al. (1997), and Lipkus et al. (2001; see also Chap. 15). Scores could range from 0 to 12. The mean numeracy score for the present sample was 8.9 (SD = 2.9). Participants in the experimental conditions did not differ in their average numeracy scores. For the sake of simplicity, we do not include numeracy in data analyses.

between-subjects factor when information about the drug was provided numerically showed a main effect of sizes of denominators. There was also a two-way interaction effect of sizes of denominators by language on the percentages of participants whose estimates of treatment risk reduction were accurate ($F_{3,128}=6.62$, $p=0.001$, and $F_{3,128}=3.12$, $p=0.01$, respectively), on confidence of estimates ($F_{3,117}=23.40$, $p=0.001$, and $F_{3,117}=3.42$, $p=0.03$, respectively), and on perceptions of treatment effectiveness ($F_{2,111}=12.48$, $p=0.001$, and $F_{2,111}=5.90$, $p=0.001$, respectively).

As Fig. 10.3a, b shows, when the overall number of treated patients was smaller than those who did not receive the treatment (i.e., in the 100 and 800 denominator condition), 75% of the participants who received information in English *overestimated* treatment risk reduction, compared to only 33% of the participants who received the risk reduction information in Polish ($p=0.003$). In line with results in the previous study, it is possible that many participants in this condition did not take proportions into account, but only absolute numbers in the numerators, especially when the information about treatment risk reduction was not provided in their native language. This might have led them to believe that the treatment had a *larger* effect than it actually did.

When the overall number of treated patients was larger than the number of those who did not receive treatment (i.e., in the 800 and 100 denominator condition), 58% of the participants *underestimated* treatment risk reduction when the information was in English, compared to only 33% of the participants who received the information in Polish ($p=0.049$). Again, participants in this condition may not have taken proportions into account, which might have led them to believe that the treatment had a smaller effect than it actually did, especially when the information about the risk reduction was not provided in their native language.

Finally, when the sizes of the denominators were equal (i.e., in the 800–800 and 100–100 conditions), estimated risk reduction was inaccurate in only 42 and 23% of those participants who received the information in English and Polish, respectively ($p=0.12$). In these conditions, participants did not necessarily have to take proportions into account to make accurate estimates but could rely on only the absolute numbers in the numerators.

Fig. 10.4 shows average confidence in estimates of treatment risk reduction. Participants who received the information in their non-native language, English, showed more confidence when the number of treated patients was equal to the number of untreated patients (i.e., in the 800 and 800 and the 100 and 100 denominator conditions) than when the denominators were different in size (i.e., in the 100 and 800 and the 800 and 100 denominator conditions; $p=0.001$). In contrast, when the risk information was provided in participants' native language, Polish, confidence judgments were similar in all sizes of denominator conditions ($p=0.25$) and greater than when the risk information was provided in English ($p=0.047$).

Finally, Fig. 10.5 shows average perceptions of treatment effectiveness. Participants who received the risk information in English perceived the treatment to be much more effective in the 100 and 800 condition than in the 800 and 100 condition ($p=0.001$). In contrast, when the denominators of the two ratios were the same and the risk information was provided in English or Polish, participants' perceptions of treatment effectiveness were similar and in-between those of the other conditions.

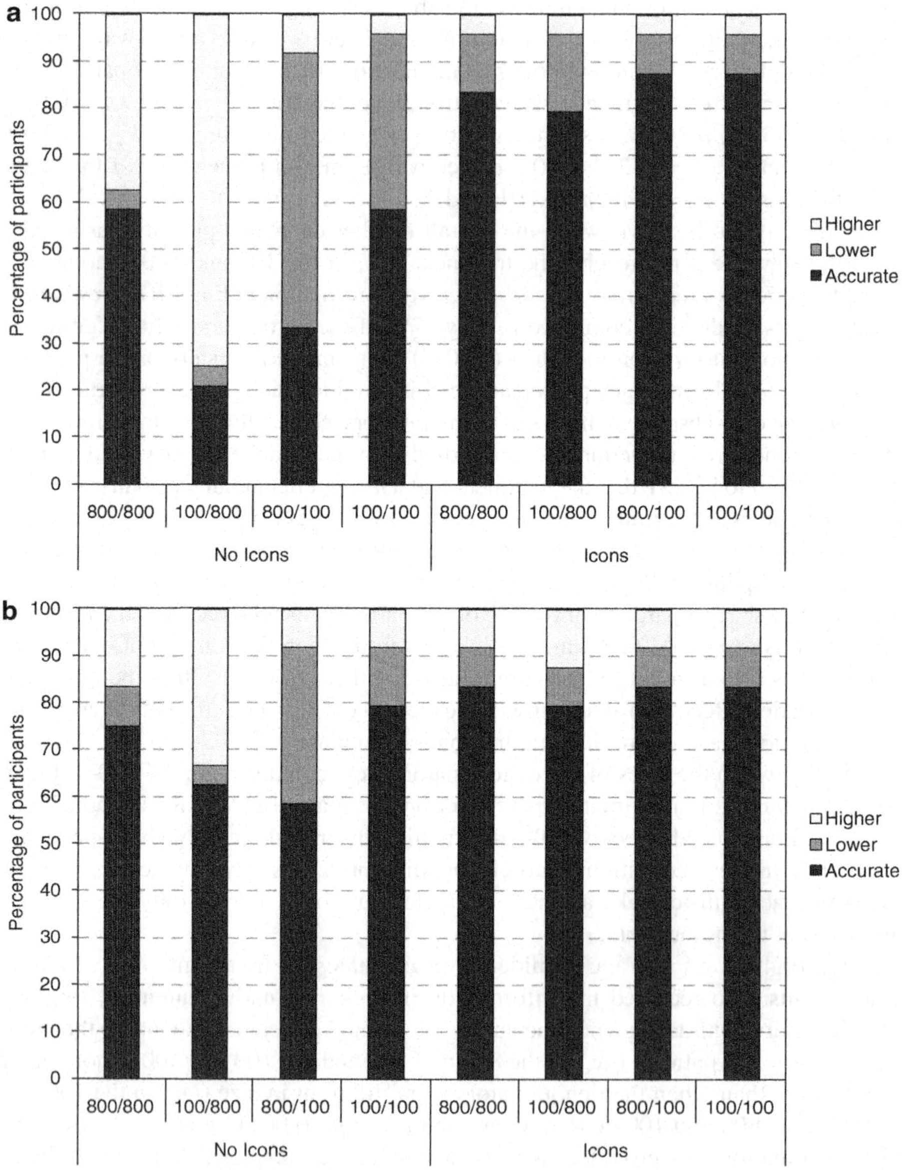

Fig. 10.3 Estimates of treatment risk reduction in Study 2: (**a**) Percentage of participants whose estimates of risk reduction were either accurate, lower, or higher than the exact value as a function of the sizes of the denominators and icon arrays when information about risk reduction was provided in *English*. (**b**) Percentage of participants whose estimates of risk reduction were either accurate, lower, or higher than the exact value as a function of the sizes of the denominators and icon arrays when information about risk reduction was provided in *Polish*

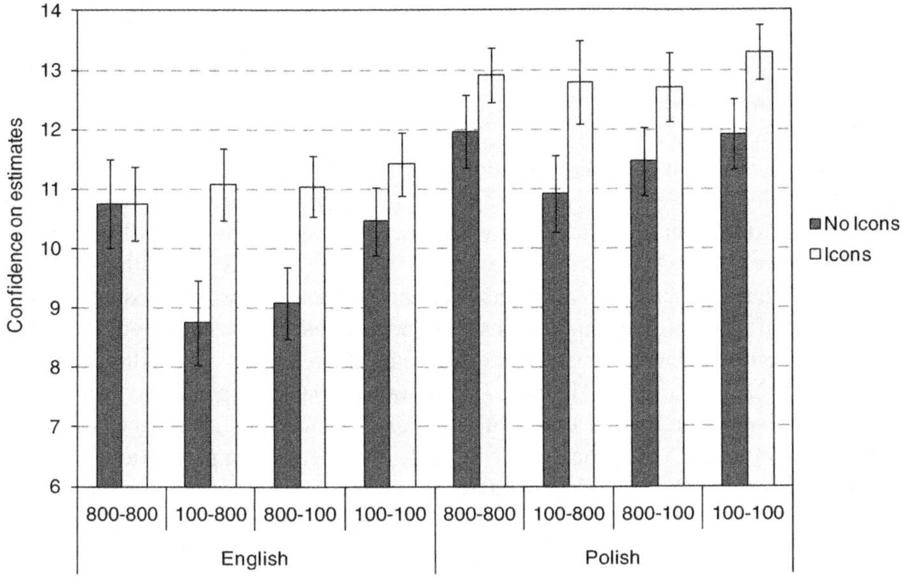

Fig. 10.4 Average confidence judgment as a function of the sizes of the denominators, icon arrays, and language in Study 2. Error bars indicate one standard error

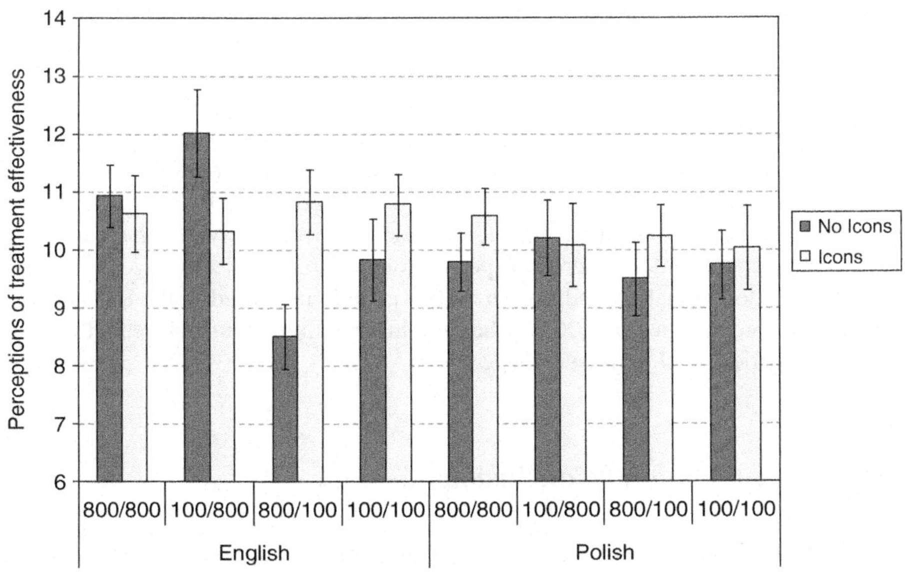

Fig. 10.5 Average perceptions of risk reduction as a function of the sizes of the denominators, icon arrays, and language in Study 2. Error bars indicate one standard error

Do icon arrays help reduce denominator neglect? And are icon arrays especially helpful when the information about risk reduction was not in participants' native language? In line with the results in Study 1, when icon arrays were added to the numerical information about treatment risk reduction, denominator neglect effectively disappeared (see Fig. 10.3a, b). This was particularly the case when treatment risk reduction was not provided in participants' native language, presumably because they discarded the verbal description of the numerical information and focused solely on information in the icon array. Again, this effect holds for all three dependent measures. The ANOVAs with sizes of denominators as the within-subjects factor, and language and icon arrays as between-subjects factors showed an interaction effect of sizes of denominators by icon arrays and of language by icon arrays on percentages of participants whose estimates of treatment risk reduction were accurate, $F_{3,272}=3.55$, $p=0.015$ and $F_{1,92}=4.66$, $p=0.03$, respectively. There was also a three-way interaction effect of sizes of denominators, language, and icon arrays on confidence in estimates, $F_{3,252}=2.61$, $p=0.04$, and on perceptions of treatment effectiveness, $F_{2,224}=4.75$, $p=0.01$.

When the sizes of the denominators were different and icon arrays were added to the numerical information, the percentage of participants who provided inaccurate estimates of treatment risk reduction decreased from 73% to 17% ($p=0.001$) and from 40% to 19% ($p=0.06$) when the information about the risk reduction was provided in English and Polish, respectively. In fact, these percentages (i.e., 17 and 19%) are similar to those when the sizes of the denominators were equal (i.e., 15%, $p=0.85$, and 17%, $p=0.76$, respectively).

In a similar vein, when icon arrays were added to the numerical information, participants who received the information in their non-native language, English, increased their confidence in their estimates of treatment risk reduction, especially when the sizes of the denominators were different ($p=0.001$; see Fig. 10.4).

Finally, when icon arrays were added to the numerical information, participants' perceptions of treatment effectiveness were similar in all sizes of denominator conditions both when risk reduction was provided in English and Polish ($p=0.55$ and $p=0.60$, respectively; see Fig. 10.5). Thus, adding icon arrays to the numerical information appropriately decreased perceptions of treatment effectiveness in the 100 and 800 denominator condition ($p=0.008$), while increased in the 800 and 100 denominator condition ($p=0.005$), when the information about risk reduction was not in the participants' native language.

10.4 Discussion and Conclusions

In two studies, we addressed the effect of denominator neglect in estimates and perceptions of treatment risk reduction, and analyzed whether this effect can be eliminated by using icon arrays to enhance people's comprehension. Our results showed that many participants disregarded the overall number of treated and non-treated patients in favor of the number of treated and non-treated patients who died.

That is, they showed denominator neglect. This result held especially for those participants with low numeracy and limited non-native language proficiency when the information about treatment risk reduction was not expressed in their native language.

The results of the studies reported in this chapter are compatible with previous evidence found by Epstein and colleagues in lottery gambles (Denes-Raj and Epstein 1994; Denes-Raj et al. 1995; Pacini and Epstein 1999a, b). Our results are also in line with the research by Chapman (1975; see also Hoemann and Ross 1982; Surber and Haines 1987), who showed that problems in which a denominator is shared (one-sample problems) or equal (two-sample equal sample size problems) are easier to solve than problems in which denominators differ across options. Finally, Yamagishi (1997) has similarly shown that causes of death with greater absolute numbers are perceived as more risky even if they have smaller proportions than others with smaller absolute numbers. Our studies, however, are unique in their effort to understand how denominator neglect is affected by numeracy and language proficiency. Our studies are also the first to investigate the effect of denominator neglect using probabilistic national samples in different countries and a large immigrant patient sample. This is in clear contrast to previous studies, in which respondents were self-selected, preventing statistical inference to broader populations, and to patients at highest risk. Moreover, our results held in accuracy of estimates of treatment risk reduction, confidence in these estimates, and perceptions of treatment effectiveness.

Our findings show that patients with low numeracy and ethnic minorities with limited non-native language proficiency are at greatest risk of illness (see also James et al. 2007; Keller and Stevens 1997; Vaughan 1995). Epidemiologic research has long shown that these populations suffer disproportionately from several diseases (Apter et al. 2006; Estrada et al. 2004; National Center for Health Statistics 2001). Immigrant groups also differ from the indigenous population in their reports of pain, the way they communicate symptoms, their beliefs about the cause of illness, and their understanding of concepts such as "risk factors" or "being at risk" (Fry et al. 2007; Groman and Ginsburg 2004; Haomiao et al. 2004; Huerta and Macario 1999; Mohai and Bryant 1998).

Similarly, patients with low numeracy have less accurate perceptions of the risks and benefits of screening (see Chaps. 2 and 8; Davids et al. 2004; Donelle et al. 2008; Galesic and Garcia-Retamero, 2010; Schwartz et al. 1997; Woloshin et al. 1999), and are more susceptible to errors in judgments and decisions than those with high numeracy (Reyna and Brainerd 2007, 2008), which reduces their medication compliance and impairs risk communication (Reyna et al. 2009). Patients with low numerical ability are also especially vulnerable to having difficulty following a complicated dosing regimen (Estrada et al. 2004), have a higher history of hospitalization (Apter et al. 2006), are more susceptible to being influenced by the way the health information is framed (see Chap. 11; see also Peters et al. 2006), and have more difficulties accurately recalling numerical information about health (Garcia-Retamero and Galesic 2011).

Our findings add to this literature showing that patients with low numeracy and limited language skills could also disregard crucial information when assessing treatment risk reduction, and suggest that one likely explanation is that pertinent health messages do not reach these groups effectively. In immigrant populations, translated resources offer a promising approach to communicating health information to immigrants, but are not always sufficient (Andrulis et al. 2007; Locke 1992; Ward et al. 1997).

The result that people—especially those with low-numeracy skills and limited non-native language proficiency—could disregard crucial information when making important decisions about their health is a trouble finding. We show, however, an effective method to eliminate denominator neglect: Providing icon arrays in addition to numerical information drew participants' attention to the denominators and helped them make more accurate assessments. Icon arrays improved accuracy of both estimates of risk reduction and perceptions of treatment effectiveness and increased participants' confidence in their estimates.

These results support and extend our own and others' findings about the usefulness of visual aids in communicating medical risks (see Chaps. 9 and 11; see also Fagerlin et al. 2007; Garcia-Retamero and Galesic 2010a, b; Paling 2003; Stone et al. 2003; Zikmund-Fisher et al. 2008). Specifically, they provide experimental support of Ancker et al. (2006) hypothesis that visual aids making part-to-whole relationships visually available, help people attend to the relationship between the numerator (i.e., the number of treated or non-treated patients who are affected) and the denominator (i.e., the entire population at risk; see also Lipkus 2007). These findings also extend the literature on denominator neglect as they provide experimental support of Reyna and Brainerd's (2008) hypothesis that visual displays can help people represent superordinate classes (i.e., the overall number of patients who did and did not receive a treatment; see also Ancker et al. 2006).

Finally, our results have implications for medical practice as they suggest suitable ways to communicate quantitative medical data to people who are disadvantaged by their lack of numerical and language skills. In fact, our findings support the medical convention of reporting risks using ratios with the same denominator (International Patient Decision Aid Standards 2005). Patients, however, not only receive health-related information from their physicians, they very often obtain this information from a number of other sources such as the media, the Internet, and their friends and relatives (Manning 1999; Waters et al. 2007). These alternative sources often do not use the most convenient formats for presenting the health information (Sedrakyan and Shih 2007; Voeten et al. 2009). When the common practice of communicating risks using ratios with the same denominator is not feasible, adding visual displays to the information about risks would be an effective method of enhancing comprehension in populations disadvantaged by their lack of non-native language skills. In contrast, if the goal is to persuade patients rather than enhance their informed decision making (e.g., cessation of smoking), using ratios with different denominators would be most effective. This seemingly exploitative approach may be considered justifiable in situations aiming to achieve health gain.

The strengths of our studies are the use of a large sample size, and a careful execution of the same study on both probabilistic national samples in two countries and in an immigrant sample (i.e., Polish people living in the UK). A limitation of our research, however, is that icon arrays were added to the numerical information about treatment risk reduction that participants received in all conditions. A second presentation of the same information might have reinforced understanding of risk reduction—regardless of the information format. Previous research by Galesic et al. (2009), however, showed that icon arrays are effective even when no additional numerical information is provided, supporting our conclusions about the usefulness of these methods for communicating medical risks. Additionally, we focused on studying the usefulness of icon arrays because they seem to be particularly promising for communicating risk reductions in the medical context (Fagerlin et al. 2005; Galesic et al. 2009; Paling 2003), and require no familiarity with scientific conventions (Ancker et al. 2009). A number of other visual formats have been proposed as useful aids for communicating with patients such as bar graphs and pie charts (Ancker et al. 2006; Edwards et al. 2002; Lipkus 2007). It would be interesting to explore the effectiveness of these alternative visual formats in reducing difficulties with ratio concepts in vulnerable populations. Finally, our study did not involve real patient–doctor interactions. Future research in more externally valid clinical settings may show additional benefits of icon arrays when physicians communicate risks directly to patients with limited language skills.

Our findings support the notion that problems in communicating risks occur because inappropriate information formats are often used and not because of biases in people's minds (Gigerenzer et al. 2007). Similar reductions in what superficially looked like biased thinking were observed in the case of conditional probabilities (Gigerenzer and Hoffrage 1995), relative risk reductions (Covey 2007), and single-event probabilities (Gigerenzer et al. 2005). In the same vein, we show that denominator neglect in estimations about treatment risk reduction disappears when both the numerator and the denominator are presented in a transparent way.

References

Ancker, J. S., Chan, C., & Kukafka, R. (2009). Interactive graphics for expressing health risks: Formative development and qualitative evaluation. *Journal of Health Communication, 14*, 461–475.

Ancker, J. S., Senathirajah, Y., Kukafka, R., & Starren, J. B. (2006). Design features of graphs in health risk communication: A systematic review. *Journal of the American Medical Informatics Association, 13*, 608–618.

Andrulis, D. P., Siddiqui, N. J., & Gantner, J. L. (2007). Preparing racially and ethnically diverse communities for public health emergencies. *Health Affairs, 26*, 1269–1279.

Apter, A. J., Cheng, J., Small, D., Bennett, I. M., Albert, C., Fein, D. G., et al. (2006). Asthma numeracy skill and health literacy. *The Journal of Asthma, 43*, 705–710.

BBC News (2009). *Nearly 600,000 new EU migrants*. http://news.bbc.co.uk/1/hi/uk_politics/5273356.stm, accessed July 30, 2012.

Burrell, K. (2009). *Polish migration to the UK in the 'new' European Union, after 2004*. Surrey: Ashgate.

Chapman, R. H. (1975). The development of children's understanding of proportions. *Child Development, 46*, 141–148.

Cleary, P. D., & Angel, R. (1984). The analysis of relationships involving dichotomous dependent variables. *Journal of Health and Social Behavior, 25*, 334–348.

Covey, J. (2007). A meta-analysis of the effects of presenting treatment benefits in different formats. *Medical Decision Making, 27*, 638–654.

Cuite, C. L., Weinstein, N. D., Emmons, K., & Colditz, G. (2008). A test of numeric formats for communicating risk probabilities. *Medical Decision Making, 28*, 377–384.

Davids, S. L., Schapira, M. M., McAuliffe, T. L., & Nattinger, A. B. (2004). Predictors of pessimistic breast cancer risk perceptions in a primary care population. *Journal of General Internal Medicine, 19*, 310–315.

Denes-Raj, V., & Epstein, S. (1994). Conflict between intuitive and rational processing: When people behave against their better judgment. *Journal of Personality and Social Psychology, 66*, 819–829.

Denes-Raj, V., Epstein, S., & Cole, J. (1995). The generality of the ratio-bias phenomenon. *Personality and Social Psychology Bulletin, 21*, 1083–1092.

Donelle, L., Arocha, J. F., & Hoffman-Goetz, L. (2008). Health literacy and numeracy: Key factors in cancer risk comprehension. *Chronic Diseases in Canada, 29*, 1–8.

Edwards, A., Elwyn, G., & Mulley, A. (2002). Explaining risks: Turning numerical data into meaningful pictures. *British Medical Journal, 324*, 827–830.

Estrada, C. A., Martin-Hryniewicz, M., Peek, B. T., Collins, C., & Byrd, J. C. (2004). Literacy and numeracy skills and anticoagulation control. *The American Journal of the Medical Sciences, 328*, 88–93.

Eurostat (2009). *Eurostat yearbook 2009: Europe in figures*. http://epp.eurostat.ec.europa.eu/portal/page/portal/product_details/publication?p_product_code=KS-CD-09-001, accessed July 30, 2012.

Fagerlin, A., Ubel, P. A., Smith, D. M., & Zikmund-Fisher, B. J. (2007). Making numbers matter: Present and future research in risk communication. *American Journal of Health Behavior, 31*(supp. 1), S47–S56.

Fagerlin, A., Wang, C., & Ubel, P. A. (2005). Reducing the influence of anecdotal reasoning on people's health care decisions: Is a picture worth a thousand statistics? *Medical Decision Making, 25*, 398–405.

Fry, R. B., Ray, M. N., Cobaugh, D. J., Weissman, N. W., Kiefe, C. I., Shewchuk, R. M., et al. (2007). Racial/ethnic disparities in patient-reported nonsteroidal antiinflammatory drug (NSAID) risk awareness, patient-doctor NSAID risk communication, and NSAID risk behavior. *Arthritis and Rheumatism, 57*, 1539–1545.

Galesic, M., & Garcia-Retamero, R. (2010). Statistical numeracy for health: A cross-cultural comparison with probabilistic national samples. *Archives of Internal Medicine, 170*, 462–468.

Galesic, M., Garcia-Retamero, R., & Gigerenzer, G. (2009). Using icon arrays to communicate medical risks: Overcoming low numeracy. *Health Psychology, 28*, 210–216.

Garcia-Retamero, R., & Dhami, M. K. (2011). Pictures speak louder than numbers: On communicating medical risks to immigrants with non-native language proficiency. *Health Expectations, 14*, 46–57.

Garcia-Retamero, R., & Galesic, M. (2009). Communicating treatment risk reduction to people with low numeracy skills: A cross-cultural comparison. *American Journal of Public Health, 99*, 2196–2202.

Garcia-Retamero, R., & Galesic, M. (2010a). How to reduce the effect of framing on messages about health. *Journal of General Internal Medicine, 25*, 1323–1329.

Garcia-Retamero, R., & Galesic, M. (2010b). Who profits from visual aids: Overcoming challenges in people's understanding of risks. *Social Science and Medicine, 70*, 1019–1025.

Garcia-Retamero, R., & Galesic, M. (2011). Using plausible group sizes to communicate information about medical risks. *Patient Education and Counseling, 84*, 245–250.

Garcia-Retamero, R., Galesic, M., & Gigerenzer, G. (2010). Do icon arrays help reduce denominator neglect? *Medical Decision Making, 30*, 672–684.

Garcia-Retamero, R., Okan, Y., & Cokely, E. T. (2012). Using visual aids to improve communication of risks about health: A review. The Scientific World Journal, 2012. Article ID 562637.

Gigerenzer, G., Gaissmaier, W., Kurz-Milcke, E., Schwartz, L. M., & Woloshin, S. (2007). Helping doctors and patients make sense of health statistics. *Psychological Science in the Public Interest, 8*, 53–96.
Gigerenzer, G., Hertwig, R., Van den Broek, E., Fasolo, B., & Katsikopoulos, K. V. (2005). "A 30% chance of rain tomorrow:" How does the public understand probabilistic weather forecasts? *Risk Analysis, 25*, 623–629.
Gigerenzer, G., & Hoffrage, U. (1995). How to improve Bayesian reasoning without instruction: Frequency formats. *Psychological Review, 102*, 684–704.
Greenhouse, S. W., & Geisser, S. (1959). On methods in the analysis of profile data. *Psychometrika, 24*, 95–112.
Groman, R., & Ginsburg, J. (2004). Racial and ethnic disparities in health care: A position paper of the American college of physicians. *Annals of Internal Medicine, 141*, 226–232.
Grossarth-Maticek, R., & Ziegler, R. (2008). Randomized and non-randomized prospective controlled cohort studies in matched pair design for the long-term therapy of corpus uteri cancer patients with a mistletoe preparation. *European Journal of Medical Research, 13*, 107–120.
Haomiao, J., Santana, A., & Lubetkin, E. I. (2004). Measuring risk perception among low-income minority primary care patients. *The Journal of Ambulatory Care Management, 27*, 314–327.
Hoemann, H. W., & Ross, B. M. (1982). Children's concepts of chance and probability. In C. Brainerd (Ed.), *Children's logical and mathematical cognition* (pp. 93–121). New York: Springer.
Huerta, E. E., & Macario, E. (1999). Communicating health risk to ethnic groups: Reaching Hispanics as a case study. *Journal of the National Cancer Institute Monographs, 25*, 23–26.
International Patient Decision Aid Standards (2005). *Criteria for judging the quality of patient decision aids*. http://www.ipdas.ohri.ca/IPDAS_checklist.pdf, accessed July 30, 2012.
James, X., Hawkins, A., & Rowel, R. (2007). An assessment of the cultural appropriateness of emergency preparedness communication for low income minorities. *Journal of Homeland Security and Emergency Management, 4*, 1–24.
Keller, C. S., & Stevens, K. R. (1997). Cultural considerations in promoting wellness. *Journal of Cardiovascular Nursing, 11*, 15–25.
Larkey, L. K., & Gonzalez, J. (2007). Storytelling for promoting colorectal cancer prevention and early detection among Latinos. *Patient Education and Counseling, 67*, 272–278.
Lipkus, I. M. (2007). Numeric, verbal, and visual formats of convening health risks: Suggested best practices and future recommendations. *Medical Decision Making, 27*, 695–713.
Lipkus, I. M., Samsa, G., & Rimer, B. K. (2001). General performance on a numeracy scale among highly educated samples. *Medical Decision Making, 21*, 37–44.
Lloyd, F. J., & Reyna, V. F. (2001). A web exercise in evidence-based medicine using cognitive theory. *Journal of General Internal Medicine, 16*, 94–99.
Lloyd, F. J., Reyna, V. F., & Whalen, P. (2001). Accuracy and ambiguity in counseling patients about genetic risk. *Archives of Internal Medicine, 161*, 2411–2413.
Locke, D. C. (1992). *Increasing multicultural understanding: A comprehensive model*. Newbury Park: Sage.
Lunney, G. H. (1970). Using analysis of variance with a dichotomous dependent variable: An empirical study. *Journal of Educational Measurement, 7*, 263–269.
Manning, A. (1999, April 27). Minorities miss out on health news. *USA Today*, 10D.
Mohai, P., & Bryant, B. (1998). Is there a "race" effect on concern for environmental quality? *Public Opinion Quarterly, 62*, 475–505.
Montori, V. M., & Rothman, R. L. (2005). Weakness in numbers. *Journal of General Internal Medicine, 20*, 1071–1072.
National Center for Health Statistics (2001). *Healthy people 2000. National health promotion and disease prevention objectives*. Washington, DC: Department of Health and Human Services.
Pacini, R., & Epstein, S. (1999a). The interaction of three facets of concrete thinking in a game of chance. *Thinking and Reasoning, 5*, 303–325.
Pacini, R., & Epstein, S. (1999b). The relation of rational and experiential information processing styles to personality, basic beliefs, and the ratio-bias phenomenon. *Journal of Personality and Social Psychology, 76*, 972–987.

Paling, J. (2003). Strategies to help patients understand risks. *British Medical Journal, 327*, 745–748.
Peters, E., Vastfjall, D., Slovic, P., Mertz, C. K., Mozzocco, K., & Dickert, S. (2006). Numeracy and decision making. *Psychological Science, 17*, 406–413.
Reyna, V. F. (2004). How people make decisions that involve risk: A dual-processes approach. *Current Directions in Psychological Science, 13*, 60–66.
Reyna, V. F., & Brainerd, C. J. (2007). The importance of mathematics in health and human judgment: Numeracy, risk communication, and medical decision making. *Learning and Individual Differences, 17*, 147–159.
Reyna, V. F., & Brainerd, C. J. (2008). Numeracy, ratio bias, and denominator neglect in judgments of risk and probability. *Learning and Individual Differences, 18*, 89–107.
Reyna, V. R., Nelson, W. L., Han, P., & Dieckmann, N. F. (2009). How numeracy influences risk comprehension and medical decision making. *Psychological Bulletin, 135*, 943–973.
Schwartz, L. M., Woloshin, S., Black, W. C., & Welch, H. G. (1997). The role of numeracy in understanding the benefit of screening mammography. *Annals of Internal Medicine, 127*, 966–972.
Sedrakyan, A., & Shih, C. (2007). Improving depiction of benefits and harms: Analyses of studies of well-known therapeutics and review of high-impact medical journals. *Medical Care, 45*, 23–28.
Shaw, A., & Hurst, J. A. (2009). 'I don't see any point in telling them': Attitudes to sharing genetic information in the family and carrier testing of relatives among British Pakistani adults referred to a genetics clinic. *Ethnicity and Health, 14*, 205–224.
Stanovich, K. E., & West, R. F. (2008). On the relative independence of thinking biases and cognitive ability. *Journal of Personality and Social Psychology, 94*, 672–695.
Stone, E. R., Sieck, W. R., Bull, B. E., Yates, J. F., Parks, S. C., & Rush, C. J. (2003). Foreground: background salience: Explaining the effects of graphical displays on risk avoidance. *Organizational Behavior and Human Decision Processes, 90*, 19–36.
Surber, C. F., & Haines, B. A. (1987). The growth of proportional reasoning: Methodological issues. In R. Vasta & G. Whitehurst (Eds.), *Annals of child development* (Vol. 4, pp. 35–87). Greenwich: JAI.
Taylor-Clark, K., Koh, H., & Viswanath, K. (2007). Perceptions of environmental health risks and communication barriers among low-SEP and racial/ethnic minority communities. *Journal of Health Care for the Poor and Underserved, 18*, 165–183.
Vaughan, E. (1995). The significance of socioeconomic and ethnic diversity for the risk communication process. *Risk Analysis, 15*, 169–180.
Voeten, H. A., de Zwart, O., Veldhuijzen, I. K., Yuen, C., Jiang, X., Elam, G., et al. (2009). Sources of information and health beliefs related to SARS and avian influenza among Chinese communities in the United Kingdom and The Netherlands, compared to the general population in these countries. *International Journal of Behavioral Medicine, 16*, 49–57.
Walitza, S., Werner, B., Romanos, M., Warnke, A., Gerlach, M., & Stopper, H. (2007). Does methylphenidate cause a cytogenetic effect in children with attention deficit hyperactivity disorder? *Environmental Health Perspectives, 115*, 936–940.
Ward, B., Bertera, E. M., & Hoge, P. (1997). Developing and evaluating a Spanish TEL-MED message on breast cancer. *Journal of Community Health, 22*, 127–135.
Waters, M. C., Ueda, R., & Marrow, H. B. (2007). *The new Americans: A guide to immigration since 1965*. Cambridge: Harvard University Press.
Woloshin, S., Schwartz, L. M., Black, W. C., & Welch, H. G. (1999). Women's perceptions of breast cancer risk: How you ask matters. *Medical Decision Making, 19*, 221–229.
Yamagishi, K. (1997). When a 12.86% mortality is more dangerous than 24.14%: Implications for risk communication. *Applied Cognitive Psychology, 11*, 495–506.
Zikmund-Fisher, B. J., Ubel, P. A., Smith, D. M., Derry, H. A., McClure, J. B., Stark, A., et al. (2008). Communicating side effect risks in a tamoxifen prophylaxis decision aid: The debiasing influence of pictographs. *Patient Education and Counseling, 73*, 209–214.

Chapter 11
Reducing the Effect of Framed Messages About Health*

Rocio Garcia-Retamero, Edward T. Cokely, and Mirta Galesic

Abstract Patients must be informed about risks before any treatment can be implemented. Yet serious problems in communicating these risks occur because of framing effects. In this chapter, we describe two studies conducted in the USA, Germany, and Spain, investigating the effects of different information frames when communicating health risks. Study 1 focused on people with low and high numeracy and investigated framing effects in perceptions of medical risks expressed in positive (i.e., chances of surviving after surgery) and negative (i.e., chances of dying after surgery) terms. Study 2 focused on a large sample of sexually active young adults and investigated framing effects in affective reactions, risk perceptions,

---

*In this chapter, we partially reproduced the articles Garcia-Retamero, R., & Galesic, M. (2010). How to reduce the effect of framing on messages about health. *Journal of General Internal Medicine*, *25*, 1323–1329, and Garcia-Retamero, R., & Cokely, E. T. (2011). Effective communication of risks to young adults: Using message framing and visual aids to increase condom use and STD screening. *Journal of Experimental Psychology: Applied*, *17*, 270–287.

R. Garcia-Retamero, Ph.D. (✉)
Departamento de Psicología Experimental, Facultad de Psicología,
University of Granada, Campus Universitario de Cartuja s/n, Granada 18071, Spain

Center for Adaptive Behavior and Cognition, Max Planck Institute
for Human Development, Lentzeallee 94, Berlin 14195, Germany
e-mail: rretamer@ugr.es

E.T. Cokely, Ph.D.
Department of Cognitive and Learning Sciences, Michigan Technological University,
211 Meese Center, Houghton, MI, USA

Center for Adaptive Behavior and Cognition, Max Planck Institute
for Human Development, Lentzeallee 94, Berlin 14195, Germany
e-mail: ecokely@mtu.edu

M. Galesic, Ph.D.
Center for Adaptive Behavior and Cognition, Max Planck Institute
for Human Development, Lentzeallee 94, Berlin 14195, Germany
e-mail: galesic@mpib-berlin.mpg.de

R. Garcia-Retamero and M. Galesic (eds.), *Transparent Communication of Health Risks: Overcoming Cultural Differences*, DOI 10.1007/978-1-4614-4358-2_11,

attitudes, behavioral intentions, and reported behaviors relating to the prevention and detection of sexually transmitted diseases. Results in both studies showed that people are susceptible to framing effects and illustrate that these effects can be countered or eliminated by using different types of visual displays.

11.1 Introduction and Background

Health messages can have profound effects on economically and personally significant health-related choices and behaviors. The investigation of the influence and efficacy of health messages is a topic of considerable interest in the cognitive and decision sciences (Bruine de Bruin and Fischhoff 2000; Kuhberger 1998; Wilson et al. 1988). A prominent example concerns the impact of *message framing* on people's attitudes, risk perceptions, and risky behaviors (Levin et al. 1998; Rothman and Salovey 1997). Following the work of Kahneman and Tversky in the 1970s and early 1980s (Kahneman and Tversky 1979, 1982; McNeil et al. 1982; Tversky and Kahneman 1981), framing is defined as the presentation of two logically equivalent situations, where one is presented in positive or gain terms and the other in negative or loss terms.

Levin et al. (1998) classified different types of framing effects according to their underlying mechanisms and consequences. Two major examples are attribute framing and goal framing. In *attribute framing*, a characteristic of an object or event serves as the focus of the framing manipulation. Examples of attribute framing are presenting risk information about surgery as chances of mortality versus survival and a focus on the risks or disadvantages of not agreeing to a medical screening versus the benefits or advantages of doing so (Des Jarlais et al. 2006; Edwards et al. 2001). In contrast, in *goal framing*, the goal of an action or behavior is framed. To illustrate, a brochure promoting condom use can emphasize the benefits of this practice (e.g., using condoms helps prevent sexually transmitted diseases, STDs), or the costs of avoiding this practice (e.g., failing to use condoms increases your risk of contracting STDs; Rothman and Salovey 1997; Rothman et al. 1999, 2003a).

In this chapter, we report two studies in which we sought to address the effect of framed messages in risk communication about health. Study 1 involved probabilistic national US and German samples of participants with different levels of numeracy and investigated the effect of attribute framing in perceptions of medical risks expressed in positive (i.e., chances of surviving after surgery) and negative (i.e., chances of dying after surgery) terms. Study 2 involved a large sample of sexually active young adults and investigated the effect of goal framing in affective reactions, risk perceptions, attitudes, behavioral intentions, and reported behaviors relating to the prevention and detection of STDs. In addition, in both studies, we considered a potential method for reducing or eliminating the framing effect. Specifically, we document the power of well-constructed visual aids for improving decision making in high stakes, risky decisions.

11.2 Study 1: On the Effect of Framed Messages in People with High and Low Numeracy

Previous research has documented important individual differences in susceptibility to framing. For instance, several studies have provided empirical support for the thesis that dispositional sensitivity to favorable or unfavorable outcomes moderates the impact of framed health appeals. To illustrate, in a study by Mann et al. (2004) designed to encourage dental flossing, undergraduate students who had a strong avoidance orientation (as indexed by a difference between their behavioral activation and their behavioral inhibition scores; Carver and White 1994) reported flossing more after having read a loss-framed message, whereas those who had a relatively stronger approach orientation reported flossing more after having read a gain-framed message (see also Gerend and Shepherd 2007; Sherman et al. 2008).

Research has also shown that individuals who have low educational attainment or lower general cognitive ability scores tend to show a stronger susceptibility to message framing than do highly educated individuals (Armstrong et al. 2002) or those who have higher cognitive ability scores (Cokely and Kelley 2009; Stanovich and West 1998; but see also Corbin et al. 2010 for counter-examples). Similarly, people with low numeracy are more susceptible to framing than those with high numeracy (Fagerlin et al. 2007; Peters and Levin 2008; Peters et al. 2006). Other studies, however, reported no influence of individual differences in susceptibility to framing or even found framing effects in the opposite direction to that hypothesized (Lerman et al. 1992; Llewellyn-Thomas et al. 1995; O'Connor et al. 1985, 1996; Siminoff and Fetting 1989; Steffen et al. 1994; Tykocinski et al. 1994; see O'Keefe and Jensen 2007, 2009 for reviews), leaving open a number of important questions related to the effects of individual differences on health message frames.

First, to the best of our knowledge framing studies have only been conducted on convenience samples of specific groups of participants (e.g., patients with particular diseases or students; Edwards et al. 2001; Kuhberger 1998; Rothman and Salovey 1997; Wilson et al. 1988). These studies provide valuable information about the influence of framing in these participants. Framing variations, however, have different effects depending on factors such as participants' demographic characteristics and previous experiences (Apanovitch et al. 2003; Edwards et al. 1996, 2001; Salovey and Williams-Piehota 2004). Differences between studies in these factors might explain the contradictory results in the literature. Moreover, due to nonprobabilistic sampling methods, we cannot be confident that results in the published literature will be generalized to a wider population. Therefore, in Study 1, we examined the effect of different information frames on probabilistic, nationally representative samples. To test the generalizability of our findings, we conducted this study in two countries—the USA and Germany.

Second, several authors have suggested that using framing to enhance the effects of health messages is not consistent with truly informed decision making and, consequently, should be avoided (Edwards et al. 2001, 2002). Few researchers, however, have sought to develop so-called debiasing techniques to reduce the potential problems associated with the effects of framing. Two prominent techniques are stating the rationale for a choice (e.g., Kim et al. 2005; Miller and Fagley 1991; Sieck and Yates 1997), and describing the decision situation to another person before making a choice (Simon et al. 2004), which both promote more detailed thinking about the decision options. In addition, asking decision makers to list the advantages and disadvantages of the decision options, as well as providing a rationale for the option they plan to choose, has been shown to eliminate the framing effect (e.g., Almashat et al. 2008). In Study 1, we considered another potential method for promoting deep cognitive processing that can reduce or eliminate the framing effect. Specifically, we examine the effect of presenting the information in a visual format, and investigate whether visual aids are more effective in eliminating framing effects in individuals who are more vulnerable when making decisions about health. In particular, we investigate whether visual aids are especially effective in eliminating the effect of framing messages for individuals with low numeracy.

11.2.1 Method

11.2.1.1 Participants

The study was conducted on probabilistic national samples in the USA and Germany as part of the project "Helping people with low numeracy understand medical information" funded by the Foundation for Informed Medical Decision Making. The project involved a survey that gathered data for a number of studies related to understanding and communicating risks (see also Chaps. 2, 4, 7–10, and 13). In particular, we selected large national samples of participants ($n = 1{,}009$ in the USA and $n = 1{,}001$ in Germany) for the overarching project. Randomly selected groups of 492 participants in the USA and of 495 in Germany were asked to answer the questions presented in this study. The sample structure is presented in Table 4.1 in Chap. 4 (see Chap. 2 for more details about the methodology of the survey).

11.2.1.2 Stimuli and Procedure

All participants completed a computerized questionnaire that was developed in English and translated into German (see Chap. 2 for more details about the translation of the materials and the programmed questionnaire). The Ethics Committee of the Max Planck Institute for Human Development approved the methodology of the study. At the beginning of the survey, all participants consented to participation through an online consent form.

All of the participants in the study completed a numeracy scale consisting of nine items developed by Schwartz et al. (1997) and Lipkus et al. (2001); see Chaps. 2 and 15. In the analyses that follow, we split the participants into two groups according to their group's median numeracy scores. The low-numeracy group includes participants with six or fewer correct answers, while the high-numeracy group includes those with seven or more correct answers (see Peters et al. 2006 for a similar procedure).

Participants were presented with two medical scenarios expressing the risk associated with a surgical procedure in either negative (i.e., chances of dying) or positive (i.e., chances of surviving) terms. Following Schwartz et al. (2005), participants received the following information when the risk was expressed in *negative* terms: "Mr. Roe needs surgery: 9 in 1,000 people die from this surgery." When the risk was expressed in *positive* terms, participants were told: "Mr. Smythe needs surgery: 991 in 1,000 people survive this surgery." The participants were then asked to evaluate the perceived risk of the surgical procedure on a 4-point scale, ranging from 1 (not risky at all) to 4 (very risky). Half of the participants were randomly assigned to answer the negatively framed question first, while the remaining participants answered the positively framed question first. Between the two scenarios, all participants answered a set of unrelated problems involving risks (for more details on these problems, see Chap. 9). The order of the questions did not have any effect on the results and the orderings were combined for further analyses.

The provision of visual aids—in addition to the numerical information about the risk—was manipulated between subjects across five conditions. In the four visual aids conditions, participants were told that the numerical information was also represented in the picture that appeared on the same page, and the number of patients who died and survived from surgery was represented using an icon array, a horizontal bar graph, a vertical bar graph, or a pie chart (see Fig. 11.1). Finally, participants in the numerical condition did not receive visual aids but got only the numerical information.

To assess the effect of visual aids and their interaction with numeracy and country on the difference between perceptions of the medical risk expressed in positive and negative terms, we conducted mixed analyses of variance (ANOVAs), following Lunney (1970) and Cleary and Angel (1984). Tukey's HSD (honest significant difference) test was used for post hoc analyses.

11.2.2 Results

Do People Show Framing Effects in Their Risk Perceptions? Do People with Low Numeracy Show More Susceptibility to Framing than Those with High Numeracy? Fig. 11.2 shows the average difference between perceptions of the medical risk expressed in positive and negative terms in participants with high and low numeracy. The larger the difference, the stronger is the framing effect. When only numerical information was provided, participants with low numeracy often perceived the surgical procedure as less risky when the associated risk was presented in positive (i.e., chances of surviving) than in negative (i.e., chances of dying) terms. In contrast, participants with high numeracy often provided equal estimates when the risks were expressed in positive and negative terms. Participants with low numeracy, therefore, were more susceptible to framing than those with high numeracy. Consistent with this result, the ANOVA with numeracy and country as a between-subjects factor on

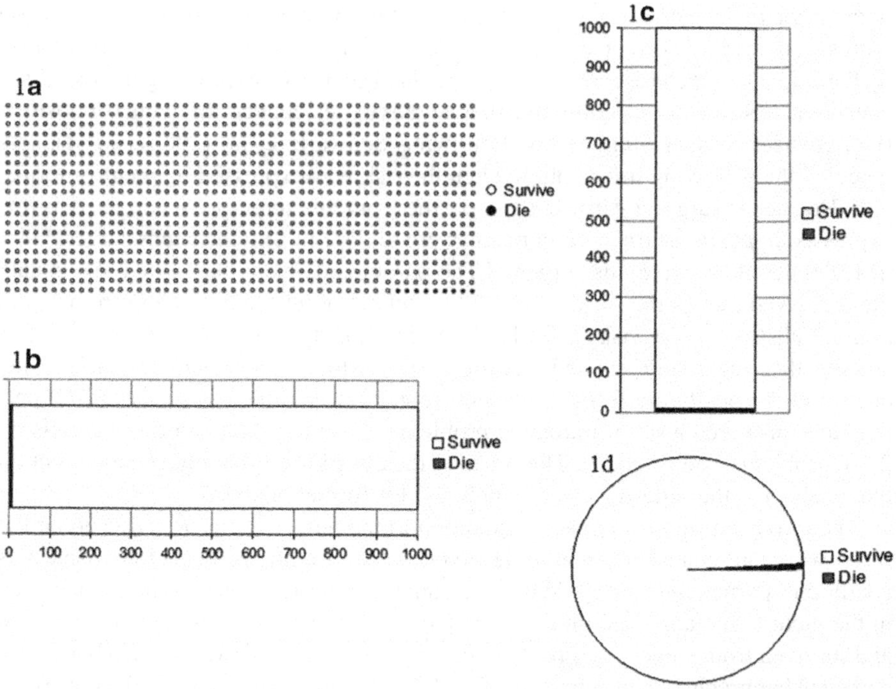

Fig. 11.1 Visual aids in Study 1: (**a**) Icon array presented in Condition 1, (**b**) horizontal bar graph presented in Condition 2. (**c**) Vertical bar graph presented in Condition 3. (**d**) Pie chart presented in Condition 4. All figures represented the number of people who died (i.e., 9) and survived (i.e., 991) from the surgery. Original material was in either German or English

the average difference between perceptions of the medical risk expressed in positive and negative terms only showed a significant main effect of numeracy, $F_{1,166}=34.19$, $p=0.001$. This effect held in both the sample in the USA and Germany.

Do Visual Aids Help Reduce the Framing Effect? Are Visual Aids Especially Helpful for Participants with Low Numeracy? As Fig. 11.2 shows, when visual aids were added to the numerical information, the effect of framing was reduced or disappeared in low-numeracy participants. Not all visual aids, however, were equally effective: Pie charts and vertical and horizontal bars almost completely removed the effect of framing. Icon arrays, however, led to a smaller decrease in the reduction of the framing effect. Furthermore, in contrast to participants with low numeracy, participants more skilled in using quantitative information benefitted less from visual aids: For these participants, the average difference between perceptions of the risk expressed in positive and negative terms was similar when they received and did not receive visual aids. Similar results were obtained regardless of which visual aid was provided. Consistent with these findings, the ANOVA with visual aids, country, and numeracy as between-subjects factors on the average difference between perceptions of the risk expressed in positive and negative terms showed a main effect of visual aids, $F_{4,967}=8.15$, $p=0.001$, and a significant interaction between numeracy

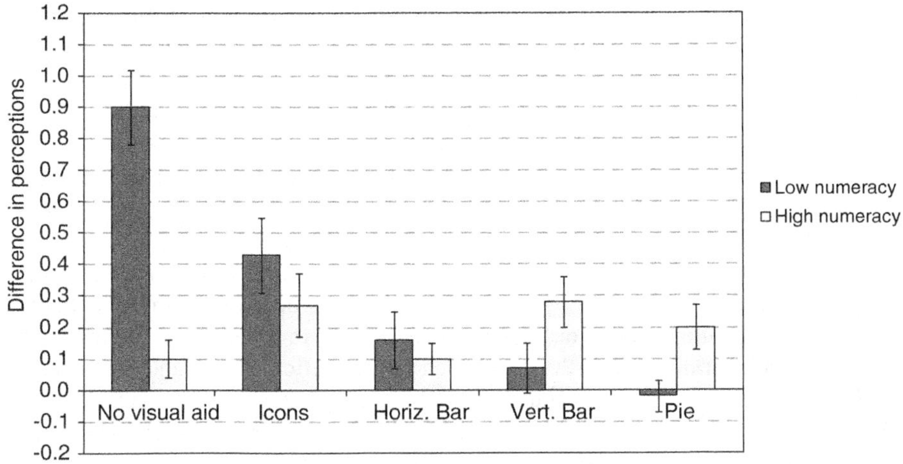

Fig. 11.2 Results in Study 1: Average difference between perceptions of the medical risk expressed in positive and negative terms, by visual aid condition and numeracy. The larger the difference, the stronger is the framing effect and vice versa. Error bars represent one standard error

and visual aids, $F_{4,967} = 12.23$, $p = 0.001$. These effects were present in both the USA and Germany. For all the analyses, the inclusion of participants' sex, age, and level of education as covariates did not systematically influence the pattern of results. We discuss the implications of these results in Sect. 11.4.

11.3 Study 2: Using Message Framing and Visual Aids to Increase Condom Use and STD Screening

A wide range of research investigating the effect of goal framing focused on whether the *function* of the health-related behavior moderates the impact of the framed messages (Rothman and Salovey 1997; see Rothman et al. 2003b, 2006 for reviews). This premise was motivated by prospect theory (Kahneman and Tversky 1979; Tversky and Kahneman 1981). According to Prospect Theory, people are relatively more likely to act to avoid risks when considering the potential gains afforded by their decisions, but are relatively more willing to take risks when considering the potential losses caused by their decisions (i.e., they are risk averse for gains but risk seeking for losses). Hence the influence of a given health message on people's behavior would depend on whether the behavior is perceived to reflect a risk-averse or a risk-seeking course of action (Rothman and Salovey 1997). To the extent that a decision affords a relatively low risk of an unpleasant outcome (e.g., it might help prevent the onset of health problems; "exercising everyday helps your heart stay healthy"), gain-framed appeals would tend to be more persuasive. Conversely, to the extent that a decision to engage in a behavior involves some risk of an unpleasant outcome (e.g., it may detect a health problem; "early detection of cancer can save your life"), loss-framed appeals would tend to be more persuasive (Rothman et al. 2006; Salovey and Wegener 2003).

Consistent with these hypotheses, gain-framed appeals tend to be more effective than loss-framed appeals in promoting health-affirming (prevention) behaviors such as physical exercise (Latimer et al. 2008), parental use of children's car seat restraints (Treiber 1986), safe driving behaviors (Millar and Millar 2000), reduced alcohol use (Gerend and Cullen 2008), smoking cessation (Toll et al. 2007, 2010), and skin cancer prevention behaviors (Detweiler et al. 1999). In contrast, loss-framed messages tend to be more effective than gain-framed appeals in promoting illness-detecting (screening) behaviors such as engaging in breast self-examination (Meyerowitz and Chaiken 1987; Williams et al. 2001), skin cancer detection (Block and Keller 1995; Rothman et al. 1993), mammography screenings (Abood et al. 2002, 2005), blood-cholesterol screenings (Maheswaran and Meyers-Levy 1990), and HIV screenings (Apanovitch et al. 2003). Some of the most compelling evidence that framing effects are contingent on the function of the advocated behavior comes from several studies in which a single health behavior served either as a prevention or detection function. For example, Rothman et al. (1999, 2003a) presented participants with framed messages advocating the use of a mouth rinse that was designed either to prevent the accumulation of plaque (i.e., a prevention behavior) or to detect the presence of plaque (i.e., a detection behavior). The results of the study indicated that participants were more likely to request a free sample of the plaque-preventing mouth rinse after having read a gain-framed message while participants were more likely to request a free sample of the plaque-detecting mouth rinse after having read a loss-framed message.

To further investigate factors influencing the efficacy of health-related messages we conducted a study with three main goals. The first goal was investigating the influence of framed messages in promoting prevention and detection of STDs in young adults. Of note, STDs—including the human immunodeficiency virus (HIV)/AIDS—are among the most common infectious diseases (European Commission 2003). Young adults aged 15–24 are the group of people at highest risk (Dehne and Riedner 2005) with one in four sexually active young adults contracting a STD every year (Child Trends 2006). Investigating the content and structure of health messages about STDs targeting this population could have important implications. In Study 2, we aimed to document the effect of framing messages (i.e., by presenting either gain- or loss-framed appeals), and the effect of the function of the health behavior (i.e., by focusing on the use of condoms to prevent STDs and the promotion of screening to detect STDs). In line with the reviewed research, we hypothesized that gain-framed messages would be most effective in promoting the use of condoms to prevent STDs, whereas loss-framed messages would be very useful in promoting STDs screening.

The second aim of our research was to document influential factors mediating the effect of gain- and loss-framed messages. As noted by Rothman and Salovey (1997; see also Rothman et al. 1999), risk perceptions along with cognitive and affective processes can mediate the influence of framed messages on people's behavior. To the best of our knowledge, this hypothesis has yet to be investigated in prevention

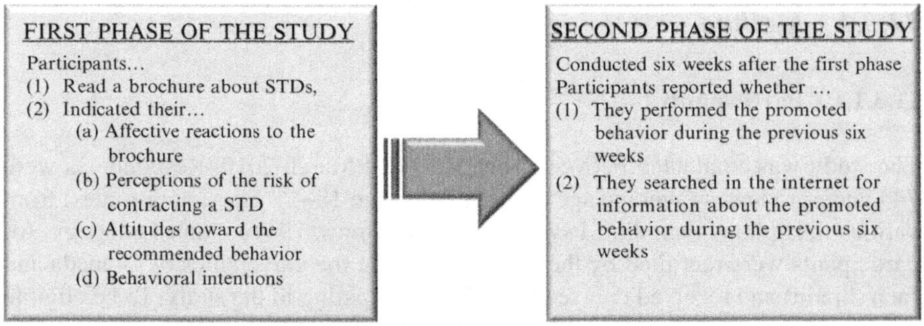

Fig. 11.3 Design of Study 2 showing the time sequence, the phases in the study, and the variables measured in each phase

and detection of STDs. In Study 2, we measured (1) young adults' affective reactions to health messages about STDs, (2) their perceptions of the risk of suffering these diseases, (3) their attitudes toward the recommended behavior, and (4) their behavioral intentions. We then evaluated the extent to which these factors served as mediators of the effect of framed messages on reported behaviors (i.e., condom use or screening for STDs). We hypothesized that young adults' attitudes and behavioral intentions would be powerful mediators of this effect.

Lastly, we aimed to investigate the efficacy of visual aids on sexual health risk communication. To the best of our knowledge, there is no published research investigating whether visual aids (e.g., bar graphs representing health information about STDs) make gain- and loss-framed messages more effective in promoting both prevention and detection behaviors as compared to presenting the same information only in written text. We hypothesized that this might be the case and reasoned that the impact of bar graphs might not be due solely to the fact that graphs provide numerical information about STDs. On the contrary, adding bar graphs to health messages might make these messages more effective because they represent the health information in a more transparent and accessible way (e.g., a format that facilitates information search, memory encoding, and representation). Accordingly, we manipulated the format of the health message about STDs by presenting information in (a) written text, (b) in written text and numerically (by adding statistics about STDs), and (c) in written text and graphically (by representing the statistics via bar graphs).

In sum, we conducted a study to investigate the factors influencing the effectiveness of message framing. We manipulated three between-subjects variables including *message frame* (gain vs. loss), *function of behavior* (prevention vs. detection), and *message format* (text based only vs. text and numerically based vs. text and graphically based). The study had two phases (see Fig. 11.3). In the first phase, participants read a brochure about STDs and indicated their affective reactions to the brochure, their perceptions of the risk of contracting a STD, their attitudes toward the recommended behavior in the brochure, and their behavioral intentions. In the second phase—conducted 6 weeks after the first—participants reported whether they performed any of several behaviors during this period.

11.3.1 Method

11.3.1.1 Participants

The study was conducted between May 2009 and March 2010. Respondents were 744 undergraduates (average age of 19 years, range 18–21 years; 46% males) from various disciplines including Psychology, Economics, History, and Pedagogy. All participants were recruited by the first author from the universities of Granada and Jaén (Spain) and received course credit for participating in the study. To be eligible for recruitment, participants had to report that they had at least one sexual encounter involving sexual intercourse during the 3 months before the study (as was the case for 86% of all individuals who wanted to participate in the study). Participants were assigned randomly to the groups (*n* per group=62). Male and female participants were evenly distributed in the groups. Of the young adults who participated in the first phase of the study, 662 (89%; average age of 19 years, range 18–21 years; 45% males) came to our lab to participate in the second phase. We only considered these participants' responses in data analyses. Sixty-five percent of these participants said that they had at least one sexual encounter in which they did not use condoms during the year before the study, and only 9% of these participants reported that they had participated in a screening test to detect STDs during that period. At the beginning of the study, all participants consented to participation via a written consent form.

11.3.1.2 Stimuli and Procedure

The information about STDs was presented in a six-page brochure. Half of the participants received a version of the brochure that promoted the use of condoms to *prevent* STDs, while the rest received a version of the brochure that promoted screening to *detect* STDs. Half of the participants who received the brochure promoting the use of condoms read the benefits afforded by adopting the health behavior (i.e., a *gain-framed* version of the brochure), while the other half of the participants read the costs associated with failing to adopt the health behavior (i.e., a *loss-framed* version of the brochure). Similarly, half of the participants who received the brochure promoting screening read the gain-framed message and half read the loss-framed message. We ensured that the gain- and loss-framed versions of the brochure were comparable in terms of length and general content.

The brochure was divided into the following three sections:

1. *General information about STDs*. Participants were provided with information defining frequent STDs and the consequences and incidence rates of these diseases in young adults. We emphasized that STDs are important problems in people aged 15–24. This information was taken from American Social Health Association (ASHA 2005) and Dehne and Riedner (2005).

2. *Information about the behavior*. Participants who received the version of the brochure promoting the use of condoms read that doctors strongly recommend that everyone use condoms when engaged in sexual intercourse. The brochure also described different types of condoms and how they should be used. Participants who received the version of the brochure promoting screening read that doctors strongly recommend that everyone make at least one appointment to do screening to detect STDs every year. The brochure also described different screening tests for STDs and how they are conducted.
3. *Message framing manipulation*. The brochure included three framed appeals: The title and two sections (see Garcia-Retamero and Cokely 2011 for more information). The gain-framed version of the brochure promoting the use of condoms emphasized that using condoms reduced the chance of both contracting STDs and of suffering several severe health symptoms (particularly when sexual intercourse involved an infected partner). In contrast, the loss-framed version of the brochure promoting the use of condoms emphasized that not using condoms increased the chance of both contracting a STD and of suffering several severe health symptoms (particularly when sexual intercourse involved an infected partner). The gain-framed version of the brochure promoting screening emphasized that conducting screening increased the chance of receiving an effective treatment and decreased the chance of suffering several, severe health symptoms (particularly if the screening was conducted at an early stage of STD infection). Finally, the loss-framed version of the brochure promoting screening emphasized how not conducting screening reduced the chance of receiving effective treatment and increased the chance of suffering several, severe health symptoms (particularly if the screening was not conducted at an early stage, but instead was conducted at a late stage of infection).[1]

In addition to the health message, one-third of the participants who received the version of the brochure promoting the use of condoms read representative numerical information about the estimated chances of contracting a STD in people who had sexual intercourse with an infected partner and used (or did not use) condoms. Specifically, participants were informed that scientists found that 17% of people who engaged in sexual intercourse with an infected partner and used condoms contracted a STD, whereas 38% of people who had sexual intercourse with an infected partner and did not use condoms contracted a STD. Similarly, one-third of the participants who received the version of the brochure promoting screening read representative information about one's chance of receiving effective treatment for those who contracted some STD and conducted (or did not conduct) a screening test at an early stage of the disease. These participants were informed that scientists found that 95% of people who contracted a STD and participated in a screening test at an early stage of the disease were effectively treated, whereas 67% of people who have

[1] We focused on the consequences of conducting screening at different stages of a STD as this factor substantially influences both the impact of the symptoms and treatment effectiveness (Centers for Disease Control and Prevention 2003; Wortley et al. 1995).

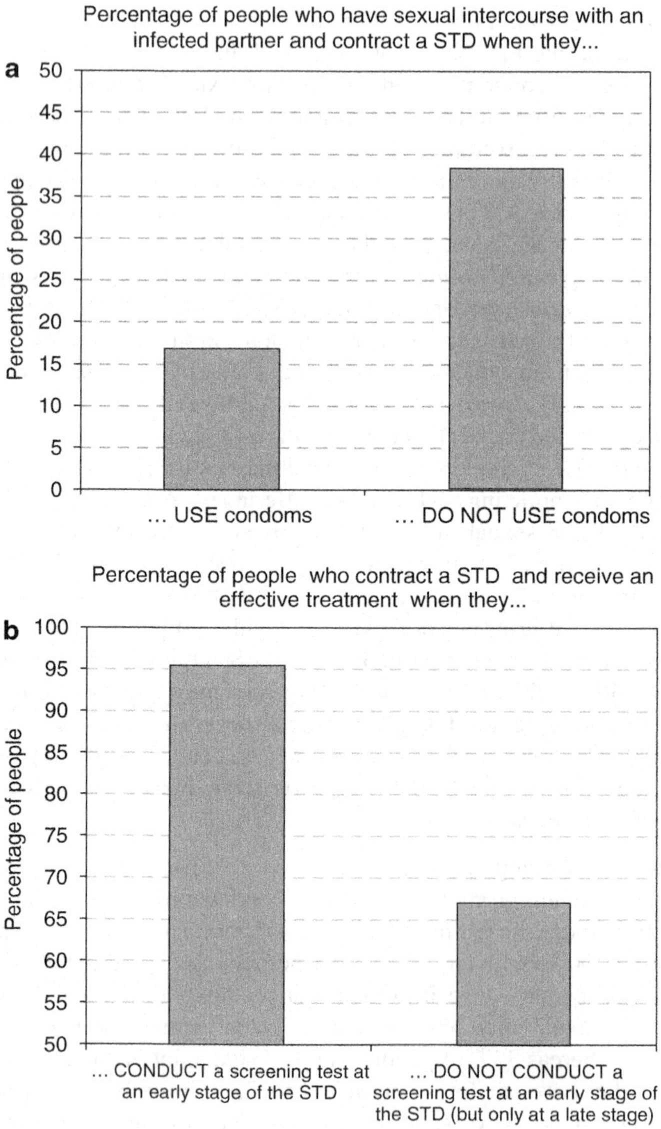

Fig. 11.4 Visual aids in Study 2. (**a**) Example of the bar graph presented to participants when they read the version of the brochure promoting the use of condoms with visual aids (translated from Spanish). (**b**) Example of the bar graph presented to participants when they read the version of the brochure promoting screening for STDs with visual aids (translated from Spanish)

contracted a STD and did not participate in a screening test at an early stage of the disease (but only at a late stage) were effectively treated. Another third of the participants received the same numerical information represented in a bar graph (see Fig. 11.4). All other participants only received the health message (i.e., they did not receive the numerical or graphical information). The numerical information was taken from the National Institute of Statistics in Spain (see Instituto Nacional de Estadística [INE] 2003; for comparable data in other countries see published studies about the issue; e.g., Palella et al. 2003; Shlay et al. 2004; Vidanapathirana et al. 2005; Weller and Davis-Beaty 2002).

Finally, the brochure described several web pages with information about the promoted behavior (condom use or screening for STDs) and suggested that the reader should search for further information on those web pages if he or she was interested in learning more about the topic.

Measures. In the first phase of the study and before reading the brochure, participants reported their age, gender, educational level, and ethnic background. They also reported whether they had at least one sexual encounter involving sexual intercourse in the 3 months before the study. Finally, participants reported whether they used condoms consistently in the year before the study and whether they did at least one screening test to detect a possible STD during that period. Four groups of dependent variables were measured after participants read the brochure in the first phase of the study (see also Rothman et al. 1999 for a similar method).

1. *Risk perceptions.* On 9-point scales ranging from 1 (very unlikely) to 9 (very likely), participants evaluated how likely they were to contract a STD if they continued behaving as they did in the past. On 9-point scales ranging from 1 (not at all) to 9 (very much) participants also rated how worried they were about contracting a STD and how serious the consequences of contracting a STD would be for them. These questions were combined into a single index (Cronbach $\alpha=0.78$).
2. *Affective reactions to the brochure.* Participants indicated how they felt while they were reading the brochure. On 9-point scales ranging from 1 (not at all) to 9 (very much), participants indicated to what extent they felt assured, calm, cheerful, happy, hopeful, relaxed, and relieved (positive adjectives). On 9-point scales ranging from 1 (not at all) to 9 (very much), they also indicated the extent to which they felt anxious, afraid, discouraged, disturbed, sad, troubled, and worried (negative adjectives). Scores in negative adjectives were reversed and combined with positive adjectives into a single composite score (Cronbach $\alpha=0.91$).
3. *Attitudes toward the behavior.* On 9-point scales ranging from 1 (not at all) to 9 (very much), participants evaluated the effectiveness of the behavior (i.e., using condoms or conducting screening for STDs), how important it was for them to perform the behavior, how beneficial it was to perform the behavior, and how favorable they felt toward engaging in the behavior. These questions were combined into a single index (Cronbach $\alpha=0.79$).
4. *Behavioral intentions.* On 9-point scales ranging from 1 (I have no intention of doing this) to 9 (I am certain that I will do this), participants who received the brochure promoting the use of condoms indicated how likely it was that they would use condoms within the next few weeks. They also indicated how likely it was that they would search on the Internet for further information about condom use. On 9-point scales ranging from 1 (I have no intention of doing this) to 9 (I am certain that I will do this), participants who received the brochure promoting screening indicated how likely it was that they would make an appointment with

their doctor to ask about screening for STDs within the next few weeks. They also indicated how likely it was that they would search on the Internet for further information about screening for STDs.

Reported behaviors. In the second phase of the study—conducted 6 weeks after the first—participants who received the brochure promoting the use of condoms indicated whether they used condoms in every sexual encounter involving sexual intercourse in the previous 6 weeks. They also reported whether they searched for information on the Internet about condom use during that period. Participants who received the brochure promoting screening for STDs indicated whether they made an appointment with their doctor to ask about such screening in the previous 6 weeks. They also reported whether they searched on the Internet for information about screening for STDs during that period.

Procedure. The study was conducted in two phases 6 weeks apart and in groups of 6–12 participants. In the first phase, all participants signed an informed consent form and provided their demographics. Next, the experimenter explained that the purpose of the study was to evaluate the effectiveness of a brochure about STDs. Participants read the brochure and answered several questions. In the second phase of the study, participants indicated whether they performed any of several behaviors in the previous 6 weeks (see reported behaviors). Participant responses were self-reported in an anonymous response booklet. The Ethics Committee of the University of Granada approved the methodology of the study. At the beginning of the survey, all participants consented to participation through an online consent form.

To test our hypothesis that the manipulation of message frame and format can improve prevention and detection of STDs, we conducted ANOVAs with message frame (gain v. loss), function of behavior (prevention vs. detection), and message format (text based only vs. text and numerically based vs. text and graphically based) as between-subjects factors on participants' reported behaviors. Tukey's honestly significant difference test was used for all post hoc analyses. To test our hypothesis about the factors that mediated the effects of framed messages on the prevention and detection of STDs, we conducted mediational analyses.

11.3.2 Results

Are gain-framed (loss-framed) messages most effective in promoting condom use (STDs screening)? Do visual aids help reduce the framing effect? The ANOVA on the percentage of participants who indicated that they had performed the behavior promoted in the brochure during the first and the second phase of the study showed an effect of message format, $F_{2,650}=8.07$, $p=0.0003$, $\eta^2=0.02$, and an interaction between message frame, function of behavior, and message format, $F_{2,650}=6.97$, $p=0.001$, $\eta^2=0.02$. In line with our predictions, when the risk information was provided *in written text only* or *in written text and numerically*, more participants reported using condoms when they read the gain-framed message than the loss-framed

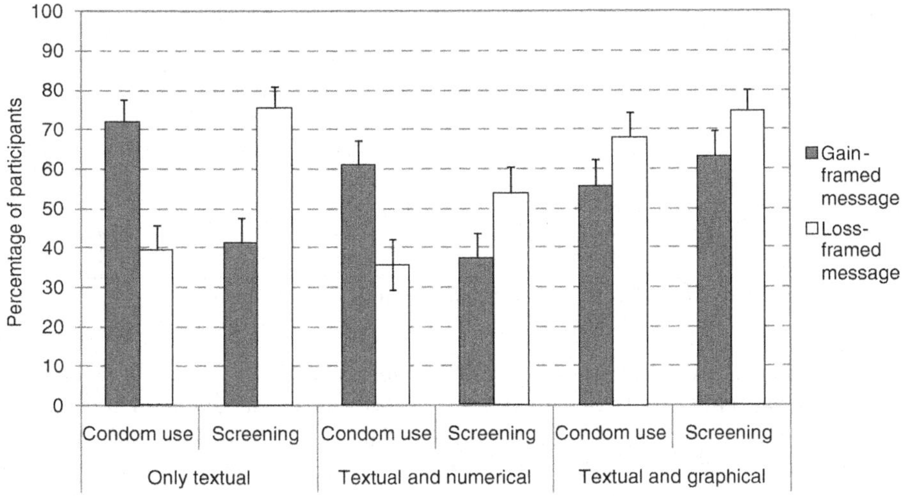

Fig. 11.5 Results in Study 2: Percentage of participants who reported performing the promoted behavior during the 6 weeks between the first and the second phase of the experiment as a function of message frame, function of behavior, and message format. Error bars indicate one standard error

message promoting the behavior ($p=0.0006$ for written text, and $p=0.008$ for written text and numerically; see Fig. 11.5). In contrast, more participants reported making an appointment with their doctor to ask about screening when they read the loss-framed message than the gain-framed message ($p=0.0003$ for written text, and $p=0.063$ for written text and numerically). Finally, when the risk information was provided *in written text and graphically*, both the gain- and loss-framed messages equally and highly influenced participants' reported behaviors ($p=0.188$ for condom use, and $p=0.218$ for screening). In other words, gain-framed (loss-framed) messages no longer induced greater adherence for prevention (detection) behaviors.

The ANOVA on the percentage of participants who indicated that they had searched for further information about the behavior on the Internet during the first and the second phase of the study revealed an effect of message format, $F_{2,650}=4.61$, $p=0.01, \eta^2=0.01$, and an interaction between message frame and function of behavior, $F_{1,650}=7.01$, $p=0.008, \eta^2=0.01$, and between function of behavior and message format, $F_{2,650}=5.21$, $p=0.006, \eta^2=0.02$. The interaction between message frame, function of behavior, and message format approached the conventional significance level, $F_{2,650}=2.33$, $p=0.09, \eta^2=0.01$. In line with the previous results, when the risk information was provided *in written text only*, more participants indicated that they searched on the Internet for information about condom use when they read the gain-framed message than the loss-framed message promoting the behavior ($p=0.009$; see Table 11.1). In contrast, more participants indicated that they searched on the Internet for information about screening when they read the loss-framed message than the gain-framed message promoting the behavior ($p=0.004$). The trend in the data suggested that results were similar when the risk

Table 11.1 Percentage of participants who reported searching for information on the Internet as a function of message frame, function of behavior, and message format

	Condom use				Screening for STDs			
	Gain-framed message		Loss-framed message		Gain-framed message		Loss-framed message	
	M	*SEM*	*M*	*SEM*	*M*	*SEM*	*M*	*SEM*
Text based only	40.71	6.46	21.43	5.53	37.04	6.63	64.29	6.46
Text and numerically based	50.00	6.74	32.14	6.30	37.04	6.63	45.71	6.46
Text and graphically based	51.85	6.86	53.57	6.72	48.15	6.86	51.85	6.86

Note. For behavioral intentions, larger values indicate stronger intentions

information was provided *in written text and numerically*. However, the loss-framed message promoting the use of screening for STDs was less appealing than when the risk information was provided in written text only (i.e., it was only slightly better than the gain-framed message). Finally, when the risk information was provided *in written text and graphically*, both the gain- and loss-framed messages equally and highly influenced participants' reported search behavior ($p = 0.858$ for condom use, and $p = 0.703$ for screening; see Table 11.1).

11.3.2.1 Mediational Analyses

We conducted mediational analyses to investigate whether the effect of the framed message on reported behaviors was mediated by their perceptions of the risk of suffering a STD, their affective reactions to the message, their attitudes toward the behavior recommended in the message, or their behavioral intentions. Because the effect of message frame on reported behaviors interacted with function of behavior and message format, we conducted the analyses for each behavior (condoms use or screening) when information was provided both in written text only and in written text and numerically, and when the information was provided in written text and graphically. In addition, we combined participants' intentions to perform the behavior promoted in the brochure and to search for information into a single, averaged score. Similarly, we combined reported behaviors (i.e., whether participants indicated that they had performed the behavior or had searched for further information on the Internet) in a single score ranging from 0 (if they did none) to 2 (if they did both).

As Rothman et al. (1999, p. 1366) suggested, to test for mediation, message frame should have influenced participants' behaviors, and the potential mediators (i.e., risk perceptions, affective reactions, attitudes towards engaging in the behavior, and behavioral intentions) must be both affected by message frame and related to participants' behaviors (see also Baron and Kenny 1986).

Condom use when providing written only or written and numerical risk information. When the risk information was provided in written text only or in written text and numerically, regression analyses showed that message frame strongly influenced participants' behavioral intentions. Participants who read the gain-framed message promoting the use of condoms had stronger intentions to perform the behaviors than

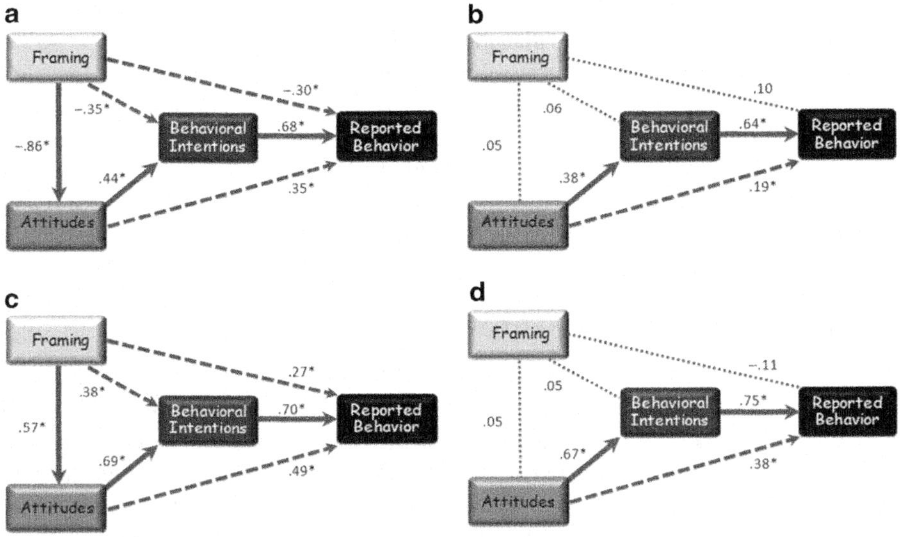

Fig. 11.6 Path analysis of the effect of message frame on reported behaviors, and the mediational effect of attitudes and behavioral intentions in Study 2. (**a**) Results for condom use when the health information was provided in written text and when numerical information was added to the written text. (**b**) Results for screening for STDs when the health information was provided in written text and when numerical information was added to the written text. (**c**) Results for condom use when the visual aid was added to the written text. (**d**) Results for screening for STDs when the visual aid was added to the written text. Note: Standardized coefficients are shown. $*p<0.05$

those who read the loss-framed message, $\beta=-0.35$, $t_{222}=-5.57$, $p=0.001$ (see Fig. 11.6a). Similarly, message frame strongly influenced participants' attitudes toward the behavior, $\beta=-0.86$, $t_{222}=-25.46$, $p=0.001$, with participants showing more favorable attitudes toward using condoms when they read the gain-framed than the loss-framed message. Message frame, however, did not affect participants' affective reactions, $\beta=-0.06$, $t_{222}=-0.96$, $p=0.34$, or their risk perceptions, $\beta=-0.11$, $t_{222}=-1.66$, $p=0.10$.

When participants' attitudes toward using condoms were included in the regression analysis, the effect of message frame on participants' intentions to perform the behaviors was significantly reduced, $\beta=0.11$, $t_{221}=0.90$, $p=0.37$. In addition, the result of the Sobel test[2] suggests that participants' attitudes toward the behavior fully mediated the influence of message frame on participants' behavioral intentions, $z=-7.06$, $p=0.001$.

Similarly, message frame strongly influenced reported behaviors. More participants indicated that they had performed the behaviors (i.e., used condoms in their

[2]The Sobel test (see Sobel 1982) indicates whether the mediator significantly carries the influence of an independent variable to a dependent variable. That is, whether the indirect effect of the independent variable on the dependent variable through the mediator variable is significant.

sexual encounters and searched on the Internet for information about the topic) after reading the gain-framed message than the loss-framed message, $\beta=-0.30$, $t_{222}=-4.73$, $p=0.001$. Participants' attitudes toward using condoms also influenced their reported behaviors, $\beta=0.35$, $t_{222}=5.56$, $p=0.001$ (i.e., more positive attitudes toward using condoms increased the chances of performing the behaviors). Interestingly, when participants' behavioral intentions were included in the regression analysis, the effect of both message frame, $\beta=-0.01$, $t_{221}=-1.42$, $p=0.16$, and attitudes toward using condoms, $\beta=0.07$, $t_{221}=1.22$, $p=0.22$, on reported behaviors was significantly reduced. Again, the results of the Sobel test suggest that participants' behavioral intentions fully mediated the effect of message frame, $z=-5.16$, $p=0.001$, and participants' attitudes, $z=6.48$, $p=0.001$, on their reported behaviors.

Screening when providing written only or written and numerical risk information. Regression analyses on screening for STDs showed similar results to those described above (see Fig. 11.6b). In particular, when the risk information was provided in written text only and in written text and numerically, message frame strongly influenced behavioral intentions: Participants who read the loss-framed message promoting screening for STDs showed stronger intentions to perform the behaviors (i.e., make an appointment with their doctor to ask about screening for STDs and search for information about screening on the Internet) than those who read the gain-framed message, $\beta=0.38$, $t_{218}=6.15$, $p=0.001$. Message frame also influenced participants' attitudes toward the behavior, $\beta=0.57$, $t_{218}=10.15$, $p=0.001$, with participants showing more favorable attitudes toward conducting screening when they read the loss-framed than the gain-framed message. Message frame, however, did not affect participants' affective reactions, $\beta=-0.06$, $t_{218}=-0.94$, $p=0.35$, or their risk perceptions, $\beta=0.001$, $t_{218}=0.01$, $p=0.99$.

When participants' attitudes toward screening were included in the regression analysis, the effect of message frame on participants' intentions to perform the behaviors was significantly reduced, $\beta=-0.01$, $t_{217}=-0.12$, $p=0.90$. Consistent with this result, the result of the Sobel test indicated that participants' attitudes toward screening fully mediated the influence of message frame on their behavioral intentions, $z=8.25$, $p=0.001$.

Mediational analyses were also conducted on reported behaviors. Regression analyses showed that message frame strongly influenced these behaviors. More participants indicated that they had performed the behaviors after having read the loss-framed message than the gain-framed message, $\beta=0.27$, $t_{218}=4.09$, $p=0.001$. Reported behaviors were also influenced by participants' attitudes toward screening, $\beta=0.49$, $t_{218}=8.34$, $p=0.001$. More positive attitudes toward screening increased the chances of indicating that they had performed the behaviors. When participants' behavioral intentions were included in the regression analysis, however, the effect of message frame, $\beta=-0.003$, $t_{217}=-0.08$, $p=0.94$, and participants' attitudes toward screening, $\beta=0.02$, $t_{217}=0.25$, $p=0.80$, on reported behaviors was significantly reduced. The results of the Sobel test indicated that participants' behavioral intentions fully mediated the influence of message frame, $z=5.57$, $p=0.001$, and participants' attitudes toward screening, $z=10.13$, $p=0.001$, on their reported behaviors.

Condom use and screening when providing written and visual risk information. When the risk information was provided in written text and graphically, only participants' attitudes toward the behavior influenced their behavioral intentions ($\beta=0.38$, $t_{108}=4.29$, $p=0.001$ for condom use, and $\beta=0.67$, $t_{106}=9.42$, $p=0.001$ for screening for STDs) and reported behaviors ($\beta=0.19$, $t_{108}=2.05$, $p=0.04$ for condom use, and $\beta=0.38$, $t_{106}=4.35$, $p=0.001$ for screening for STDs; see Fig. 11.6c, d). When participants' behavioral intentions were included in the regression analysis, the effect of participants' attitudes toward the behavior on their reported behaviors was significantly reduced ($\beta=-0.06$, $t_{107}=-0.76$, $p=0.45$ for condom use, and $\beta=-0.21$, $t_{105}=-2.49$, $p=0.014$ for screening). The results of the Sobel test suggested that participants' behavioral intentions fully mediated the influence of their attitudes on their reported behaviors ($z=3.84$, $p=0.001$ for condom use, and $z=7.29$, $p=0.001$ for screening for STDs).

11.4 Discussion and Conclusions

Our research confirms that problems in communicating medical risks can result from the effects of using different information frames, especially in people who are more vulnerable to having difficulty when making decisions. Study 1 showed that low-numeracy participants both in the USA and Germany perceived a surgical procedure as less risky when the associated risk was expressed as chance of surviving than of dying, whereas participants with high numeracy did not differ in their perceptions. These results are in line with previous research showing that people with low numeracy also have less accurate perceptions of the risks and benefits of screening and medical treatments (see Chap. 9; see also Davids et al. 2004; Schwartz et al. 1997; Woloshin et al. 1999) and are more susceptible to biases in judgments and decisions than those with high numeracy (see Chap. 10; see also Reyna and Brainerd 2007, 2008; Reyna et al. 2009), which reduces medication compliance, impedes access to treatments, impairs risk communication, and adversely affects medical outcomes (Reyna et al. 2009). Our results in Study 1 are also consistent with previous literature supporting the notion that gain frames induce greater compliance for surgical procedures than loss frames (Haward et al. 2008; Levin et al. 1988; Marteau 1989; McNeil et al. 1982; Wilson et al. 1987). Our research also extends these literatures in several notable ways. In particular, we revealed a significant influence of people's numeracy skills on the effects of framing information about health, which could shed light on previous mixed results in the literature on the issue. Differences between studies in participants' numeracy skills due to the use of convenience samples and nonprobabilistic sampling methods seem likely to explain, at least in part, why some research failed to observe framing effects (Lerman et al. 1992; Llewellyn-Thomas et al. 1995; O'Connor et al. 1985, 1996; Siminoff and Fetting 1989; Steffen et al. 1994; Tykocinski et al. 1994), whereas others found strong effects of message frames (Haward et al. 2008; Levin et al. 1988; Marteau 1989; McNeil et al. 1982; Wilson et al. 1987).

Study 2 examined a large sample of young adults at high risk of contracting a STD. Many of these participants had at least one sexual encounter in which they did not use condoms during the year before the study and very few of them reported any screening for STDs during that period. Consistent with our hypotheses, results in this study indicated that gain-framed messages induced greater adherence for condom use, whereas loss-framed messages were more effective in promoting screening for STDs when health information about STDs was provided in written text, or when numerical information was added to the text. These findings build on the conceptual framework of Rothman and Salovey (1997) as they reveal some key aspects of the processes that underlie the impact of message frame on participants' prevention and detection behaviors. In particular, participants who read the positive-framed message promoting condom use more often performed this behavior because the framed message caused their attitudes towards the behavior to become more favorable. Similarly, participants who read the loss-framed message promoting screening for STDs more often made an appointment with their doctor to ask about screening because the framed message caused their attitudes toward the behavior to become more favorable. These attitudes ultimately strengthened their intentions toward engaging in the behavior, which in turn affected participants' health behaviors.

More importantly, our studies are unique in their efforts to investigate whether visual aids can overcome framing effects when communicating important health information: Study 1 showed that framing was reduced or disappeared for participants with low numeracy when visual aids were added to the numerical information about the risk of the surgical procedure. Similarly, Study 2 showed that the gain- and loss-framed messages were equally and highly effective in promoting condom use and screening for STDs when a visual aid was added to the health information. That is, gain-framed (loss-framed) messages no longer induced greater adherence for prevention (detection) behaviors. In short, adding visual aids to health messages made both gain- and loss-framed messages equally and highly effective, conferring benefits without any noteworthy costs. Several theoretical and clinical implications follow from these findings.

First, our research helps to explain how and why visual aids eliminate the effect of framed messages. The results of the mediational analyses indicated that attitudes were again key variables: When the risk information was reported visually, participants' attitudes toward engaging in detection and prevention behaviors were often very positive and were not influenced by framed messages. These positive attitudes strongly influenced participants' behavioral intentions, which in turn affected their reported behaviors. In line with research examining debiasing of framing effect (e.g., Almashat et al. 2008; Simon et al. 2004), we hypothesize that visual aids may increase the likelihood of better or more elaborative encoding of the relevant risk information. Visual aids might lead to a more thorough encoding of potential benefits of adopting the promoted behavior and drawbacks associated with failing to adopt such behavior. We speculate that more accurate memory for information about potential costs and benefits would tend to overshadow the impact of framed messages on people's attitudes. Previous research is consistent with our expectations.

Visual aids improve reasoning by making part-to-whole relations in the data visually available (e.g., the number of sick patients who received a medical treatment and the overall number of treated people; see Chap. 9; see also Ancker et al. 2006) or by helping people to clearly understand and represent superordinate classes (e.g., the overall number of treated people; see Chap. 10; see also Reyna and Brainerd 2008). In a similar vein, individuals with higher cognitive abilities—who are known to more elaboratively encode and thoroughly process information during learning and risky decision making (Cokely and Kelley 2009; Cokely et al. 2006)—also tend to be less susceptible to the effects of message framing (Stanovich and West 1998; but see also Corbin et al. 2010 for boundary conditions), and benefit less from visual aids (Galesic et al. 2009). It is then possible that the more proximal mechanisms that might give rise to the observed changes in participants' attitudes toward the promoted behavior are cognitive (e.g., changes in information search and encoding or changes to specific content in memory; Ajzen and Gilbert Cote 2008; Johnson et al. 2007; Weber and Johnson 2006; Weber et al. 2007; Reyna and Brainerd 2007, 2008). Ongoing research is currently using cognitive process tracing techniques (e.g., eye-tracking, memory assessments, reaction time analyses, and protocol analyses) to assess the validity of these and alternative memory based theoretical accounts.

Second, our results offer a potentially effective method for communicating health information in a way that is consistent with informed decision making: Health information could be framed in positive or negative terms as long as visual aids representing the risk information are provided. Our findings also support and extend our own and others' previous findings about the usefulness of visual aids to enhance comprehension of health messages (see Chaps. 9 and 10; see also Fagerlin et al. 2005, 2007; Galesic et al. 2009; Garcia-Retamero et al. 2010, 2011; Lipkus 2007; Lipkus and Hollands 1999; Paling 2003). Critically, these findings provide evidence for the notion that problems in communicating medical risks do not simply result because biases prevent good decision making. In contrast, errors occur because inappropriate information formats complicate and mislead adaptive decision makers (Gigerenzer and Edwards 2003; Gigerenzer et al. 2007).

Finally, results in Study 2 have implications for medical practice and public policy. Although young people aged 15–24 represent 25% of the sexually active population, they account for about half of all new cases of STDs, including HIV infections (ASHA 2005; Weinstock et al. 2004). This means that nearly four million cases of STDs occur annually among teens in the USA alone (see Bermudez and Teva-Álvarez 2003; European Commission 2003; World Health Organization, Europe 2005 for similar results in Europe). In particular, human papillomavirus (HPV), trichomoniasis, and chlamydia were and continue to be the most prevalent—causing 88% of the new STDs cases in those between the ages of 15 and 24 (ASHA 2005). In the USA, the associated lifetime medical treatment costs were estimated to be approximately $6.5 billion annually (Chesson et al. 2004; see also Walensky et al. 2007). Therefore, our results suggest an efficient and effective way to communicate health information about STDs promoting prevention and detection behaviors to the group of people at highest risk (Dehne and Riedner 2005; Downs et al. 2006; European Commission 2003) without any noteworthy costs.

In summary, health messages can save lives and reduce the cost of health care. As several authors have argued, investigating the content and the structure of these health messages is crucial (e.g., Kirby 2008; Kirby and Laris 2009; Kohler et al. 2008). The current results highlight the potential impact of both message framing and visual aids (i.e., the influence of appropriately framed brochures that include well-constructed visual aids). Larger scale implementation of the method used in the studies reported in this chapter holds the promise of large and meaningful benefits (e.g., money, health, and time) that are relatively inexpensive and ethically desirable.

References

Abood, D. A., Black, D. R., & Coster, D. C. (2005). Loss-framed minimal intervention increases mammography use. *Women's Health Issues, 15*, 258–264.

Abood, D. A., Coster, D. C., Mullis, A. K., & Black, D. R. (2002). Evaluation of a "loss-framed" minimal intervention to increase mammography utilization among medically un- and under-insured women. *Cancer Detection and Prevention, 26*, 394–400.

Ajzen, I., & Gilbert Cote, N. (2008). Attitudes and the prediction of behavior. In W. D. Crano & R. Prislin (Eds.), *Attitudes and attitude change* (pp. 289–311). New York: Psychology Press.

Almashat, S., Ayotte, B., Edelstein, B., & Margrett, J. (2008). Framing effect debiasing in medical decision making. *Patient Education and Counseling, 71*, 102–107.

American Social Health Association (ASHA). (2005). *State of the nation 2005: Challenges facing STD prevention in youth*. Research Triangle Park, NC: ASHA.

Ancker, J. S., Senathirajah, Y., Kukafka, R., & Starren, J. B. (2006). Design features of graphs in health risk communication: A systematic review. *Journal of the American Medical Informatics Association, 13*, 608–618.

Apanovitch, A. M., McCarthy, D., & Salovey, P. (2003). Using message framing to motivate HIV testing among low-income, ethnic minority women. *Health Psychology, 22*, 60–67.

Armstrong, K., Schwartz, J. S., Fitzgerald, G., Putt, M., & Ubel, P. A. (2002). Effect of framing as gain versus loss on understanding and hypothetical treatment choices: Survival and mortality curves. *Medical Decision Making, 22*, 76–83.

Baron, R. M., & Kenny, D. A. (1986). The moderator-mediator variable distinction in social psychological research: Conceptual, strategic, and statistical consideration. *Journal of Personality and Social Psychology, 51*, 1173–1182.

Bermudez, M. P., & Teva-Álvarez, I. (2003). Situación actual del VIH/SIDA en Europa: Análisis de las diferencias entre países. *International Journal of Clinical and Health Psychology, 3*, 89–106.

Block, L. G., & Keller, P. A. (1995). When to accentuate the negative: The effects of perceived efficacy and message framing on intentions to perform a health-related behavior. *Journal of Marketing Research, 32*, 192–203.

Bruine de Bruin, W., & Fischhoff, B. (2000). The effect of question format on measured HIV/AIDS knowledge: Detention center teens, high school students, and adults. *AIDS Education and Prevention, 12*, 187–198.

Carver, C. S., & White, T. L. (1994). Behavioral inhibition, behavioral activation, and affective responses to impending reward and punishment. *Journal of Personality and Social Psychology, 67*, 319–333.

Centers for Disease Control and Prevention (2003). Late versus early testing of HIV—16 sites, United States, 2000–2003. *MMWR Weekly Report, 52*, 581–586. http://www.cdc.gov/mmwr/preview/mmwrhtml/mm5225a2.htm, accessed July 30, 2012.

Chesson, H. W., Blandford, J. M., Gift, T. L., Tao, G., & Irwin, K. L. (2004). The estimated direct medical cost of sexually transmitted diseases among American youth, 2000. *Perspectives on Sexual and Reproductive Health, 36*, 11–19.

Child Trends (2006). *Facts at a glance. Publication # 2006-03*. http://www.childtrends.org/files/faag2006.pdf, accessed July 30, 2012.

Cleary, P. D., & Angel, R. (1984). The analysis of relationships involving dichotomous dependent-variables. Journal of Health and Social Behavior, 25, 334–348.

Cokely, E. T., & Kelley, C. M. (2009). Cognitive abilities and superior decision making under risk: A protocol analysis and process model evaluation. *Judgment and Decision Making, 4*, 20–33.

Cokely, E. T., Kelley, C. M., & Gilchrist, A. H. (2006). Sources of individual differences in working memory: Contributions of strategy to capacity. *Psychonomic Bulletin and Review, 13*, 991–997.

Corbin, J., McElroy, T., & Black, C. (2010). Memory reflected in our decisions: Higher working memory capacity predicts greater bias in risky choice. *Judgment and Decision Making, 5*, 110–115.

Davids, S. L., Schapira, M. M., McAuliffe, T. L., & Nattinger, A. B. (2004). Predictors of pessimistic breast cancer risk perceptions in a primary care population. *Journal of General Internal Medicine, 19*, 310–315.

Dehne, K. L., & Riedner, G. (2005). *Sexually transmitted infections among adolescents: The need for adequate health services*. Geneva: World Health Organization and Deutsche Gesellschaft fuer Technische Zusammenarbeit. http://whqlibdoc.who.int/publications/2005/9241562889.pdf, accessed July 30, 2012.

Des Jarlais, D. C., Sloboda, Z., Friedman, S. R., Tempalski, B., McKnight, C., & Braine, N. (2006). Diffusion of the D.A.R.E. and syringe exchange programs. *American Journal of Public Health, 96*, 1354–1358.

Detweiler, J. B., Bedell, B. T., Salovey, P., Pronin, E., & Rothman, A. J. (1999). Message framing and sunscreen use: Gain-framed messages motivate beach-goers. *Health Psychology, 18*, 189–196.

Downs, J. S., Bruine de Bruin, W., Murray, P. J., & Fischhoff, B. (2006). Specific STI knowledge may be acquired too late. *Journal of Adolescent Health, 38*, 65–67.

Edwards, A., Elwyn, G., Covey, J., Matthews, E., & Pill, R. (2001). Presenting risk information: A review of the effects of "framing" and other manipulations on patient outcomes. *Journal of Health Communication, 6*, 61–82.

Edwards, A., Elwyn, G., & Mulley, A. (2002). Explaining risks: Turning numerical data into meaningful pictures. *British Medical Journal, 324*, 827–830.

Edwards, A. G. K., Pill, R. M., & Stott, N. C. H. (1996). Communicating risk: Use of standard terms is unlikely to result in standard communication. *British Medical Journal, 313*, 1483.

European Commission (2003). *Health statistics: Key data on health 2002. Luxembourg: Office for Official Publications of the European Communities*. http://epp.eurostat.ec.europa.eu/cache/ITY_OFFPUB/KS-08-02-002/EN/KS-08-02-002-EN.PDF, accessed July 30, 2012.

Fagerlin, A., Ubel, P. A., Smith, D. M., & Zikmund-Fisher, B. J. (2007). Making numbers matter: Present and future research in risk communication. *American Journal of Health Behavior, 31*, 47–56.

Fagerlin, A., Wang, C., & Ubel, P. A. (2005). Reducing the influence of anecdotal reasoning on people's health care decisions: Is a picture worth a thousand statistics? *Medical Decision Making, 25*, 398–405.

Galesic, M., Garcia-Retamero, R., & Gigerenzer, G. (2009). Using icon arrays to communicate medical risks: Overcoming low numeracy. *Health Psychology, 28*, 210–216.

Garcia-Retamero, R., & Cokely, E. T. (2011). Effective communication of risks to young adults: Using message framing and visual aids to increase condom use and STD screening. *Journal of Experimental Psychology. Applied, 17*, 270–287.

Garcia-Retamero, R., Galesic, M., & Gigerenzer, G. (2010). Do icon arrays help reduce denominator neglect? *Medical Decision Making, 30*, 672–684.

Garcia-Retamero, R., Galesic, M., & Gigerenzer, G. (2011). Enhancing understanding and recall of quantitative information about medical risks: A cross-cultural comparison between Germany and Spain. *Spanish Journal of Psychology, 14*, 213–221.

Gerend, M. A., & Cullen, M. (2008). Effects of message framing and temporal context on college student drinking behavior. *Journal of Experimental Social Psychology, 44*, 1167–1173.

Gerend, M. A., & Shepherd, J. E. (2007). Using message framing to promote acceptance of the human papillomavirus vaccine. *Health Psychology, 26*, 745–752.
Gigerenzer, G., & Edwards, A. (2003). Simple tools for understanding risks: From innumeracy to insight. *British Medical Journal, 327*, 741–744.
Gigerenzer, G., Gaissmaier, W., Kurz-Milcke, E., Schwartz, L. M., & Woloshin, S. (2007). Helping doctors and patients make sense of health statistics. *Psychological Science in the Public Interest, 8*, 53–96.
Haward, M. F., Murphy, R. O., & Lorenz, J. M. (2008). Message framing and perinatal decisions. *Pediatrics, 122*, 109–118.
Instituto Nacional de Estadística (INE) (2003). *Encuesta de salud y hábitos sexuales, 2003: Resultados*. http://www.ine.es/jaxi/menu.do?type=pcaxis&path=/t15/p455&file=inebase&L=0, accessed July 30, 2012.
Johnson, E. J., Haubl, G., & Keinan, A. (2007). Aspects of endowment: A query theory of value construction. *Journal of Experimental Psychology: Learning, Memory, and Cognition, 33*, 461–474.
Kahneman, D., & Tversky, A. (1979). Prospect theory: An analysis of decision making under risk. *Econometrica, 6*, 621–630.
Kahneman, D., & Tversky, A. (1982). The psychology of preferences. *Scientific American, 46*, 160–173.
Kim, S., Goldstein, D., Hasher, L., & Zacks, R. T. (2005). Framing effects in younger and older adults. *Journals of Gerontology Series B: Psychological Sciences and Social Sciences, 60B*, P215–P218.
Kirby, D. B. (2008). The impact of abstinence and comprehensive sex and STD/HIV education programs on adolescent sexual behavior. *Sexuality Research and Social Policy: A Journal of the NSRC, 5*, 18–27.
Kirby, D., & Laris, B. A. (2009). Effective curriculum-based sex and STD/HIV education programs for adolescents. *Child Development Perspectives, 3*, 21–29.
Kohler, P. K., Manhart, L. E., & Lafferty, W. E. (2008). Abstinence-only and comprehensive sex education and the initiation of sexual activity and teen pregnancy. *Journal of Adolescent Health, 42*, 344–351.
Kuhberger, A. (1998). The influence of framing on risky decisions: A meta-analysis. *Organizational Behavior and Human Decision Processes, 75*, 23–55.
Latimer, A. E., Rivers, S. E., Rench, T. A., Katulak, N. A., Hicks, A., Hodorowski, J. K., et al. (2008). A field experiment testing the utility of regulatory fit messages for promoting physical activity. *Journal of Experimental Social Psychology, 44*, 826–832.
Lerman, C., Ross, E., Boyce, A., Gorchov, P. M., McLaughlin, R., Rimer, B., et al. (1992). The impact of mailing psychoeducational materials to women with abnormal mammograms. *American Journal of Public Health, 82*, 729–730.
Levin, I. P., Schneider, S. L., & Gaeth, G. J. (1998). All frames are not created equal: A typology and critical analysis of framing effects. *Organizational Behavior and Human Decision Processes, 76*, 149–188.
Levin, I. P., Schnittjer, S. K., & Thee, S. L. (1988). Information framing effects in social and personal decisions. *Journal of Experimental Social Psychology, 24*, 520–529.
Lipkus, I. M. (2007). Numeric, verbal, and visual formats of conveying health risks: Suggested best practices and future recommendations. *Medical Decision Making, 27*, 696–713.
Lipkus, I. M., & Hollands, J. G. (1999). The visual communication of risk. *Journal of the National Cancer Institute. Monographs, 25*, 149–163.
Lipkus, I. M., Samsa, G., & Rimer, B. K. (2001). General performance on a numeracy scale among highly educated samples. *Medical Decision Making, 21*, 37–44.
Llewellyn-Thomas, H. A., McGreal, M. J., & Thiel, E. C. (1995). Cancer patients' decision making and trial-entry preferences: The effects of "framing" information about short-term toxicity and long-term survival. *Medical Decision Making, 15*, 4–12.
Lunney, G. H. (1970). Using analysis of variance with a dichotomous dependent variable—Empirical study. Journal of Educational Measurement, 7, 263–269.

Maheswaran, D., & Meyers-Levy, J. (1990). The influence of message framing and issue involvement. *Journal of Marketing Research, 27*, 361–367.
Mann, T. L., Sherman, D. K., & Updegraff, J. A. (2004). Dispositional motivations and message framing: A test of the congruency hypothesis in college students. *Health Psychology, 23*, 330–334.
Marteau, T. M. (1989). Framing of information: Its influence upon decisions of doctors and patients. *British Journal of Social Psychology, 28*, 89–94.
McNeil, B. J., Pauker, S. G., Sox, H. C., & Tversky, A. (1982). On the elicitation of preferences for alternative therapies. *The New England Journal of Medicine, 306*, 1259–1262.
Meyerowitz, B. E., & Chaiken, S. (1987). The effect of message framing on breast self-examination attitudes, intentions, and behavior. *Journal of Personality and Social Psychology, 52*, 500–510.
Millar, M. G., & Millar, K. U. (2000). Promoting safe driving behaviors: The influence of message framing and issue involvement. *Journal of Applied Social Psychology, 30*, 853–866.
Miller, P. M., & Fagley, N. S. (1991). The effects of framing, problem variations, and providing rationale on choice. *Personality and Social Psychology Bulletin, 17*, 517–522.
O'Connor, A. M., Boyd, N. F., Tritchler, D. L., Kriukov, Y., Sutherland, H., & Till, J. E. (1985). Eliciting preferences for alternative cancer drug treatments: The influence of framing, medium, and rater variables. *Medical Decision Making, 5*, 453–463.
O'Connor, A. M., Pennie, R. A., & Dales, R. E. (1996). Framing effects on expectations, decisions, and side effects experienced: The case of influenza immunization [published erratum appears in Journal of Clinical Epidemiology. 1997;50:747–8]. *Journal of Clinical Epidemiology, 49*, 1271–1276.
O'Keefe, D. J., & Jensen, J. D. (2007). The relative persuasiveness of gain-framed and loss-framed messages for encouraging disease prevention behaviors: A meta-analytic review. *Journal of Health Communication, 12*, 623–644.
O'Keefe, D. J., & Jensen, J. D. (2009). The relative persuasiveness of gain-framed and loss-framed messages for encouraging disease detection behaviors: A meta-analytic review. *Journal of Communication, 59*, 296–316.
Palella, F. J., Deloria-Knoll, M., Chmiel, J. S., Moorman, A. C., Wood, K. C., Greenberg, A., et al. (2003). Survival benefit of initiating antiretroviral therapy in HIV-infected. *Annals of Internal Medicine, 138*, 620–626.
Paling, J. (2003). Strategies to help patients understand risks. *British Medical Journal, 327*, 745–748.
Peters, E., & Levin, I. P. (2008). Dissecting the risky-choice framing effect: Numeracy as an individual-difference factor in weighting risky and riskless options. *Judgment and Decision Making, 3*, 435–448.
Peters, E., Västfjäll, D., Slovic, P., Mertz, C. K., Mazzocco, K., & Dickert, S. (2006). Numeracy and decision making. *Psychological Science, 17*, 407–413.
Reyna, V. F., & Brainerd, C. J. (2007). The importance of mathematics in health and human judgment: Numeracy, risk communication, and medical decision making. *Learning and Individual Differences, 17*, 147–159.
Reyna, V. F., & Brainerd, C. J. (2008). Numeracy, ratio bias, and denominator neglect in judgments of risk and probability. *Learning and Individual Differences, 18*, 89–107.
Reyna, V. R., Nelson, W. L., Han, P., & Dieckmann, N. F. (2009). How numeracy influences risk comprehension and medical decision making. *Psychological Bulletin, 135*, 943–973.
Rothman, A. J., Bartels, R. D., Wlaschin, J., & Salovey, P. (2006). The strategic use of gain- and loss-framed messages to promote healthy behavior: How theory can inform practice. *Journal of Communication, 56*, S202–S220.
Rothman, A. J., Martino, S. C., Bedell, B. T., Detweiler, J. B., & Salovey, P. (1999). The systematic influence of gain- and loss-framed messages on interest in and use of different types of health behavior. *Personality and Social Psychology Bulletin, 25*, 1355–1369.
Rothman, A. J., Martino, S. C., Bedell, B. T., Detweiler, J. B., & Salovey, P. (2003a). The systematic influence of gain- and loss-framed messages on interest in and use of different types of health behavior. In P. Salovey & A. J. Rothman (Eds.), *Social psychology of health* (pp. 286–299). New York, NY: Psychology Press.

Rothman, A. J., & Salovey, P. (1997). Shaping perceptions to motivate healthy behaviour: The role of message framing. *Psychological Bulletin, 121*, 3–19.

Rothman, A. J., Salovey, P., Antone, C., Keough, K., & Martin, C. (1993). The influence of message framing on health behavior. *Journal of Experimental Social Psychology, 29*, 408–433.

Rothman, A., Stark, E. N., & Salovey, P. (2003b). Using message framing to promote healthful behaviors: A guide to best practices. In J. A. Trafton & W. P. Gordon (Eds.), *Best practices in the behavioral management of chronic disease* (pp. 31–45). Los Altos: Institute for Brain Potential.

Salovey, P., & Wegener, D. T. (2003). Communicating about health: Message framing, persuasion and health behavior. In J. Suls & K. Wallston (Eds.), *Social psychological foundations of health and illness* (pp. 54–81). Malden, MA: Blackwell.

Salovey, P., & Williams-Piehota, P. (2004). Field experiments in social psychology: Message framing and the promotion of health protective behaviors. *American Behavioral Scientist, 47*, 488–505.

Schwartz, L. M., Woloshin, S., Black, W. C., & Welch, H. G. (1997). The role of numeracy in understanding the benefit of screening mammography. *Annals of Internal Medicine, 127*, 966–972.

Schwartz, L. M., Woloshin, S., & Welch, G. (2005). Can patients interpret health information? An assessment of the medical data interpretation test. *Medical Decision Making, 25*, 290–300.

Sherman, D. K., Updegraff, J. A., & Mann, T. (2008). Improving oral health behavior. *Journal of the American Dental Association, 139*, 1382–1387.

Shlay, J. C., McClung, M. W., Patnaik, J. L., & Douglas, J. M. (2004). Comparison of sexually transmitted disease prevalence by reported condom use: Errors among consistent condom users seen at an urban sexually transmitted disease clinic. *Sexually Transmitted Diseases, 31*, 526–532.

Sieck, W., & Yates, J. F. (1997). Exposition effects on decision making. *Organizational Behavior and Human Decision Processes, 70*, 207–219.

Siminoff, L. A., & Fetting, J. H. (1989). Effects of outcome framing on treatment decisions in the real world: Impact of framing on adjuvant breast cancer decisions. *Medical Decision Making, 9*, 262–271.

Simon, A. F., Fagley, N. S., & Halleran, J. G. (2004). Decision framing: Moderating effects of individual differences and cognitive processing. *Journal of Behavioral Decision Making, 17*, 77–93.

Sobel, M. E. (1982). Asymptotic confidence intervals for indirect effects in structural models. In S. Leinhardt (Ed.), *Sociological methodology* (pp. 290–312). San Francisco: Jossey-Bass.

Stanovich, K. E., & West, R. F. (1998). Individual differences in framing and conjunction effects. *Thinking and Reasoning, 4*, 289–317.

Steffen, V. J., Sternberg, L., Teegarden, L. A., & Shepherd, K. (1994). Practice and persuasive frame: Effects on beliefs, intention, and performance of a cancer self-examination. *Journal of Applied Social Psychology, 24*, 897–925.

Toll, B. A., Martino, S., Latimer, A., Salovey, P., O'Malley, S., Calin-Menter, S., et al. (2010). Randomized trial: Quitline specialist training in grain-framed vs standard-care messages for smoking cessation. *Journal of the National Cancer Institute, 102*, 96–106.

Toll, B. A., O'Malley, S. S., Katulak, N. A., Wu, R., Dubin, J. A., Latimer, A., et al. (2007). Comparing gain- and loss-framed messages for smoking cessation with sustained-release bupropion: A randomized controlled trial. *British Journal of Health Psychology, 13*, 659–681.

Treiber, F. A. (1986). A comparison of positive and negative consequences approaches upon car restraint usage. *Journal of Pediatric Psychology, 11*, 15–24.

Tversky, A., & Kahneman, D. (1981). The framing of decisions and the psychology of choice. *Science, 211*, 453–458.

Tykocinski, O. E., Higgins, T., & Chaiken, S. (1994). Message framing, self-discrepancies, and yielding to persuasive messages: The motivational significance of psychological situations. *Personality and Social Psychology Bulletin, 20*, 107–115.

Vidanapathirana, J., Abramson, M. J., Forbes, A., & Fairley, C. (2005). Mass media interventions for promoting HIV testing. *Cochrane Database of Systematic Reviews, 3*, Art. No.: CD004775.

Walensky, R. P., Freedberg, K. A., Weinstein, M. C., & Paltiel, A. D. (2007). Cost-effectiveness of HIV testing and treatment in the United States. *Clinical Infectious Diseases, 45*, S248–S254.

Weber, E. U., & Johnson, E. J. (2006). Constructing preferences from memories. In S. Lichtenstein & P. Slovic (Eds.), *The construction of preferences* (pp. 397–410). New York: Cambridge University Press.

Weber, E. U., Johnson, E. J., Milch, K. F., Chang, H., Brodscholl, J. C., & Goldstein, D. G. (2007). Asymmetric discounting in intertemporal choice: A query theory account. *Psychological Science, 18*, 516–523.

Weinstock, H., Berman, S., & Cates, W. (2004). Sexually transmitted diseases among American youth: Incidence and prevalence estimates. *Perspectives on Sexual and Reproductive Health, 36*, 6–10.

Weller, S. C., & Davis-Beaty, K. (2002). Condom effectiveness in reducing heterosexual HIV transmission. *Cochrane Database of Systematic Reviews, 1*, Art. No.: CD003255.

Williams, T., Clarke, V., & Borland, R. (2001). Effects of message framing on breast-cancer-related beliefs and behaviors: The role of mediating factors. *Journal of Applied Social Psychology, 31*, 925–950.

Wilson, D. K., Kaplan, R. M., & Schneiderman, L. J. (1987). Framing of decisions and selections of alternatives in health care. *Social Behavior, 2*, 51–59.

Wilson, D. K., Purdon, S. E., & Wallston, K. A. (1988). Compliance to health recommendations: A theoretical overview of message framing. *Health Education Research, 3*, 161–171.

Woloshin, S., Schwartz, L. M., Black, W. C., & Welch, H. G. (1999). Women's perceptions of breast cancer risk: How you ask matters. *Medical Decision Making, 19*, 221–229.

World Health Organization, Europe. (2005). *The health of children and adolescents in Europe: Fact sheet EURO/06/05*. Copenhagen: WHO Regional Office for Europe.

Wortley, P. M., Chu, S. T., Diaz, T., Ward, J. W., Doyle, B., Davidson, A. J., et al. (1995). HIV testing patterns: Where, why, and when were persons with AIDS tested for HIV? *AIDS, 9*, 487–492.

Part III
Overcoming Cultural Differences in Decision Making About Health

Chapter 12
Transparent Health Information in the Media*

Stephanie M. Müller, Nicolai Bodemer, Yasmina Okan, Rocio Garcia-Retamero, and Angela Neumeyer-Gromen

Abstract When it comes to medical decisions, people have to deal with a wide range of information from different sources. Information from the media is a prominent example: It increasingly addresses health-related issues and communicates benefits and risks of medical treatments and prevention programs. Is the media a

---

*In this chapter, we partially reproduce the article Bodemer, N., Müller, S. M., Okan, Y., Garcia-Retamero, R., & Neumeyer-Gromen, A. (2012). *Do the media provide transparent health information? A cross-cultural comparison of public information about the HPV vaccine*. Vaccine, *30*, 3747–3756.

S.M. Müller, Ph.D. (✉)
Center for Empirical Research in Economics and Behavioral Science (CEREB),
University of Erfurt, Nordhäuser Str. 63, 99089 Erfurt, Germany
e-mail: stephanie.mueller.01@uni-erfurt.de

N. Bodemer, Ph.D.
Harding Center for Risk Literacy, Center for Adaptive Behavior and Cognition,
Max Planck Institute for Human Development, Lentzeallee 94, Berlin 14195, Germany
e-mail: bodemer@mpib-berlin.mpg.de

Y. Okan
Departamento de Psicología Experimental, Facultad de Psicología, University of Granada,
Campus Universitario de Cartuja s/n, Granada 18071, Spain
e-mail: yasminaokan@gmail.com

R. Garcia-Retamero, Ph.D.
Departamento de Psicología Experimental, Facultad de Psicología, University of Granada,
Campus Universitario de Cartuja s/n, Granada 18071, Spain

Center for Adaptive Behavior and Cognition,
Max Planck Institute for Human Development, Lentzeallee 94, Berlin 14195, Germany
e-mail: rretamer@ugr.es

A. Neumeyer-Gromen, M.D., M.P.H., Dr.P.H.
Harding Center for Risk Literacy, Center for Adaptive Behavior and Cognition,
Max Planck Institute for Human Development, Lentzeallee 94, Berlin 14195, Germany
e-mail: angela_neumeyer@yahoo.de

R. Garcia-Retamero and M. Galesic (eds.), *Transparent Communication of Health Risks: Overcoming Cultural Differences*, DOI 10.1007/978-1-4614-4358-2_12,

reliable and objective source of health information? To investigate this issue, we conducted a media analysis of the widely promoted vaccination against human papillomavirus (HPV) in newspaper reports and Internet sources in Germany and Spain. These two countries differ in vaccination compliance rates and in the extent to which their health systems are directive. This chapter describes information categories in the media analyses. These categories included prevalence of cervical cancer and risk at baseline of suffering this disease, etiology, effectiveness of the vaccination, possible side effects, and costs. We compared media coverage and how balanced reports were in the two countries and investigated cross-cultural differences in medical communication.

12.1 Introduction and Background

Risk communication in health has become increasingly important due to two major developments: First, there has been a shift from a paternalistic relationship between doctors and their patients—where physicians primarily make decisions for their patients—toward a mutual process in which doctors and patients make conjoint decisions (Edwards and Elwyn 2009), as evidenced by the relatively new terms shared decision making and informed consent. Second, evidence-based medicine—the application of scientific principles to evaluate health treatments—constitutes a basis for policy decision makers, doctors, and patients to ground their health decisions on the best scientific evidence available. Scientific evidence should therefore be translated into language that helps patients understand the benefits, harms, and risks of health treatments so they can make informed decisions.

The channels through which the public can be informed about health treatments are manifold, including doctors, friends, patients, pamphlets, newspapers, and the Internet. Our key question in this chapter is whether the media—specifically, Internet sources and newspapers—offers reliable and balanced information about the vaccination against human papillomavirus (HPV).[1] Gigerenzer and Gray (2011) criticized the current information policy in health care and claimed that patients are consistently misled. Misinformation of patients is the consequence of a number of factors: biased reporting in medical journals, pamphlets, and the media; commercial conflicts of interest; defensive medicine; doctors' lack of understanding of health statistics; and innumeracy in the general public (see Chap. 1). We will focus on examining the reliability of information provided in the media. We first give a general overview of our understanding of *biased reporting* and offer a brief summary of the contribution of the media to the misunderstanding of risk information. We then focus on the analysis of media coverage of the HPV vaccine in Germany and Spain.

---

[1] The vaccine by Gardasil® protects against HPV 16 and 18, which have been found in 70% of all cervical cancers (Zechmeister et al. 2007).

As a model of balanced reporting, we developed a "facts box" that includes essential scientific facts about the HPV vaccine and used it as the criterion against which to evaluate media reports. Our main results concern etiological and epidemiological information about cervical cancer, effectiveness of the vaccine, and generally balanced reporting. We conclude that the media in Germany and Spain have offered unbalanced reporting about the HPV vaccine. We provide solutions to improve balanced reporting, which in turn may facilitate shared decision making.

12.1.1 Biased Reporting

The media is one of the most prominent channels through which the public is informed about health issues and innovations (James et al. 1999; Johnson 1997; Meissner et al. 1992). However, media reports are often biased: First, information can be one-sided, omitting potential harms. Second, risk information is often reported using nontransparent formats and is often framed in a way that misleads the target audience. Let us illustrate this phenomenon with an example. When the U.K. Committee on Safety for Medicine stated that the risk of life-threatening blood clots in legs or lungs increases by 100% when using the third generation of the oral contraceptive pill, the public was appalled. Consequently, many women stopped taking the pill, which resulted in undesired pregnancies and abortions. But what did this 100% actually mean? Studies revealed that 1 in 7,000 women taking the second generation of the contraceptive pill suffered blood clots; women taking the third generation pill suffered blood clots at a rate of 2 in 7,000. Obviously, the *relative risk* increased by 100%; the *absolute risk*, however, increased by only 1 in 7,000 (example taken from Gigerenzer et al. 2007). This example demonstrates that risk increase (and treatment risk reduction) can be framed in either relative or absolute terms. Although relative and absolute risk formats are equivalent, people often overestimate treatment benefits when they are framed in relative instead of absolute numbers (e.g., Sarfati et al. 1998; see also Chap. 9).

Another example of biased reporting is the use of *verbal probability estimates* rather than *numerical probability estimates*. A medical practitioner may use a verbal estimate to inform a patient about the "rare" occurrence of a side effect or, alternatively, a numerical estimate about the occurrence of a side effect in 1 out of 1,000 patients. Verbal probability estimates carry the risk of large inter- and intra-individual variation in interpretation (Brun and Teigen 1988; Budescu and Wallsten 1985). For instance, Knapp et al. (2004) presented participants with information about the probability of a side effect in either a verbal or a numerical format. The verbal description followed the European guidelines on the "readability of the label and package leaflets of medical products for human use" (European Commission 1998). Participants who received verbal estimates showed higher overestimations of the respective side effect than those who received numerical estimates. Overall, verbal estimates are likely to result in a mismatch between the intended and the perceived probability information.

12.1.2 Risk Communication in the Media

A content analysis of news-media stories concerning new drug therapies revealed that they often lack complete information about risks, benefits, harms, and costs of drugs (Moynihan et al. 2000). Further content analyses that investigated media coverage of health issues (e.g., Kurzenhäuser 2003; Schwartz et al. 2001) supported the conclusion that the media does not inform the public sufficiently. For instance, Kurzenhäuser (2003) evaluated 26 pamphlets informing women about mammography screening. Thirty-seven percent of the pamphlets contained information about lifetime risk of developing breast cancer, and only 4% informed about the lifetime risk of dying of breast cancer. Only 7% of the pamphlets reported benefits of mammography in the form of relative risk reduction (RRR); in another 7%, this information was presented as absolute risk reduction (ARR). Finally, only 11% of the pamphlets mentioned potential harms, such as overdiagnosis (e.g., false positive test result) and related psychological distress.

An analysis of pamphlets and websites informing about mammography in eight countries revealed a similar pattern (Gigerenzer et al. 2007): Less than 50% of the 27 pamphlets and websites contained information about lifetime risks and harms of breast cancer screening. The proportion of pamphlets and websites mentioning risk reduction of death from breast cancer was higher, although predominantly in relative formats (56%) as opposed to absolute formats (19%). In the same vein, a content analysis of pamphlets about colon cancer screening (Steckelberg et al. 2001) revealed that these pamphlets rarely present information about the risk of developing and dying from colon cancer or how colon cancer screening reduces incidence and mortality rates. In sum, the media often lacks critical information about risk in health contexts – and even when this information is included, its presentation in nontransparent formats makes it difficult for consumers to balance benefits and harms (Gigerenzer et al. 2007; see also Frost et al. 1997).

In Chap. 5, we described a study illustrating some prominent consequences of biased reporting in the media. In this study, Gigerenzer, Mata, and Frank asked a representative sample of women and men in nine European countries about the benefits of mammography and prostate cancer screening to measure the perceived benefit of these screening procedures. Participants estimated how many of 1,000 women and men who regularly participate in mammography and prostate-specific antigen (PSA) tests, respectively, would die, compared with women and men not participating in these screening procedures. The majority of women and men greatly overestimated the benefits, which amount to a mortality reduction of around 1 in 1,000 for both mammography and PSA screening. Overestimations were higher among those who indicated the media or pamphlets as one of their major information sources of medical information. This finding highlights that providing health information in formats that can mislead patients might affect the perception of risks, benefits, and harms in important ways. Additionally, as illustrated by the contraceptive pill scare example reviewed above (see Gigerenzer and Gray 2011), biased reporting in the media can motivate people to health-related behavioral changes leading to unwanted consequences.

12.2 What Information Should Be Reported in the Media?

To evaluate health-related media coverage, it is necessary to define what information is required for making informed decisions. Gigerenzer et al. (2007) proposed the notion of *minimal statistical literacy* to refer to what patients should know before making a decision. First, patients have to learn to live with uncertainty. While most laypeople and experts try to maintain an illusion of certainty (see Chap. 1), a first step toward statistical literacy is to accept that in medicine there is no certainty. Second, patients should have the capacity to evaluate the risks associated with a disease and a respective health treatment. For example, a risk can refer to a lifetime risk of developing a disease or a lifetime risk of dying from a disease. Additionally, risks can refer to different periods, such as lifetime incidence or incidence within 10 years. Risks also differ for various subpopulations, such as those based on age, gender, or region. It is therefore important to understand the actual threat for an individual. Third, to evaluate screening programs adequately, Fourth, diagnostic tests and treatments also include benefits and harms. patients should be familiar with the concepts of sensitivity, specificity, and false alarms. Patients should know how much a treatment reduces the risk of dying from a particular disease and what the probability of suffering side effects is. Minimal statistical literacy provides a guideline for deciding what should be taken into account when informing patients about their health. In terms of the HPV vaccine, patients should be in a position to evaluate, for instance, how safe the vaccine is and what its potential side effects are; to what extent the vaccine reduces the risk of developing cervical cancer; how many lives can be saved when women are vaccinated; and which target population the vaccine primarily addresses. We used these guidelines to evaluate media health coverage in a study.

12.2.1 Media Coverage of the HPV Vaccine

We conducted a content analysis of the media coverage of the HPV vaccine in Germany and Spain. The vaccine has received extensive media coverage in several countries due to its innovative application for cancer prevention, its public health relevancy (all girls 12–17 years old are targeted), and the critical voices that have questioned the vaccine's introduction (Dören et al. 2008; Martín-Llaguno and Álvarez-Dardet 2010).

In September 2006, the European Medicines Agency (2008b) approved the vaccine Gardasil in Europe. The vaccine protects against four HPV types (6, 11, 16, 18), which can cause cervical cancer and genital warts. According to the manufacturers' and governmental health institutions' recommendations, the vaccine should be administered before the first sexual contact. Although the Committee for Medicinal Products for Human Use (European Medicines Agency 2008a) concluded that Gardasil's benefits are greater than its risks and recommended market authorization, scientists have raised doubts about whether the vaccine has been sufficiently evaluated. Dören et al. (2008) criticized the admission of Gardasil in Germany, as the Standing Committee on Vaccination at the Robert Koch Institute (STIKO) had approved the vaccination before the publication of two major evaluation studies (FUTURE I Investigators 2007; FUTURE II Study Group 2007). According to Dören et al. (2008), the efficacy of the vaccine was still unclear. In Spain, criticism of the vaccine was scientifically communicated by a group of physicians who questioned the implementation of the vaccine given the lack of definitive evidence about its effectiveness (Martín-Llaguno and Álvarez-Dardet 2010).

How does the media report about the HPV vaccine? Previous media analyses of the HPV vaccine have already pointed out the lack of basic information about risk factors, transmission, and symptoms of HPV (Abdelmutti and Hoffman-Goetz 2009; Habel et al. 2009; Kelly et al. 2009). In addition, many campaigns (e.g., "tell someone" by Sanofi Pasteur MSD GmbH 2010) promote the vaccine and encourage young girls to get vaccinated—often without providing basic information about treatment risks or benefits and harms.

We extended previous research by comparing reports of two different media types, newspapers and Internet websites, in two countries, Germany and Spain. We evaluated *what* information was provided to the public (i.e., the *content*) and *how* the information was communicated (i.e., the *format*). Health reporting in these types of media might differ in important aspects because (1) their target groups differ in age, income, and education, and (2) Internet sources often provide information tailored to specific groups, whereas newspaper reports address a broader audience (Cotton and Gupta 2004; Schönbach et al. 2005). We compared public information about the HPV vaccine in Germany and Spain because these countries and their citizens differ in important aspects that affect decision making about health.

12.2.2 Intercultural Comparison of Media Coverage in Germany and Spain

We focused our analysis on Germany and Spain for several reasons. First, Spaniards are less proactive than Germans in seeking health information and making medical decisions (Delgado et al. 2010). Germans often report higher expectations about being involved in treatment decisions and are more often involved in decisions about their health, compared to Spaniards (Coulter and Jenkins 2005). Second, computer and Internet use in Spain is more than twice as low as in Germany (World Health Organization [WHO] 2012). Third, the two countries differ on mortality rates of cervical cancer, with lower rates in Spain (WHO 2011). Finally, the countries' immunization rates differ: Whereas Germany reported vaccination rates of 32% for girls aged 12–17 years in October 2009 (Fricke 2010), Spain reported vaccination rates of 77% for girls aged 11–14 years in the same period, achieved through school-based vaccination programs. In contrast, the German vaccination programs are opportunistic and girls have to actively seek to receive the vaccination. The administration of the vaccine by the public authorities and in schools might have increased the acceptance of the vaccine in Spain. Such cultural differences can substantially affect the communication of information concerning HPV, the HPV vaccine, and people's health-related behaviors.

12.2.3 Developing a Facts Box About HPV

Prior to conducting the media analysis, we developed a "facts box," which included essential scientific facts about the HPV vaccine based on the concept of minimal statistical literacy. The facts box served as a basis for coding media reports and summarized the medical literature on cervical cancer and the HPV vaccine (Table 12.1; see also Bodemer et al. 2012; Neumeyer-Gromen et al. 2011). Scientific evidence was taken from findings for Gardasil in May 2009—since Gardasil was the first approved vaccine and had the highest market share. Statistics about the vaccine's effectiveness refer to studies performed for the vaccine's approval (see reference list for the facts box). To understand the mechanism of an intervention and the likelihood of its effectiveness, one requires basic knowledge about the etiology of virus dynamics, pathology, including spontaneous remission rates of HPV infection and dysplasia, the base rate of infection, as well as approaches and recommendations about prevention. The base rate resembles the basic probability of getting the disease. Additionally, one should also have comparative numerical information about other known diseases (i.e., other types of cancer). Information about the benefits, side effects, and costs of the vaccine is also important.

12.2.4 Evaluation of Reports and Coding Scheme

To identify media reports from newspapers and the Internet, we conducted a two-step systematic literature search. First, we searched for relevant articles on websites from governmental institutions, health authorities, medical societies and associations, insurance providers, and pharmaceutical companies in Germany and Spain. We used the following search criteria for the Internet: "HPV" and (1) "vaccination," or (2) "human papillomavirus vaccination," or (3) "Papanicolaou," or (4) "Pap smear test." Second, we performed a LexisNexis search to identify newspaper articles about HPV and cervical cancer in each country. To document media reporting during implementation of the vaccine as an innovative approach to preventing cancer and its critical scientific discussion, the search covered the period from March 2007 to June 2009 for newspaper reports and from January 2009 to May 2009 for websites. We had to restrict the period for the Internet search to those websites that were accessible during our search process.

Predefined inclusion criteria restricted our analysis to reports that (a) intended to inform about the HPV vaccine, (b) had a minimum length of 200 words (to exclude brief notes about cervical cancer or material about general prevention programs), and (c) primarily addressed laypeople (i.e., the general public) as the target population.

Table 12.1 Facts box for the HPV vaccine

Human papillomavirus (HPV) vaccination with Gardasil					
What is the aim of the vaccine?[1,2]	Preventing infection with HPV type 16 and 18 to decrease the risk of cervical cancer; additional protection against genital warts				
How is HPV transmitted?[1,2]	By sexual contact				
What are the consequences of an infection?[3–6]	Infections with potentially 18 different types of HPV over decades can lead to changes in the tissue, which may (1) cause preliminary stages of cancer in the cervix, which may develop into (2) cervical cancer. Seventy of 100 cases of cervical cancer are due to HPV 16/18.				
How prevalent is cervical cancer?	*In 100,000 women per year*			*In all women per year*	
		Germany[7]	Spain[8]	Germany[7]	Spain[8]
Deaths	Cervical cancer	*3*	*2.5*	1,500	718
	All types of cancer	*230*	*236*	*101,000*	*6,565*
Incidence	Cervical cancer	*15*	*7.6*	6,200	1,965
	All types of cancer	*500*	*450*	*200,000*	*121,176*
Is there a chance that the infection will disappear without treatment?[3,5,6]	Yes. There is spontaneous recovery in over 90 of 100 cases for infections and in 50 of 100 cases for preliminary stages of cancer.				
For whom is it recommended *and* covered by public insurance?[1,2]	Girls 12–17 years (Germany) and 11–14 years (Spain), preferably before any first sexual contact. Some Spanish communities also recommend vaccination for girls 9–15 years.				
How long does the vaccine last?[1,2]	Minimum 5 years.				
Are there other types of HPV that could increase and/or decrease after the vaccination?[1]	According to theoretical assumptions, potentially yes. This is called replacement and cross protection.				
Are there other methods preventing cervical cancer?[1,9]	Yes. Early detection with Papanicolaou/Pap test "for woman aged 20 years and older" (Germany) or "between 15 and 25 until 49–65 years" (Spain, differing by community), which should also be applied for vaccinated women. Use of condoms.				

How effective was Gardasil in scientific studies?[a, 10–12]		
	Of 1,000 women	
1) Incidence of risky, preliminary stages of cervical cancer (due to all HPV viruses)	*Vaccinated*	*Not vaccinated*
At the beginning of the study, all participants had not been infected with the types of HPV that are covered by the vaccine/all were virgins[10]	20	28
All participants (at the beginning of the study, infection with HPV possible)[10–12]	42	49
2) Incidence of cervical cancer[12]	Not clear, no scientific evidence	
Are there side effects of Gardasil? (based on the European release)[12–14]		
Very frequent–frequent	*Occasional–rare*	*Very rare*
>1,000– 10,000 of 100,000	*10–1,000 of 100,000*	*<10 of 100,000*
Fever; injection site: redness, pain, swelling, effusion, itching	Unspecific arthritis, joint trouble Severe allergic reaction, urticaria	Bronchoconstriction with severe shortness of breath
On the basis of spontaneous reports after the release of the vaccine (size and estimated number of unreported cases is unclear). These reports are in temporal relation to the vaccine; it is unclear whether the vaccine caused these incidences.		
Serious neurological illness (Guillain–Barré Syndrome), signs of paralysis, paralysis of the face, seizure		
Vomiting, muscle pain, lymphadenopathy, allergic reaction		
Sporadic cases of death		
What are the vaccination costs?		
	Germany[15–17]	*Spain*[18, 19]
Costs for one complete vaccination	*465 euros*	*465 euros*
Total cost for one cohort of girls	*about 200 million euros*	*about 63 million euros*
Total cost of all annual public health programs (for all diseases)	*about 1,883 million euros*	*about 946 million euros*

(continued)

Table 12.1 (continued)

Note: When numerical information about risk reduction and concrete side effects was reported, we always allowed for slight deviations due to variability of measures in the medical literature. We focused on risk reductions given for all dysplasia because those surrogate parameters are more likely to reflect the disease burden than measures for HPV-specific dysplasia.

[a]The numbers of the first effectiveness data can be found on page 1922, second paragraph, in the Future II study; this result corresponds to the a priori defined "unrestricted susceptible population," which is similar to the combined analyses of the Future I and Future II studies[11, 12] of the "modified intention-to-treat-analyses" (MITT-2) in the European Medicines Agency (2008) report on page 22 in Table 15.[12] The numbers of the second effectiveness data can be found on page 22, last paragraph, and in Table 15 as the a priori defined "MITT-3" analysis; it is also a combined analysis of the Future I and Future II studies.[11, 12]

1. Robert Koch Institut. (2007). Mitteilung der Ständigen Impfkommission/STIKO am RKI (Stand: März 2007) [Notification of the German Standing Vaccination Committee/STIKO am RKI (March 2007)]. *Epidemiologisches Bullettin, 12*, 97–103.
2. Robert Koch Institut. (2010). Empfehlungen der Ständigen Impfkommission/STIKO am RKI (Stand: Juli 2010) [Recommendation of the German Standing Vaccination Committee/STIKO am RKI (July 2007)]. *Epidemiologisches Bullettin, 30*, 235–250.
3. Wentzensen, N., & Klug, S. J. (2009). Früherkennung des Zervixkarzinoms: Suche nach einem Gesamtkonzept [Screening of the cervical carcinoma: Searching for a general concept]. *Deutsches Ärzteblatt, 105*, 617–622.
4. Muñoz, N., Bosch, X., de Sanjose, S., Herrero, R., Castellsagué, X., Shah, K. V., et al. (2003). Epidemiologic classification of human papillomavirus types associated with cervical cancer. *New England Journal of Medicine, 348*, 518–527.
5. Schiffman, M. (2007). Integration of human papillomavirus vaccination, cytology, and human papillomavirus testing. *Cancer, 111*, 145–153.
6. Ostor, A. G. (1993). Natural history of cervical intraepithelial neoplasia: A critical review. *International Journal of Gynecological Pathology, 12*, 186–192.
7. Statistisches Bundesamt. (2009). *Gesundheitsberichterstattung des Bundes (2009)* [Health reporting of the state]. http://www.destatis.de, accessed July 30, 2012.
8. Ferlay, J., Parkin, D. M., & Steliarova-Foucher, E. (2008). Estimates of cancer incidence and mortality in Europe in 2008. *European Journal of Cancer, 46*, 765–781.
9. Winer, R. L., Hughes, J. P., Feng, Q., O'Reilly, S., Kiviat, M. B., Holmes, K. K., et al. (2006). Condom use and the risk of genital human papillomavirus infection in young women. *New England Journal of Medicine, 354*, 2645–2654.
10. FUTURE II Study Group. (2007). Quadrivalent vaccine against human papillomavirus to prevent high-grade cervical lesions. *New England Journal of Medicine, 356*, 1915–1927.
11. FUTURE I Investigators. (2007). Quadrivalent vaccine against human papillomavirus to prevent anogenital diseases. *New England Journal of Medicine, 356*, 1928–1943.
12. European Medicines Agency. (2008). *Europ. Beurteilungsbericht [European evaluation report] (EPAR) GARDASIL* (31/10/2008 Gardasil-H-C-703- II-13). http://www.ema.europa.eu/ema/index.jsp?curl=pages/medicines/human/medicines/000703/human_med_000805.jsp&mid=WC0b01ac058001d125&murl=menus/medicines/medicines.jsp, accessed July 9, 2012 and http://www.ema.europa.eu/docs/en_GB/document_library/EPAR_-_Procedural_steps_taken_and_scientific_information_after_authorisation/human/000703/WC500021147.pdf, accessed July 30, 2012.

13. Centers for Disease Control and Prevention. (2008). *Vaccine Adverse Event Reporting System (VAERS) 2008*. http://www.vaers.hhs.gov/, accessed July 30, 2012.
14. European Medicines Agency. (2010). *Gardasil: EPAR—Summary for the public (14/09/2010)*. http://www.ema.europa.eu/docs/en_GB/document_library/EPAR_-_Summary_for_the_public/human/000703/WC500021146.pdf, accessed July 30, 2012 and http://www.ema.europa.eu/docs/en_GB/document_library/EPAR_-_Procedural_steps_taken_and_scientific_information_after_authorisation/human/000703/WC500021147.pdf, accessed July 9, 2012.
15. a-t (Arznei-Telegramm). (2008). *1997 und 2007 im Vergleich—die Umsatzstärksten Arzneimittel* [1997 and 2007 in comparison—the top-selling drugs]. *a-t, 39*, 65–66.
16. Rosenbrock, R. (2007). *HPV-Impfung—Durchbruch in der Krebsprävention [HPV vaccination—break-through in the prevention of cancer]?* http://www.forum-gesundheitspolitik.de/artikel/artikel.pl?artikel=0644, accessed July 30, 2012 or http://www.forum-gesundheitspolitik.de/dossier/PDF/Rosenbrock-HPV-Impfung.pdf, accessed July 30, 2012.
17. OECD. (2011). *Dataset System of Health Accounts, Country Germany*. http://www.oecd.org/document/23/0,3746,en_33873108_33873402_33884311_1_1_1_1,00.html, accessed July 9, 2012.
18. OECD. (2011.) *Dataset System of health Accounts, Country Spain*.http://www.oecd.org/document/17/0,3343,en_2649_33929_33884753_1_1_1_1,00.html, accessed July 30, 2012.
19. Lopez Alemany, J. M., Cortes Bordoy, J., & Gil de Miguel, A. (2007). Human papilomavirus tetravalent vaccine cost-effectiveness study. *Revista Española de Economia de Salud, 6*, 400–408.

We identified a total of 1,586 and 2,496 newspaper reports in Germany and Spain, respectively. Of those, 141 and 293 articles met our inclusion criteria. For Internet reports, we identified 61 and 41 reports, respectively. All were included in our analysis.

The coding scheme included four sections: (1) general information about the media reports (e.g., information source, media type, date, and length); (2) identification of authors, communicators, and the target population; (3) etiological and epidemiological information about cervical cancer; and (4) evaluation of the transparency and balance of the report (i.e., discussion of pros and cons and concrete side effects) and of the information format (i.e., absolute or relative risk reduction measures). For brevity, we will focus on results obtained for (3) and (4) in this chapter.

The coding scheme was first developed in German and then translated into Spanish by a bilingual speaker. The Spanish scheme underwent a revision by two Spanish native speakers and was translated back into German. The two versions were equivalent. The evaluation criteria for media reports included (1) the completeness of the statements regarding the benefits and drawbacks, effectiveness, side effects, test accuracy, and false positives; (2) the transparency and provision of natural frequencies and/or the translation of conditional probabilities into frequencies and trees; (3) the numerical correctness of information, uncertainties, and general information in a numerical format (Gigerenzer et al. 2007; Neumeyer-Gromen et al. 2011).

12.2.5 Etiological and Epidemiological Information About Cervical Cancer

Websites in both countries provided more numerical estimates about morbidity and mortality than the newspapers (*epidemiology*; Fig. 12.1). However, only 57% and 39% of these websites and 43% and 20% of newspapers gave correct estimates for Germany and Spain, respectively. Spanish websites reported *causes of cancer* and the *possibility of spontaneous recovery* (i.e., the possibility that the cancer disappears without treatment) more often than German websites (66% and 68%, respectively, in Spain compared with 52% and 38% in Germany). Newspapers reported this information less often than websites and similarly often for both countries (38% of Spanish newspapers reported causes of cancer and 13% the possibility of spontaneous recovery, compared with 31% and 12%, respectively, of German newspapers).

12.2.6 Evaluation of the Transparency and Balance of the Report

Benefits in form of RRR and ARR of cervical dysplasia were rarely reported in either country and estimates were incorrect in most cases. The presentation of these numbers was higher for websites than for newspapers (German websites: 20% RRR and 5% ARR; German newspapers: 11% RRR and 1% ARR; Spanish websites: 5% RRR; Spanish newspapers: 0.3% ARR).

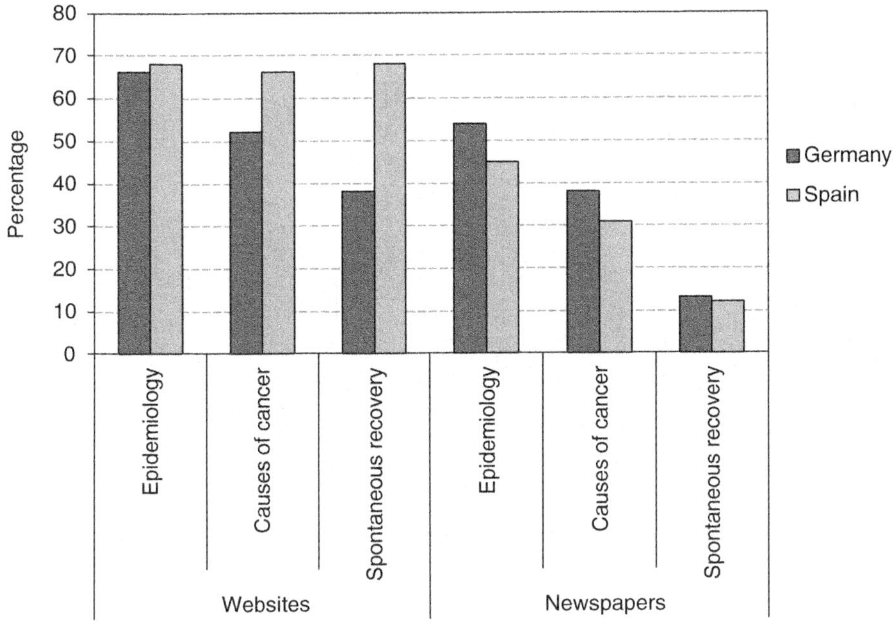

Fig. 12.1 Information about cervical cancer by country and media type in percentages

Fig. 12.2 shows that in websites, *cost estimates* of the vaccination were rarely mentioned (Germany: 28% vs. Spain: 22%). This information was reported more often in newspapers, particularly in Spanish ones (66% vs. 44% in German newspapers). Interestingly, German websites and newspapers *recommended the vaccination explicitly* (66% and 29%, respectively) more frequently than Spanish ones (17% and 10%, respectively). Finally, the majority of websites referred to the necessity for women to still do additional Pap screening, independently of whether they received the vaccination (61% and 73% for Germany and Spain, respectively), while only one-third of newspapers mentioned this piece of (36% and 33% for Germany and Spain, respectively).

Fig. 12.3 shows that German reports more often discussed both *pros and cons of the HPV vaccine* (52% of websites and 50% of newspapers) than Spanish reports (37% of websites and 17% of newspapers). *Side effects* were reported by half of all German websites and 14% of German newspapers (with 30% and 7% as numerical estimates). However, only a third of the Spanish websites (all in numerical estimates) and 11% of newspapers (with 5% in numerical estimates) included information about concrete side effects—but predominantly as isolated positive proof for the vaccine's harmlessness as compared to other common vaccines (e.g., hepatitis). A striking result is that newspapers in both countries provided less information than websites on most key aspects, such as baseline risk (see RRR and ARR of the vaccine, discussed above), cancer causes, spontaneous recovery, efficacy, and side effects.

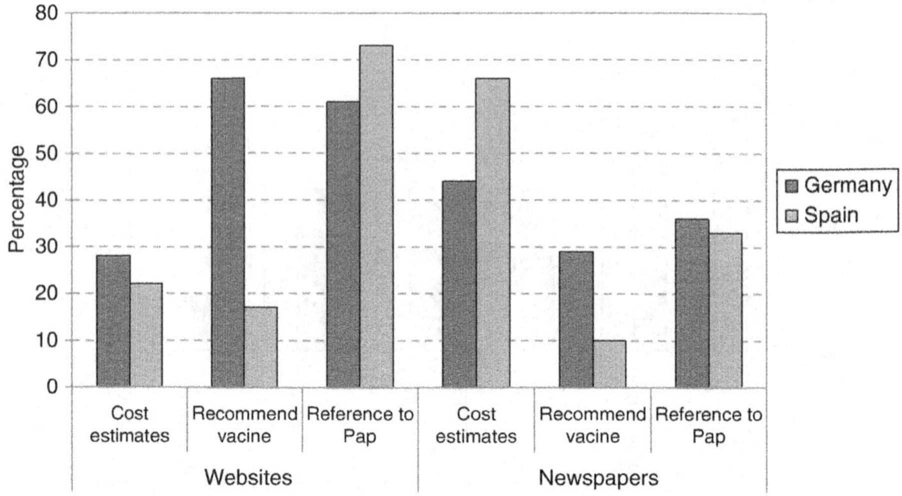

Fig. 12.2 Information about effectiveness of the HPV vaccine by country and media type in percentages

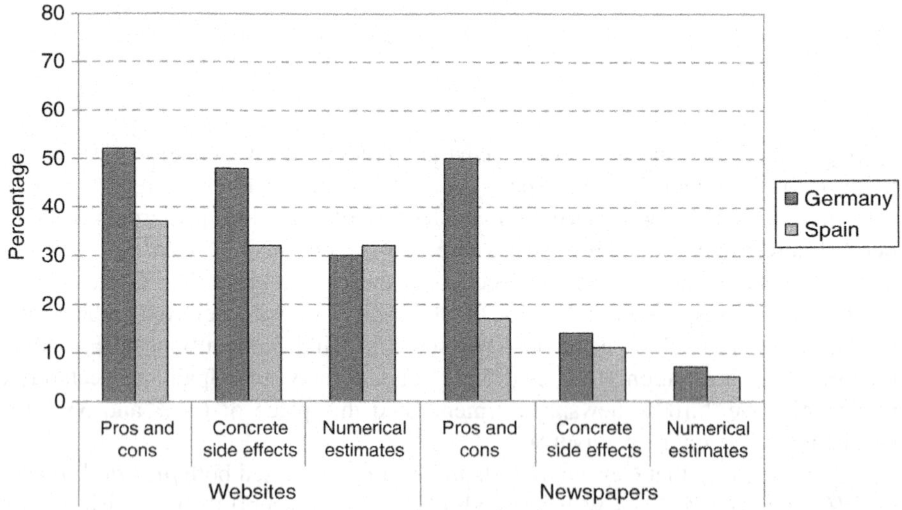

Fig. 12.3 Balanced information about the HPV vaccine by country and media type in percentages

12.3 Unbalanced Reporting in the Media

Taken together, our findings revealed that the media in Germany and Spain failed to provide balanced and transparent information. In line with previous findings (e.g., Abdelmutti and Hoffman-Goetz 2009; Habel et al. 2009; Kelly et al. 2009), the media in these two countries did not provide numerical information about pros and cons and concrete side effects of the HPV vaccination. Websites more often communicated epidemiological and etiological information, statistics about risk reduction, and concrete side effects than newspapers.

Taking a closer look at intercultural differences, we found that a higher proportion of German reports discussed pros and cons of the vaccine and included numerical estimates. German websites and newspapers also recommended vaccination more often than Spanish ones. This could be because Germans participate more in health decisions and more frequently *select* medical treatments compared with Spaniards (Coulter and Jenkins 2005). Consequently, German media reports might engage in a marketing strategy to promote the vaccination campaign in the public. Spanish media reports, however, more often referred to the possibility of spontaneous recovery and the necessity to maintain Pap screening (in websites) and cost estimates (in newspapers).[2] Yet it could be that Spaniards were informed about the limitations of vaccination, as its implementation was not questioned. Furthermore, cost estimates were often framed positively (e.g., it was often said that the Spanish community is able to afford high prevention costs), underlining the beneficial value of the vaccination.

As we mentioned above (see also Chap. 1), there are also differences between the Spanish and German health care systems. In Spain, the centrally organized national health care system offers systematic school-based vaccination programs, whereas in Germany the vaccination is offered opportunistically and in a more decentralized, self-administered system. These differences might lead to more directive and less participative health care in Spain along with fewer demands for and less active interest in transparent, balanced media reporting, whereas Germans might need to be convinced about the benefits of the vaccination. To what extent this is the case remains an open question for future research.

The present descriptive results involve the limitations of a hypothesis generating rather than a testing approach to map differences in media coverage between media sources and countries. However, the LexisNexis search and the identification of websites of the most prominent and common health authorities reflect a representative sample of current media coverage of both media sources and countries. It should also be noted that differences between media types may be a consequence of different periods of literature search (newspaper: March 2007 to June 2009; Internet: January 2009 to May 2009)—although we did not find any differences in newspaper coverage before and after the emergence of the general criticism about the vaccine.

The current findings are highly relevant as the media has the power to educate and influence the public's health behavior (Grilli et al. 2009). Yet there is a lack of transparency in the information that is reported. Why is this the case? First, research

[2] Follow-up studies that provide data to allow an evaluation of the vaccine's effectiveness in reducing cervical cancer incidence and mortality are not yet available; cancer development needs decades of observation.

is not entirely independent of medical industries' or governmental interests, which aim to promote health treatments. This conflict of interest also affects scientific journals (Weinfurt et al. 2008) and may result in biased reporting (Gigerenzer and Gray 2011). Second, health professionals often practice defensive decision making—for example, by ordering PSA tests although they are not convinced of their benefits (Steurer et al. 2009; Studdert et al. 2005)—to avert any potential legal consequences.

12.4 Discussion and Conclusions

Taken together, the public might not be able to evaluate adequately the effectiveness of the HPV vaccine. To guarantee credibility and transparency, the media should provide information about uncertainties. The vaccine's potential to reduce cervical cancer mortality, its duration of immunization, and its pros and cons for sexually active women still require further scientific evaluation. We suggest that facts boxes can provide all the relevant information (Schwartz et al. 2009)—they serve as useful tools for balanced reporting and could be included in media reports. One might argue that the facts box presented here is too complex and detailed for some patient groups. However, it allows each individual to select the information needed to make a personal decision. Similarly, health professionals and journalists could benefit from facts boxes and extract the key information needed to communicate treatment effectiveness and shortcomings to patients. Facts boxes can also be used in everyday physician–patient consultations and as decision aids for patients.

To improve future media coverage, reporting standards—such as the Consolidated Standards of Reporting Trials (2011) or the Strobe Statement (2011) for scientific communication—should be developed and made equally accessible for journalists, public-health advocates, and other health care professionals as well as interested citizens. Such standards would help consumers identify reliable and balanced information sources. In addition, standards should encourage the use of transparent formats to translate scientific knowledge into comprehensible and unbiased language (see Table 12.2). The standards proposed here are based on the results of the media analysis reported, and they constitute a refinement of International Patient Decision Aid Standards (IPDAS; Elwyn et al. 2006; Holmes-Rovner 2007). The IPDAS standards have been shown to increase people's involvement in medical decisions and to lead to informed values-based decisions (O'Connor et al. 2007). Although the media might just reproduce biased reporting that has its origin in scientific journals (Gigerenzer and Gray 2011), it could also use its power to make scientific evidence accessible to the general public.

Table 12.2 Guidelines for transparent, balanced, and unbiased communication of medical treatments for laypeople

Standards for media coverage of health issues
• Explain goal of medical treatment or prevention (e.g., primary vs. secondary prevention programs)
• Define target population
• Explain etiology (e.g., causes of cancer, possibility of spontaneous recovery)
• Provide epidemiological data (e.g., number of incidences and number of deaths) to convey an idea of baseline risk
• Communicate treatment effects in absolute numbers (e.g., absolute risk reduction). Additionally, communicate side effects in absolute numbers (e.g., risk increase, false positives) to convey information for shared decision making
• Communicate cost estimates to convey an idea of individual and public health investments in view of limited individual public resources
• Mention alternatives to treatment
• Use comparative figures (e.g., effects of other well-established prevention programs, overall cancer mortality, costs of other well-known interventions, etc.)
• Disclose uncertainties and what is not (yet) known (e.g., duration of immunization, effects on cancer since only surrogate measures are available, etc.)
• Disclose conflicts of interests

References

Abdelmutti, N., & Hoffman-Goetz, L. (2009). Risk messages about HPV, cervical cancer, and the HPV vaccine Gardasil: A content analysis of Canadian and U.S. national newspaper articles. *Women and Health, 49*, 422–440.

Bodemer, N., Müller, S. M., Okan, Y., Garcia-Retamero, R., & Neumeyer-Gromen, A. (2012). Do the media provide transparent health information? A cross-cultural comparison of public information about the HPV vaccine. *Vaccine, 30*, 3747–3756.

Brun, W., & Teigen, K. H. (1988). Verbal probabilities: Ambiguous, context-dependent, or both? *Organizational Behavior and Human Decision Processes, 41*, 390–404.

Budescu, D. V., & Wallsten, T. S. (1985). Consistency in interpretation of probabilistic phrases. *Organizational Behavior and Human Decision Processes, 36*, 391–405.

Commission, E. (1998). *A guideline on the readability of the label and package leaflet of medicinal products for human use*. Brussels: EC Pharmaceuticals Committee.

Consolidated Standards of Reporting Trials (CONSORT) (2011). http://www.consort-statement.org/consort-statement/, accessed July 30, 2012.

Cotton, S. R., & Gupta, S. S. (2004). Characteristics of online and offline health information seekers and factors that discriminate between them. *Social Science and Medicine, 59*, 1795–1806.

Coulter, A., & Jenkins, C. (2005). European patients' views on the responsiveness of health systems and healthcare providers. *European Journal of Public Health, 15*, 355–360.

Delgado, A., López-Fernández, L. A., de Dios Luna, J., Saletti Cuesta, L., Gil Garrido, N., & Puga González, A. (2010). Patient expectation of decision making for distinct health problems. *Gaceta Sanitaria, 24*, 66–71.

Dören, M., Gerhardus, A., Gerlach, F. M., Hornberg, C., Kochen, M. M., Kolip, P., et al. (2008). *Wissenschaftlier/innen fordern Neubewertung der HPV-Impfung und ein Ende der irreführenden Informationen* [Scientists request a re-evaluation of the HPV vaccination and an end to providing misleading information]. http://www.uni-bielefeld.de/gesundhw/ag3/downloads/Stellungnahme_Wirksamkeit_HPV-Impfung.pdf, accessed July 30, 2012.

Edwards, A., & Elwyn, G. (2009). *Shared decision making in health care: Achieving evidence-based patient choice*. Oxford: Oxford University Press.
Elwyn, G. J., O'Connor, A., Stacey, D., Volk, R., Edwards, A. G. K., Coulter, A., et al. (2006). Developing a quality criteria framework for patient decision aids: Online international Delphi consensus process. *British Medical Journal, 333*, 417–424.
European Medicines Agency (2008a). Committee for medical products for human use post-authorisation summary of positive opinion for Silgard. http://www.ema.europa.eu/docs/en_GB/document_library/Summary_of_opinion/human/000732/WC500059444.pdf, accessed July 30, 2012.
European Medicines Agency (2008b). *Europ. Beurteilungsbericht* [European evaluation report] (EPAR) GARDASIL (31/10/2008 Gardasil-H-C-703- II-13). http://www.ema.europa.eu/ema/index.jsp?curl=pages/medicines/human/medicines/000703/human_med_000805.jsp&mid=WC0b01ac058001d125&murl=menus/medicines/medicines.jsp, accessed July 30, 2012 and http://www.ema.europa.eu/docs/en_GB/document_library/EPAR_-_Procedural_steps_taken_and_scientific_information_after_authorisation/human/000703/WC500021147.pdf, accessed July 9, 2012.
Fricke, A. (2010). *Langfristiger Erfolg der HPV Impfung erwartet* [Long-term success of the HPV vaccination expected]. Ärztezeitung [Doctors' journal]. http://www.aerztezeitung.de/politik_gesellschaft/article/592205/langfristiger-erfolg-hpv-impfung-erwartet.html, accessed July 30, 2012.
Frost, K., Frank, E., & Maibach, E. (1997). Relative risk in the news media: A quantification of misrepresentation. *American Journal of Public Health, 87*, 842–845.
Future, I. Investigators. (2007). Quadrivalent vaccine against human papillomavirus to prevent anogenital diseases. *The New England Journal of Medicine, 356*, 1928–1943.
Future, II Study Group. (2007). Quadrivalent vaccine against human papillomavirus to prevent high-grade cervical lesions. *The New England Journal of Medicine, 356*, 1915–1927.
Gigerenzer, G., Gaissmaier, W., Kurz-Milcke, E., Schwartz, L. M., & Woloshin, S. (2007). Helping doctors and patients to make sense of health statistics. *Psychological Science in the Public Interest, 8*, 53–96.
Gigerenzer, G., & Gray, M. (2011). Launching the century of the patient. In G. Gigerenzer & M. Gray (Eds.), *Better doctors, better patients, better decisions: Envisioning health care 2020* (pp. 3–28). Cambridge, MA: MIT Press.
Grilli, R., Ramsey, C., & Minozzi, S. (2009). Mass media interventions: Effects on health care utilization. *Cochrane Database Systematical Review, 1*, CD000389.
Habel, M. A., Liddon, N., & Stryker, J. E. (2009). The HPV vaccine: A content analysis of online news stories. *Journal of Women's Health, 18*, 401–407.
Holmes-Rovner, M. (2007). International Patient Decision Aid Standards (IPDAS): Beyond decision aids to usual design of patient education materials. *Health Expectation, 10*, 103–107.
James, C., James, N., Davies, D., Harvey, P., & Tweddle, S. (1999). Preferences for different sources of information about cancer. *Patient Education and Counseling, 37*, 273–282.
Johnson, J. (1997). *Cancer-related information seeking*. Cresskill, NJ: Hampton Press.
Kelly, B. J., Leader, A. E., Mittermaier, D. J., Hornik, R. C., & Cappella, J. N. (2009). The HPV vaccine and the media: How has the topic been covered and what are the effects on knowledge about the virus and cervical cancer? *Patient Education and Counseling, 77*, 308–313.
Knapp, P., Raynor, D. K., & Berry, D. C. (2004). Comparison of two methods of presenting risk information to patients about the side effects of medicines. *Quality and Safety in Health Care, 13*, 176–180.
Kurzenhäuser, S. (2003). Welche Informationen vermitteln deutsche Gesundheitsbroschüren über die Screening-Mammographie [What information is provided by German health brochures about mammography screening]? *Zeitschrift für Ärztliche Fortbildung und Qualitätssicherung, 97*, 53–57.
Martín-Llaguno, M., & Álvarez-Dardet, C. (2010). Withdrawal of an advertising campaign to promote the quadrivalent human papilloma virus vaccine in Spain. *Gaceta Sanitaria, 24*, 75–77.
Meissner, H. I., Potosky, A. L., & Convissor, R. (1992). How sources of health information relate to knowledge and use of cancer screening exams. *Journal of Community Health, 17*, 153–165.

Ministerio de Sanidad, Politica Social e Igualidad (2011). Coberturas de vacunación (vaccination coverage). http://www.msps.es/profesionales/saludPublica/prevPromocion/vacunaciones/coberturas.htm, accessed July 30, 2012.

Moynihan, R., Bero, L., Ross-Degnan, D., Henry, D., Lee, K., Watkins, J., et al. (2000). Coverage by the news media of the benefits and risks of medications. *The New England Journal of Medicine, 342*, 1645–1650.

Neumeyer-Gromen, A., Bodemer, B., Müller, S. M., & Gigerenzer, G. (2011). Ermöglichen Medienberichte und Broschüren informierte Entscheidungen zur Gebärmutterhalskrebsprävention? [Do media reports and brochures facilitate decisions about prevention of cervical cancer?]. *Bundesgesundheitsblatt, 54*, 1197–1210.

O'Connor, A. M., Bennett, C., Stacey, D., Barry, M. J., Col, N. F., Eden, K. B., et al. (2007). Do patient decision aids meet effectiveness criteria of the international patient decision aid standards collaboration? A systematic review and meta-analysis. *Medical Decision Making, 27*, 554–574.

Sanofi Pasteur MSD GmbH (2010). *Tell someone. Eine Informationsseite über Gebärmutterhalstkrebs, seine Vorstufen und die HPV-Impfung* (An information site about cervical cancer, its preliminary stages and the HPV vaccination). http://www.tellsomeone.de/, accessed July 30, 2012.

Sarfati, D., Howden-Chapman, P., Woodward, A., & Salmond, C. (1998). Does the frame affect the picture? A study into how attitudes to screening for cancer are affected by the way benefits are expressed. *Journal of Medical Screening, 5*, 137–140.

Schönbach, K., de Waal, E., & Lauf, E. (2005). Online and print newspapers: Their impact on the extent of the perceived public agenda. *European Journal of Communication, 20*, 245–258.

Schwartz, G. G., Olsson, A. G., Ezekowitz, M. D., Ganz, P., Oliver, M. F., Waters, D., et al. (2001). Effects of atorvastatin on early recurrent ischemic events in acute coronary syndromes. The MIRACL study: A randomized controlled trial. *Journal of the American Medical Association, 285*, 1711–1718.

Schwartz, L. M., Woloshin, S., & Welch, H. G. (2009). Using a drug facts box to communicate drug benefits and harms. *Annals of Internal Medicine, 150*, 516–527.

Steckelberg, A., Balgenorth, A., & Mühlhauser, I. (2001). Analyse von deutschsprachigen Verbraucher-Informationsbroschüren zum Screening auf kolorektales Karzinom [An analysis of German consumer-information brochures about the screening of colorectal cancer]. *Zeitschrift für Ärztliche Fortbildung und Qualitätssicherung, 95*, 535–538.

Steurer, J., Held, U., Schmidt, M., Gigerenzer, G., Tag, B., & Bachman, L. M. (2009). Legal concerns trigger PSA testing. *Journal of Evaluation in Clinical Practice, 15*, 390–392.

Strobe Statement (2011). *Strengthening the reporting of observational studies in epidemiology.* http://www.strobe-statement.org/, accessed July 30, 2012.

Studdert, D. M., Mello, M. M., Sage, W. M., DesRoches, C. M., Peugh, J., Zapert, K., et al. (2005). Defensive medicine among high-risk specialist physicians in a volatile malpractice environment. *Journal of the American Medical Association, 293*, 2609–2617.

Weinfurt, K. P., Seils, D. M., Tzeng, J. P., Lin, L., Schulman, K. A., & Califf, R. M. (2008). Consistency of financial interest disclosures in the biomedical literature: The case of coronary stents. *PLoS One, 7*, e2128.

World Health Organization (2011). *Preparing for the introduction of HPV vaccine in the WHO European region.* http://www.euro.who.int/__data/assets/pdf_file/0007/98746/E91432.pdf, accessed July 9, 2012.

World Health Organization (2012). *World Health Statistics 2012.* http://www.who.int/gho/publications/world_health_statistics/2012/en/, accessed July 30, 2012.

Zechmeister, I., Freiesleben de Blasio, B., Radlberger, P., Wild, C., Kvas, E., Garnett, G., et al. (2007). *Ökonomische Evaluation der Impfung gegen humane Papillomaviren (HPV-Impfung) in Österreich. HTA-Projektbericht Nr. 009, Wien 2007.* [Economic evaluation of the vaccination against human papillomavirus (HPV vaccination) in Austria. HTA project report no. 009, Vienna 2007]. http://eprints.hta.lbg.ac.at/760/2/HTA-Projektbericht_009.pdf, accessed July 30, 2012.

Chapter 13
On the Effect of Individual Differences on Shared Decision Making*

Mirta Galesic and Rocio Garcia-Retamero

Abstract Do patients want to participate in making decisions about their health? Is there a relationship between their preferences for shared decision making and numeracy skills? Are those preferences different in countries with different medical systems, and for different age groups? Extant studies cannot answer these questions because most are based on nonprobabilistic, highly selective patient samples that prevent generalizations to a broader population. In a survey on probabilistic national samples in the USA and Germany, we interviewed participants with low and high numeracy skills. A significant number of people with low numeracy in both the USA and Germany preferred to be more passive than they currently were. High-numeracy people, in contrast, were mostly satisfied with their current role. Education efforts to increase numeracy, as well as using nonquantitative communication formats, may foster involvement of low-numeracy patients in decisions about their health.

---

*In this chapter, we partially reproduced the article Galesic, M., & Garcia-Retamero, R. (2011). Do low-numeracy people avoid shared decision making? *Health Psychology, 30*, 336–341.

M. Galesic, Ph.D. (✉)
Center for Adaptive Behavior and Cognition, Max Planck Institute for Human Development, Lentzeallee 94, Berlin 14195, Germany
e-mail: galesic@mpib-berlin.mpg.de

R. Garcia-Retamero, Ph.D.
Departamento de Psicología Experimental, Facultad de Psicología, University of Granada, Campus Universitario de Cartuja s/n, Granada 18071, Spain

Center for Adaptive Behavior and Cognition, Max Planck Institute for Human Development, Lentzeallee 94, Berlin 14195, Germany
e-mail: rretamer@ugr.es

R. Garcia-Retamero and M. Galesic (eds.), *Transparent Communication of Health Risks: Overcoming Cultural Differences*, DOI 10.1007/978-1-4614-4358-2_13,

13.1 Introduction and Background

Doctors have been increasingly encouraged to involve patients in decision making rather than pursuing the paternalistic model in which they make the decisions for their patients (Barry 1999; Frosch and Kaplan 1999; Hanson 2008). However, a number of important issues related to patients' preferences for shared decision making remain unexplored.

First, it is not clear how much patients actually want to participate in medical decision making. Although a number of studies have been conducted on different patient groups, the results are mixed: While some have found strong preferences for shared decision making (Beaver and Booth 2007; Caress et al. 2002; Deber 1994; Ende et al. 1989; Gaston and Mitchell 2005; Strull et al. 1984), other studies are less supportive, in particular those involving cancer patients (Degner and Sloan 1992; Frosch and Kaplan 1999). One reason for these mixed results might be that patients' usual role in interactions with medical doctors differs from their preferred role. Patients' usual role may be determined by a number of factors independent of their personal preferences, such as the nature of their disease, their doctor's attitude toward shared decision making, the availability and complexity of the information about different treatments, and whether the patients have health insurance. These factors can make patients either more or less active in deciding about their own health than they would like to be. Therefore, in the study we reported in this chapter we asked not only about the role patients *usually* play in their interactions with doctors, but also about the role they think they *should* play. The latter might be more revealing: The way it diverges from their usual role indicates whether they would prefer to be more active or more passive in their interactions with doctors than they currently are.

We hypothesized that many patients would prefer to play a different role than they usually play. This has important implications for programs aimed at promoting shared decision making. If patients are usually passive and believe that this is the role they should play, then such programs should focus on changing patients' attitudes toward shared decision making. If patients are passive but would like to be more active, then efforts should be made to change doctors' attitudes toward shared decision making. Finally, if patients are active but would prefer to be more passive, then steps should be taken to empower the patients—for instance, through education—to participate in deciding about their health.

The second unexplored issue is the role of numeracy in preferences for shared decision making. Patients might prefer a passive role in their interactions with doctors because they lack the skills needed to understand the risks and benefits of different medical options. One such important skill is numeracy, which is essential for the understanding and use of quantitative information about health (Ancker and Kaufman 2007; Galesic and Garcia-Retamero 2010; Galesic et al. 2009; Garcia-Retamero and Galesic 2009, 2010b; Nelson et al. 2008; Peters and Levin 2008; Peters et al. 2006). People with low-numeracy skills, for instance, have less accurate perceptions of the risks and benefits of screening and medical treatments (see

Chap. 9; see also Davids et al. 2004; Donelle et al. 2008; Schwartz et al. 1997; Woloshin et al. 1999) and are more susceptible to biases in judgments and decisions than those with high numeracy (see Chaps. 10 and 11; see also Fagerlin et al. 2007; Garcia-Retamero and Galesic 2009, 2010a; Garcia-Retamero et al. 2010; Peters et al. 2006; Reyna and Brainerd 2007, 2008). Therefore, even when patients receive accurate information about all available medical options they may not be able to understand the probabilities of outcomes associated with those options. It may be more difficult for them both to align the options with their personal preferences and to make decisions about their health (Deber 1994). There is a dearth of published research on how much patients' numeracy skills affect their preferences for shared decision making. In this chapter, we focused particularly on comparing the decision-making preferences of people with low- and high-numeracy skills. We hypothesized that even though the usual roles of low- and high-numeracy people might be similar, low-numeracy people might prefer a more passive role in interactions with their doctors.

The third issue is that, so far, most studies on shared decision making have been conducted on convenience samples of specific patient groups (Beaver and Booth 2007; Caress et al. 2002; Deber 1994; Degner and Sloan 1992; Ende et al. 1989; Gaston and Mitchell 2005; Strull et al. 1984). Although these studies provide valuable information about the preferences of these particular patients, the results cannot be generalized to a wider population due to nonprobabilistic sampling methods. This is problematic because it prevents researchers from reaching conclusions about the effects of important demographic characteristics—such as age (Cassileth et al. 1980; Degner and Russell 1988; Ende et al. 1989; Frosch and Kaplan 1999)—on preferences for shared decision making. For instance, several existing studies have suggested that there is a negative correlation between age and a preference for shared decision making (Cassileth et al. 1980; Degner and Russell 1988; Ende et al. 1989). However, most of these studies included only patients. As young people in the general population typically have less experience in interacting with doctors, they might in fact be more passive than older groups. We hypothesized that the correlation between age and shared decision-making preferences in the general population is smaller than in the patient samples. To investigate this, we studied shared decision-making preferences using probabilistic national samples that are representative of general populations.

The final unexplored issue is how shared decision-making preferences differ in countries with different medical practices. Two prominent examples are the USA and Germany. As we mentioned (see Chap. 1), most health expenditure in the USA is privately based (55%; World Health Organization 2012), and—at least before the new health reform—a significant part of the population either did not have health insurance (26%) or had sporadic or insufficient coverage (an additional 9%; Schoen et al. 2005). By contrast, in Germany only 23% of health expenditure is privately based, and most people have health insurance (More than 99%; Statistisches Bundesamt Deutschland 2011). This means that Americans might be more often than Germans required to determine whether they need a medical treatment, and which one would be best given the amount of money they can spend. In addition, patient-targeted advertising of pharmaceutical products is allowed in the USA but not in Germany, adding to the pressure on US patients to make their own decisions about their health. Because of these differences, we hypothesized that the US patients would usually play a more active role in their interactions with doctors than German patients would. We investigated whether these differences are indeed reflected in preferences for shared decision making in the two countries.

13.2 Study: Do Low-Numeracy People Avoid Shared Decision Making?

13.2.1 Method

13.2.1.1 Participants

The study was conducted on probabilistic national samples in the USA and Germany as part of the project "Helping people with low numeracy understand medical information," funded by the Foundation for Informed Medical Decision Making. The project involved a survey that gathered data for a number of studies related to understanding and communicating risks, conducted in two waves (see Chaps. 2, 4, 7 to 11). In the first wave, large national samples of participants ($n=1,009$ in the USA and $n=1,001$ in Germany) completed a numeracy scale consisting of nine items selected from Schwartz et al. (1997) and Lipkus et al. (2001; see Chap. 15). Participants with numeracy scores in the top and bottom third of the whole sample were invited to the second wave 3 weeks later. A random half of these participants were asked to answer the questions about shared decision making presented in this study, resulting in the sample structure given in Table 2.4 in Chap. 2 (see also Chap. 2 for more details about the methodology of the survey). This sample enabled us to compare people with low- and high-numeracy scores within each country, as well as each of those groups between countries.

13.2.1.2 Stimuli and Procedure

To investigate preferences for shared decision making, we used two questions adapted from the classic study by Strull et al. (1984). This method has been used often in previous research (Cassileth et al. 1980; Deber et al. 1996; Degner and Sloan 1992; Degner et al. 1997a). The first question asked about the usual role participants play in their interactions with medical doctors. The second asked about the role they believe they should play. Both used a 5-point scale ranging from "1—Doctor makes (should make) the decision" to "5—I (should) make the decision." Higher scores meant more active involvement. The questions were presented on separate pages, and the order of the questions was counterbalanced. Numeracy was measured as described above.

The questions were developed in English and translated into German (see Chap. 2 for more details about the translation of the materials and the programmed questionnaire). The Ethics Committee of the Max Planck Institute for Human Development approved the methodology, and all participants consented to participation through an online consent form at the beginning of the survey.

In data analysis, we classified participants into three groups by their role in decision making: passive, collaborative, and active (see Degner et al. 1997b, for a similar procedure). For the usual role, participants who answered that their doctor makes decisions for them, or that their doctor makes decisions but strongly considers their opinion were classified as *passive*; participants who said that they make decisions together with their doctor were classified as *collaborative*; and participants who answered that they make decisions for themselves, or that they make decisions but strongly consider their doctor's opinion were classified as *active* (see Galesic and Garcia-Retamero 2011). The answers to the question about the preferred role were classified in an equivalent way. To calculate the difference between the usual and preferred role, we deducted participants' answers to the usual role question from their answers to the question about their preferred role, and then classified the participants as those who (a) would prefer to have a more passive role, (b) were satisfied with their current role, or (c) would prefer a more active role than they usually had. To calculate the difference, we used participants' raw answers given on 5-point scales, although the pattern of results was very similar when we started from the recoded 3-point scales.

13.2.2 Results

What role do people play in medical decision making? How is it related to culture and numeracy? In line with our hypothesis, the usual role of US participants was more active than that of German participants (see Fig. 13.1). Accordingly, in a multinomial logistic regression analysis with numeracy and country predicting the usual role, the odds of Germans reporting being active were 64% lower than the odds for the US participants ($\beta=-0.45, p=0.035$). Results for the preferred role show a similar pattern (see Fig. 13.2): German participants preferred a passive role more often than the US participants ($\beta=-0.49$, $p=0.023$). Numeracy did not have an effect on answers to either of the questions: None of the differences were reliably larger than zero.

Does the role people usually play coincide with the role they wish to play in medical decision making? How is this match related to culture and numeracy? The *group-level* results shown in Figs. 13.1 and 13.2 may mask a divergence between usual and preferred roles on the individual level. We therefore calculated *for each individual* the difference between his or her answers to the two questions. Fig. 13.3 shows the proportion of participants who (a) would prefer to have a more passive role, (b) were satisfied with their current role, or (c) would prefer a more active role than they usually had. In accord with our hypothesis, approximately one-third of the low-numeracy people thought they should be more passive than they currently

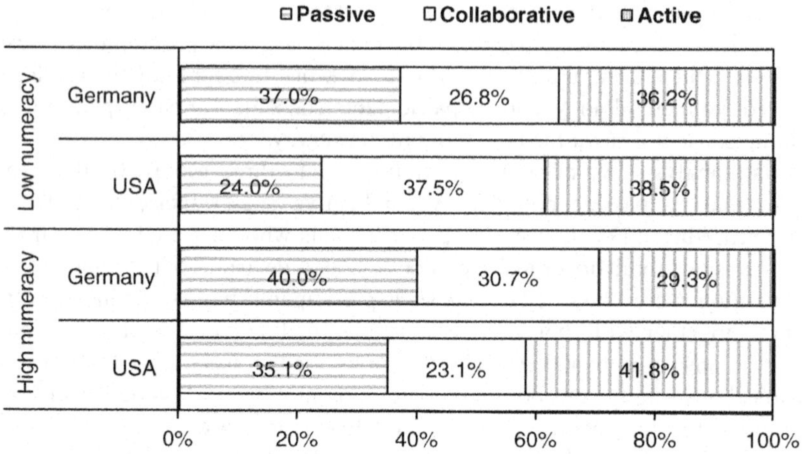

Fig. 13.1 Usual role in decision making by numeracy and country

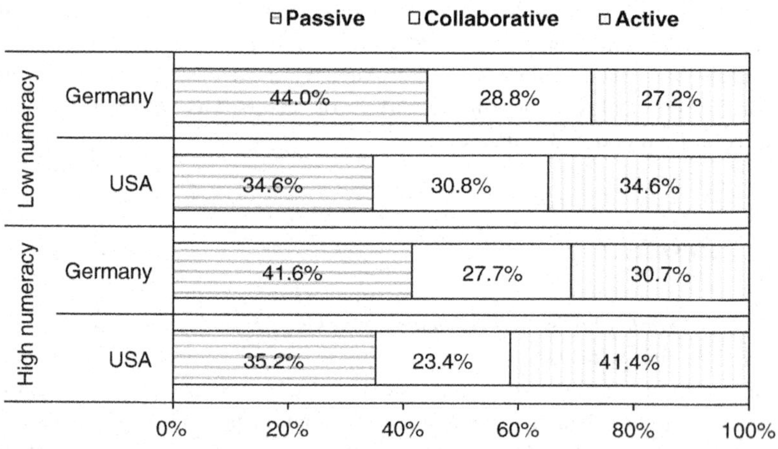

Fig. 13.2 Preferred role in decision making by numeracy and country

were (see Fig. 13.3). Among the high-numeracy people, only around 10% wanted to be more passive, with a large majority being satisfied with their role. To rule out the possibility that these differences are an artifact of individual differences in starting points—people whose usual role is already passive are less likely to show a preference toward an even more passive role—we controlled for the usual role (along with numeracy and country) in a multinomial logistic regression analysis. Even after controlling for this baseline, people with low numeracy were still more likely to report a preference for a more passive role than people with high numeracy: Their odds of preferring a more passive role were twice as high as for the high-numeracy people (β=0.72, p=0.035). This pattern of results appeared consistently in both countries.

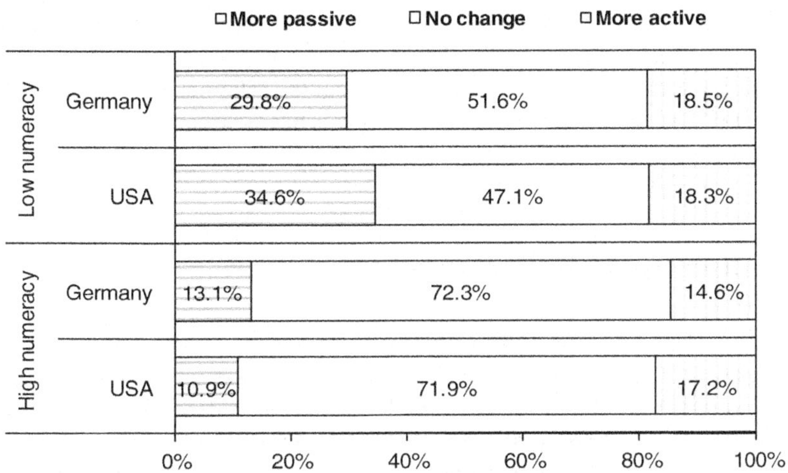

Fig. 13.3 Divergence of usual and preferred role on the individual level by numeracy and country: Percentage of participants who would like to play a more passive role than they usually play, not to change the role they usually play, or to play a more active role than they usually play

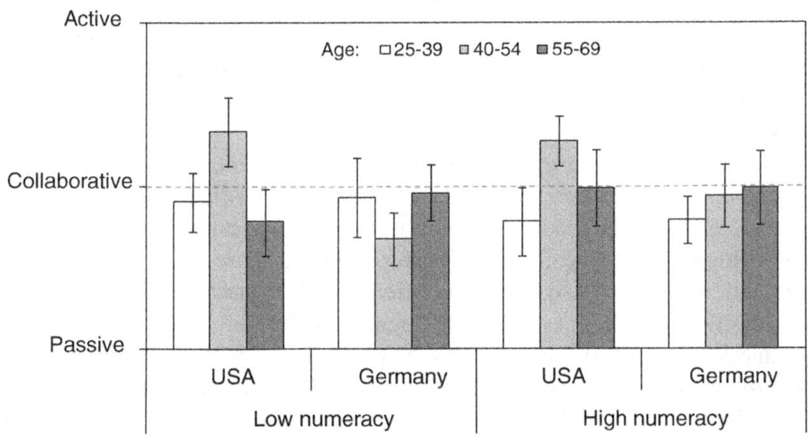

Fig. 13.4 Relationship of age and mean preference for shared decision making by numeracy and country. *Bars* show means on a 3-point condensed scale (1 = passive, 2 = collaborative, 3 = active). Error bars show ±1 *SE* of the means

Are preferences for shared decision making related to age? In contrast to the findings of patient-based studies on shared decision making (e.g., Frosch and Kaplan 1999) and in line with our expectations, our results did not show a negative correlation between age and a preferred role for shared decision making (see Fig. 13.4). On the contrary, in the USA we found a low preference for active roles in both the youngest (25–39) and oldest (55–69) age groups compared to the middle-aged (40–54) group. This holds for both low- and high-numeracy groups (with the exception of a nonsignificant difference between the two older groups in the high-numeracy group). In Germany, there were no differences between the age groups in either of the numeracy groups. We can then conclude that the relationship between patients' age and preferences for shared decision making is not as straightforward as has been previously suggested.

13.3 Discussion and Conclusions

Although we found that a significant number of both high- and low-numeracy people usually play a collaborative or even an active role in decision making about their health, a number of low-numeracy people in both the USA and Germany would prefer to play a more passive role (see Fig. 13.3). This is troublesome given the current trend that encourages patients and doctors to share decision making. It is possible that low-numeracy people do not feel prepared to make important medical decisions without fully understanding information about the risks and benefits of different options (see Chap. 2; see also Estrada et al. 2004; Fagerlin et al. 2005; Reyna and Brainerd 2007; Reyna et al. 2009; Schwartz et al. 1997). Education efforts to increase numeracy, as well as the use of communication formats that do not require high levels of numeracy, such as certain graphical displays (see Chaps. 9, 10, and 11; Galesic et al. 2009; Garcia-Retamero and Galesic 2010b), metaphors, and analogies (see Chap. 7; see also Edwards 2003) might help low-numeracy patients feel comfortable as partners in decision making.

The US participants reported a more active role in medical decision making than the German participants (see Fig. 13.1). As mentioned in the Introduction, this may reflect differences in the medical systems of the two countries. Interestingly, we did not find evidence for a negative relationship between shared decision making preferences and age (Fig. 13.4), which is often found in studies on nonprobabilistic patient samples (Cassileth et al. 1980; Degner and Russell 1988; Ende et al. 1989; Frosch and Kaplan 1999). Instead, in the USA we found that both younger and older people preferred to be less involved than the middle-aged group. Younger people in the general population are less likely to have serious illnesses and may therefore be less motivated to be involved in decisions about their health.

A limitation of the study we reported in this chapter is that we only focused on low- and high-numeracy participants. We do not know whether people with intermediate levels of numeracy are more similar to those with a low or a high level of this skill. In addition, in these nationwide surveys we were able to record only participants' reports about their usual and preferred roles in interactions with doctors. We were not able to observe their actual interactions with doctors. However, we feel that the ability to generalize our results to a broader population and to make cross-cultural comparisons compensates for this limitation. A further limitation of our study is that our participants were sampled from a general population and not from a population of patients with immediate medical problems. Therefore, prior experience with doctors may have been minimal for some participants—in particular the younger ones. This could have affected the results, especially the relationship of shared decision-making preferences and age.

The study described in this chapter is, to our knowledge, the first on preferences for shared decision making that uses probabilistic national samples in two countries. We found that numeracy is an important predictor of these preferences, highlighting the need for more patient-centered education efforts and the use of communication formats that do not require high-numeracy skills. We encourage further research on the relationship of numeracy skills and shared decision making in general populations of other countries, and in particular on the ways to overcome negative effects of low numeracy on informed and shared medical decision making in different cultural contexts.

References

Ancker, J. S., & Kaufman, D. (2007). Rethinking health numeracy: A multidisciplinary literature review. *Journal of the American Medical Informatics Association, 14*, 713–721.

Barry, M. J. (1999). Involving patients in medical decisions: How can physicians do better? *Journal of the American Medical Association, 282*, 2356–2357.

Beaver, K., & Booth, K. (2007). Information needs and decision-making preferences: Comparing findings for gynaecological, breast and colorectal cancer. *European Journal of Oncology Nursing, 11*, 409–416.

Caress, A. L., Luker, K., Woodcock, A., & Beaver, K. (2002). Qualitative exploration of treatment decision-making role preference in adult asthma patients. *Health Expectations, 5*, 223–235.

Cassileth, B. R., Zupkis, R. V., Sutton-Smith, K., & March, V. (1980). Information and participation preferences among cancer patients. *Annals of Internal Medicine, 92*, 832–836.

Davids, S. L., Schapira, M. M., McAuliffe, T. L., & Nattinger, A. B. (2004). Predictors of pessimistic breast cancer risk perceptions in a primary care population. *Journal of General Internal Medicine, 19*, 310–315.

Deber, R. B. (1994). Physicians in health care management: 8. The patient-physician partnership: Decision making, problem solving and the desire to participate. *Canadian Medical Association Journal, 151*, 423–427.

Deber, R. B., Kraetschmer, N., & Irvine, J. (1996). What role do patients wish to play in treatment decision making? *Archives of Internal Medicine, 156*, 1414–1420.

Degner, L. F., Kristjanson, L. J., Bowman, D., Sloan, J. A., Carriere, K. C., O'Neil, J., et al. (1997a). Information needs and decisional preferences in women with breast cancer. *Journal of the American Medical Association, 277*, 1485–1492.

Degner, L. F., & Russell, C. A. (1988). Preferences for treatment control among adults with cancer. *Research in Nursing and Health, 11*, 367–374.

Degner, L. F., & Sloan, J. A. (1992). Decision making during serious illness: What role do patients really want to play? *Journal of Clinical Epidemiology, 45*, 941–949.

Degner, L. F., Sloan, J. A., & Venkatesh, P. (1997b). The control preferences scale. *Canadian Journal of Nursing Research, 29*, 21–43.

Donelle, L., Arocha, J. F., & Hoffman-Goetz, L. (2008). Health literacy and numeracy: Key factors in cancer risk comprehension. *Chronic Diseases in Canada, 29*, 1–8.

Edwards, A. (2003). Communicating risks through analogies. *British Medical Journal, 327*, 749.

Ende, J., Kazis, L., Ash, A., & Moskowitz, M. A. (1989). Measuring patients' desire for autonomy: Decision making and information-seeking preferences among medical patients. *Journal of General Internal Medicine, 4*, 23–30.

Estrada, C. A., Martin-Hryniewicz, M., Peek, B. T., Collins, C., & Byrd, J. C. (2004). Literacy and numeracy skills and anticoagulation control. *The American Journal of the Medical Sciences, 328*, 88–93.

Fagerlin, A., Ubel, P. A., Smith, D. M., & Zikmund-Fisher, B. J. (2007). Making numbers matter: Present and future research in risk communication. *American Journal of Health Behavior, 31*, 47–56.

Fagerlin, A., Zikmund-Fisher, B. J., & Ubel, P. A. (2005). How making a risk estimate can change the feel of that risk: Shifting attitudes toward breast cancer risk in a general public survey. *Patient Education and Counseling, 57*, 294–299.

Frosch, D. L., & Kaplan, R. M. (1999). Shared decision making in clinical medicine: Past research and future directions. *American Journal of Preventive Medicine, 17*, 285–294.

Galesic, M., & Garcia-Retamero, R. (2010). Statistical numeracy for health: A cross-cultural comparison with probabilistic national samples. *Archives of Internal Medicine, 170*, 462–468.

Galesic, M., & Garcia-Retamero, R. (2011). Do low-numeracy people avoid shared decision making? *Health Psychology, 30*, 336–341.

Galesic, M., Garcia-Retamero, R., & Gigerenzer, G. (2009). Using icon arrays to communicate medical risks: Overcoming low numeracy. *Health Psychology, 28*, 210–216.

Garcia-Retamero, R., & Galesic, M. (2009). Communicating treatment risk reduction to people with low numeracy skills: A cross-cultural comparison. *American Journal of Public Health, 99*, 2196–2202.

Garcia-Retamero, R., & Galesic, M. (2010a). How to reduce the effect of framing on messages about health. *Journal of General Internal Medicine, 25*, 1323–1329.

Garcia-Retamero, R., & Galesic, M. (2010b). Who profits from visual aids? Overcoming challenges in people's understanding of risks. *Social Science and Medicine, 70*, 1019–1025.

Garcia-Retamero, R., Galesic, M., & Gigerenzer, G. (2010). Do icon arrays help reduce denominator neglect? *Medical Decision Making, 30*, 672–684.

Gaston, C. M., & Mitchell, G. (2005). Information giving and decision-making in patients with advanced cancer: A systematic review. *Social Science and Medicine, 61*, 2252–2264.

Hanson, J. L. (2008). Shared decision making: Have we missed the obvious? *Archives of Internal Medicine, 168*, 1368–1370.

Lipkus, I. M., Samsa, G., & Rimer, B. K. (2001). General performance on a numeracy scale among highly educated samples. *Medical Decision Making, 21*, 37–44.

Nelson, W., Reyna, V. F., Fagerlin, A., Lipkus, I., & Peters, E. (2008). Clinical implications of numeracy: Theory and practice. *Annals of Behavioral Medicine, 35*, 261–274.

Peters, E., & Levin, I. P. (2008). Dissecting the risky-choice framing effect: Numeracy as an individual-difference factor in weighting risky and riskless options. *Judgment and Decision Making, 3*, 435–448.

Peters, E., Vastfjall, D., Slovic, P., Mertz, C. K., Mozzocco, K., & Dickert, S. (2006). Numeracy and decision making. *Psychological Science, 17*, 406–413.

Reyna, V. F., & Brainerd, C. J. (2007). The importance of mathematics in health and human judgment: Numeracy, risk communication, and medical decision making. *Learning and Individual Differences, 17*, 147–159.

Reyna, V. F., & Brainerd, C. J. (2008). Numeracy, ratio bias, and denominator neglect in judgments of risk and probability. *Learning and Individual Differences, 18*, 89–107.

Reyna, V. R., Nelson, W. L., Han, P., & Dieckmann, N. F. (2009). How numeracy influences risk comprehension and medical decision making. *Psychological Bulletin, 135*, 943–973.

Schoen, C., Doty, M. M., Collins, S. R., & Holmgren, A. L. (2005). Insured but not protected: How many adults are underinsured? *Health Affairs*, W5-289–W5-302.

Schwartz, L. M., Woloshin, S., Black, W. C., & Welch, H. G. (1997). The role of numeracy in understanding the benefit of screening mammography. *Annals of Internal Medicine, 127*, 966–972.

Statistisches Bundesamt Deutschland (2011). *Sozialleistungen Angaben zur Krankenversicherung (Ergebnisse des Mikrozensus)-Fachserie 13 Reihe 1.1-2007.* https://www.destatis.de/DE/

Publikationen/Thematisch/Bevoelkerung/HaushalteMikrozensus/Krankenversicherung Mikrozensus2130110079004.html, accessed July 30, 2012.
Strull, W. N., Lo, B., & Charles, G. (1984). Do patients want to participate in medical decision making? *Journal of the American Medical Association, 252*, 2990–2994.
Woloshin, S., Schwartz, L. M., Black, W. C., & Welch, H. G. (1999). Women's perceptions of breast cancer risk: How you ask matters. *Medical Decision Making, 19*, 221–229.
World Health Organization (2012). *World Health Statistics 2012*. http://www.who.int/gho/publications/world_health_statistics/2012/en/, accessed July 30, 2012.

Part IV
Conclusions and Appendix

Chapter 14
Guidelines for Transparent Communication in a Globalized World

Rocio Garcia-Retamero and Mirta Galesic

Abstract In this book we have examined the broad theme of risk communication, distinguishing three central topics: (1) cultural differences in understanding health-related risks, (2) the use of information formats for enhancing transparent communication of these risks, and (3) methods for overcoming cultural differences in decision making about health. Each of these topics was examined in detail in several chapters analyzing specific problems across different cultures. In turn, each chapter included a review of the relevant literature, an original empirical study illuminating a specific problem, and a discussion of practical and theoretical implications. Across all these chapters and topics, results have converged to demonstrate that many problems associated with risk illiteracy are not simply the result of cognitive biases preventing good decision making. Rather, errors occur because ineffective information formats complicate and mislead adaptive decision makers. In closing, this chapter ties together the preceding chapters and synthesizes guidelines for transparent communication. Information formats that exploit people's inherent capacity to recognize relationships in naturally occurring problems (so-called transparent information formats) can dramatically enhance risk comprehension, communication, and recall and foster better decisions about health regardless of culture.

R. Garcia-Retamero, Ph.D. (✉)
Departamento de Psicología Experimental, Facultad de Psicología, University of Granada, Campus Universitario de Cartuja s/n, Granada 18071, Spain

Center for Adaptive Behavior and Cognition, Max Planck Institute for Human Development, Lentzeallee 94, Berlin 14195, Germany
e-mail: rretamer@ugr.es

M. Galesic, Ph.D.
Center for Adaptive Behavior and Cognition, Max Planck Institute for Human Development, Lentzeallee 94, Berlin 14195, Germany
e-mail: galesic@mpib-berlin.mpg.de

R. Garcia-Retamero and M. Galesic (eds.), *Transparent Communication of Health Risks: Overcoming Cultural Differences*, DOI 10.1007/978-1-4614-4358-2_14,

14.1 What We Have Learned So Far: Transparent Communication of Risks Helps Overcome Cultural Differences

Our research on risk literacy and medical decision making shows that across different cultures, people often have severe problems grasping a host of concepts that are prerequisites for understanding health-related risk information (i.e., numbers, graphs, and knowledge about basic medical facts; see Chaps. 2–6). As a consequence, they are prone to errors in risk perception and decision making (Edwards et al. 2002; Garcia-Retamero et al. 2010; Gigerenzer et al. 2010; Peters et al. 2006; Reyna et al. 2009). Prominent examples of such difficult numerical concepts are the incidence and prevalence of different diseases, risk reductions due to medical screenings and treatments, and risk increases due to side effects of treatments and unhealthy behaviors (Gigerenzer 2002; Gigerenzer and Gray 2011). In addition, informed medical decision making is heavily reinforced these days by the legal requirement for informed consent in most, if not all countries and critically depends on communication of quantitative medical information (Barry 1999; Brody et al. 1989; Frosch and Kaplan 1999; Garcia-Retamero and Galesic 2009; Hanson 2008). With this challenge, understanding how health-related risk information can be effectively communicated is more essential than ever (Fagerlin et al. 2007, 2010; Gigerenzer et al. 2007; Lipkus 2007; Lipkus and Peters 2009).

Our main hypothesis in this book is that problems with numerical concepts do not result simply because cognitive biases and lack of numeracy prevent risk understanding and good decision making. Rather, we assume that errors occur because inappropriate information formats complicate and mislead adaptive decision makers. In line with this hypothesis, our studies show that using transparent information formats enhances risk comprehension, communication, and recall and helps people make better decisions about their health. Importantly, our research also shows that information formats that work well in one culture often improve risk understanding and decision making in other cultures. Our studies produced three noteworthy findings.

First, information formats that rely on what people from different cultures know about their everyday contexts work better than formats requiring understanding of numerically expressed probabilities or arbitrary graph conventions. Prominent examples of successful formats are listed in Table 14.1 and include the use of analogies to explain predictive accuracy of medical screenings (Chap. 7), the use of specific numerical formats that can be related to everyday experiences to enhance risk communication and recall (Chap. 8), the use of visual aids to enhance risk understanding and communication (Chap. 9) or to eliminate biases such as denominator neglect (Chap. 10) and errors induced by framed messages (Chap. 11), and the use of transparent brochures explaining the current state of scientific evidence and side effects of medical treatments (Chap. 12).

Second, in all the cultures we investigated, people with low risk literacy (i.e., numeracy and graph literacy; Chaps. 2–4; Ancker and Kaufman 2007; Cokely et al.

Table 14.1 Transparent information formats diminish differences between countries: Percentage of people in the USA and Germany who accurately understood health risks presented in different formats

Health-related problem	USA (%)	Germany (%)	Absolute difference in percentage points
Understood that the base rate of a disease is needed to determine the benefit of prevention (Chap. 7)			
Without analogies	55	34	21
With analogies	70	55	15
Understood that the positive predictive value is needed to determine the benefit of screening tests (Chap. 7)			
Without analogies	68	72	4
With analogies	81	79	2
Understood the consequences of health-related behaviors (overweight and exercise; Chap. 8)			
Risk of disease in percentages	70	66	4
Life expectancy in months	87	88	1
Understood the magnitude of risk reduction (Chap. 9)			
Numerical	29	40	11
Numerical + graphical (bar graphs or icon arrays)	54	53	1
Understood that group size (denominator) is important when comparing risks in two groups of unequal size (Chap. 10)			
Numerical	47	60	13
Numerical + graphical (icon arrays)	69	74	5
Avoided being influenced by positive or negative information frames when evaluating medical risks (Chap. 11)			
Numerical	44	55	11
Numerical + graphical (icon arrays, bar, or pie charts)	67	70	3

2012; Galesic and Garcia-Retamero 2010, 2011; Lipkus et al. 2001; Peters et al. 2007; Schwartz et al. 1997) profited *more* from transparent information formats than those with high risk literacy (Chaps. 7–11). This is a promising result because it shows that low risk literacy—prevalent in all the cultures we studied (see Chaps. 2–4)—is not necessarily an obstacle to informed and shared decision making about health (Chap. 13).

The third noteworthy result is that transparent information formats reduce or eliminate differences in the understanding of risk information and decision making between cultures. To illustrate, Table 14.1 summarizes the success of the different information formats that we have investigated. As can be seen, once information is presented transparently, cross-cultural differences in understanding largely vanish, and the level of overall understanding increases substantially. It follows that cultural differences in risk perception—aside from those that produce differences in risk literacy—often have a relatively small influence on understanding of transparently communicated health risks. Thus, for effective communication in the globalized world—where the same message about a health risk may be received in different countries—it is important to use transparent information formats. Even within the

Table 14.2 Transparent information formats improved communication with nonnative speakers within a country: Percentage of Polish immigrants in the UK who accurately understood health risks presented in different formats and languages

Health-related problem	Native language (Polish) (%)	Nonnative language (English) (%)	Absolute difference in percentage points
Understood the magnitude of absolute risk reduction (Chap. 9)			
Numerical	77	58	19
Numerical + graphical	83	85	2
Understood that group size (denominator) is important when comparing risks in two groups of unequal size (Chap. 10)			
Numerical	60	27	33
Numerical + graphical	81	83	2

same country a transparent format can improve communication with different cultural groups (Garcia-Retamero and Dhami 2011). For instance, in a study described in Chap. 10, visual aids helped nonnative English speakers living in the UK understand risk information presented either in English or in their native language, Polish (Table 14.2).

14.2 Open Avenues for Future Research

To the best of our knowledge, our book is the first to present a collection of studies showing that using transparent information formats not only improves risk communication but also helps alleviate cross-cultural differences in the understanding of health risks (Douglas and Wildawsky 1983; Garcia-Retamero et al. 2011; Renn and Rohrmann 2000). These formats (see Table 14.1) can help health professionals and organizations communicate transparently in the global community that is our world today. At the same time, our work reveals some questions that remain open for further investigation. In what follows, we describe several important areas in which research still needs to be conducted. Our aim is not to present an exhaustive list of avenues for future research; rather we intend to provide some initial ideas to encourage further theoretical and empirical work.

14.2.1 Risk Understanding Across the Life-Span

What are the developmental precursors of limited numeracy and graph literacy? Future research should explore the age-related changes in numeracy and graph literacy throughout the life-span, as well as the role of cultural factors in the development of these skills. How do children acquire health-related knowledge as they age—through the media or family socialization? Is the nature of limited risk literacy in older adults different from that in younger populations? More studies are also needed on the effectiveness of interventions aimed at increasing risk literacy or reducing its impact for different age groups (e.g., Galesic et al. 2009; Zhu and Gigerenzer 2006).

14.2.2 Use of the Media to Communicate Health Risks

Risk information available in the media may have different effects on patients' communication with physicians in different cultures (Gigerenzer et al. 2009; Groman et al. 2004). More studies are needed on the use of media to inform patients who vary in cultural background, numeracy, graph literacy, age, race, ethnicity, and health status (Andrulis et al. 2007; James et al. 2007; Sudore et al. 2009). Studies should also evaluate the role of information technology in seeking, accessing, and interpreting relevant health information in patients with different cultural backgrounds and levels of numeracy (Vaughn 1995). Finally, studies are needed to examine how the design and structure of a health care system can support the information needs of patients with different levels of numeracy.

14.2.3 Cognitive Processes Underlying the Understanding of Transparent Information Formats in Patients with Different Levels of Numeracy and Graph Literacy

What cognitive processes underlie the differences in understanding of health risks in patients with different levels of numeracy and graph literacy? Can theories of graph comprehension (e.g., Carpenter and Shah 1998; Cooper et al. 2003; Friel et al. 2001) contribute to our understanding of why visual aids are particularly beneficial for communicating health risks? Do patients with low graph literacy rely more on spatial-to-conceptual mappings when interpreting graphs than those with higher graph literacy (e.g., see Okan et al. 2012)? Studies recording patients' eye movements while they explore graphs may be particularly useful in this regard (see Okan et al. 2010, Woller-Carter et al. 2012 for this approach).

14.2.4 Impact and Consequences of Limited Numeracy and Graph Literacy

Do health professionals possess adequate communication skills for adapting to the communication needs of patients with limited numeracy and graph literacy (Donelle et al. 2008)? What is the impact of patients' limited numeracy and graph literacy on their adherence to health recommendations, engagement in health care, and use of health technologies (see Amalraj et al. 2009; Apter et al. 2006; Estrada et al. 2004 for some preliminary results)? Finally, what are the costs of limited numeracy and graph literacy from the social and organizational points of view?

14.2.5 Education and Training

What is and could be the role of educational systems in different countries in increasing levels of numeracy and graph literacy and improving health communication skills? Studies are needed to implement and evaluate training programs for community health professionals to improve these skills (Murray et al. 2010). Initiatives to increase numeracy and graph literacy through adult education programs, such as promoting access to simple and free interactive information on the Internet, should also be evaluated (e.g., via sites like riskliteracy.org; Cokely et al. 2012).

14.2.6 Intervention in Health Systems

Future research should implement and evaluate interventions aimed at increasing numeracy and graph literacy in the general public and in the health care system (Paling 2003). For example, what health care system designs support the information needs of patients with different levels of numeracy and graph literacy? Research should also determine the best methods of developing and disseminating effective information sources and materials for audiences with different levels of risk literacy and from different cultural backgrounds. For instance, how should prevention campaigns be designed to effectively communicate with audiences with differing levels of numeracy and graph literacy? Finally, research should investigate the ability of patients with different levels of risk literacy to understand and navigate health insurance options and benefits and how this impacts the use of health services as well as health outcomes.

14.2.7 Research in Other Cultures

As we mentioned in Chap. 1, cultural specifics of living in a certain country can shape people's health-related knowledge and behaviors. Many studies collected in this book compared two or more countries, including a number of European and Asian countries and the USA. Research on health-risk understanding and medical decision making still remains to be conducted beyond these countries. African and Latin American countries, for instance, critically differ from the countries we considered in a number of ways that can affect risk perception and decision making about health (Huerta and Macario 1999; Larkey and Gonzalez 2007). In particular, their citizens might differ in their level of risk literacy, and websites, forums, and blogs providing health information might be less common (Taylor-Clark et al. 2007; Ward et al. 1997). Efforts investigating risk understanding and medical decision making in these countries should help scientists design even more transparent formats to communicate risks related to health across the globalized world.

14.3 Conclusions

In this book we aimed at providing a set of guidelines for (1) helping patients understand risks and make better decisions about their health, (2) helping health professionals improve the way risk information is communicated, and (3) stimulating researchers to explore a number of remaining open questions about risk perception and communication in different cultures. Our studies emphasize the importance and value of working toward the development of tailored risk communication interventions that are sensitive to the various needs and abilities of diverse individuals who must make potentially life-changing decisions about their health. In addition, our research has prescriptive implications for the design of transparent health brochures and Internet-based tools that improve the comprehension of medical information among patients across the full range of abilities (e.g., low to high levels of numeracy and graph literacy). Our recommendations for improving risk perception and communication can help promote shared decision making between doctors and patients, which has been advocated as the ideal method for medical decisions (Edwards et al. 2004; Heesen et al. 2007).

From a theoretical point of view, our studies provide additional converging evidence on the utility of the ecological approach to communicating risks, which has already led to important theoretical and practical applications in medicine, law, and education (see Gigerenzer 2000, 2007, 2008; Gigerenzer and Engel 2006; Gigerenzer and Gaissmaier 2011; Gigerenzer et al. 1999, 2010, 2011). Critically, the ecological approach suggests that problems in understanding relevant health information often do not reside in people's mind, but in the representation of the task. This approach emphasizes the importance of considering the fit between people, their cognitive processes, and task environments when designing interventions (Gigerenzer and Edwards 2003). With results supporting the ecological approach, our studies converged to demonstrate that information formats that exploit people's inherent capacity to recognize relationships in naturally occurring problems (i.e., transparent information formats) can dramatically enhance risk comprehension, communication, and recall and foster better decisions in a wide range of cultures.

Finally, the guidelines in this book have implications for other areas of everyday life in which risk information is presented to the general public. These areas include education and psychology, economics and finance, and climate science and engineering. Transparent information formats can be a starting point for improving risk communication and promoting interdisciplinary research in these domains. Designing good information formats will only be possible if scientists from these areas look beyond the boundaries of their own disciplines and share their ideas and expertise to achieve a common goal: transparent communication of risks across cultures.

We hope that our work will inspire further applied and theoretical studies on efficient and effective ways to communicate risks to a wide range of people around the world. We believe that the studies presented in this book are a good first step toward promoting risk understanding and good decision making at little cost.

References

Amalraj, S., Starkweather, C., Nguyen, C., & Naeim, A. (2009). Health literacy, communication, and treatment decision-making in older cancer patients. *Oncology, 23*, 369–375.

Ancker, J. S., & Kaufman, D. (2007). Rethinking health numeracy: A multidisciplinary literature review. *Journal of the American Medical Informatics Association, 14*, 713–721.

Andrulis, D. P., Siddiqui, N. J., & Gantner, J. L. (2007). Preparing racially and ethnically diverse communities for public health emergencies. *Health Affairs, 26*, 1269–1279.

Apter, A. J., Cheng, J., Small, D., Bennett, I. M., Albert, C., Fein, D. G., et al. (2006). Asthma numeracy skill and health literacy. *The Journal of Asthma, 43*, 705–710.

Barry, M. J. (1999). Involving patients in medical decisions: How can physicians do better? *Journal of the American Medical Association, 282*, 2356–2357.

Brody, D. S., Miller, S. M., Lerman, C. E., Smith, D. G., Lazaro, C. G., & Blum, M. J. (1989). The relationship between patients' satisfaction with their physicians and perceptions about interventions they desired and received. *Medical Care, 11*, 1027–1035.

Carpenter, P. A., & Shah, P. (1998). A model of the perceptual and conceptual processes in graph comprehension. *Journal of Experimental Psychology: Applied, 4*, 75–100.

Cokely, E. T., Galesic, M. Schulz, E., Ghazal, S., & Garcia-Retamero, R. (2012). The Berlin Numeracy Test: A three minute adaptive test of risk literacy for highly educated samples. *Judgment and Decision Making, 7*, 25–47.

Cooper, R. J., Schriger, D. L., Wallace, R. C., Mikulich, V. J., & Wilkes, M. S. (2003). The quantity and quality of scientific graphs in pharmaceutical advertisements. *Journal of General Internal Medicine, 18*, 294–297.

Donelle, L., Arocha, J. F., & Hoffman-Goetz, L. (2008). Health literacy and numeracy: Key factors in cancer risk comprehension. *Chronic Diseases in Canada, 29*, 1–8.

Douglas, M., & Wildawsky, A. (1983). *Risk and culture: An essay on the selection of technological and environmental dangers*. Berkely, CA: University of California Press.

Edwards, A., Elwyn, G., Hood, K., Atwell, C., Robling, M., Houston, H., et al. (2004). Patient-based outcome results from a cluster randomized trial of shared decision making skill development and use of risk communication aids in general practice. *Family Practice, 21*, 347–354.

Edwards, A., Elwyn, G., & Mulley, A. (2002). Explaining risks: Turning numerical data into meaningful pictures. *British Medical Journal, 324*, 827–830.

Estrada, C. A., Martin-Hryniewicz, M., Peek, B. T., Collin, C., & Byrd, J. C. (2004). Literacy and numeracy skills and anticoagulation control. *The American Journal of the Medical Sciences, 328*, 88–93.

Fagerlin, A., Sepucha, K. R., Couper, M., Levin, C. A., Singer, E., & Zikmund-Fisher, B. J. (2010). Patients' knowledge about 9 common health conditions: The DECISIONS survey. *Medical Decision Making, 30*, 35S–52S.

Fagerlin, A., Ubel, P. A., Smith, D. M., & Zikmund-Fisher, B. J. (2007). Making numbers matter: Present and future research in risk communication. *American Journal of Health Behavior, 31*, 47–56.

Friel, S. N., Curcio, F. R., & Bright, G. W. (2001). Making sense of graphs: Critical factors influencing comprehension and instructional implications. *Journal for Research in Mathematics Education, 32*, 124–158.

Frosch, D. L., & Kaplan, R. M. (1999). Shared decision making in clinical medicine: Past research and future directions. *American Journal of Preventive Medicine, 17*, 285–294.

Galesic, M., & Garcia-Retamero, R. (2010). Statistical numeracy for health: A cross-cultural comparison with probabilistic national samples. *Archives of Internal Medicine, 170*, 462–468.

Galesic, M., & Garcia-Retamero, R. (2011). Graph literacy: A cross-cultural comparison. *Medical Decision Making, 31*, 444–457.

Galesic, M., Gigerenzer, G., & Straubinger, N. (2009). Natural frequencies help older adults and people with low numeracy to evaluate medical screening tests. *Medical Decision Making, 29*, 368–371.

Garcia-Retamero, R., & Dhami, M. K. (2011). Pictures speak louder than numbers: On communicating medical risks to immigrants with limited non-native language proficiency. *Health Expectations, 14*, 46–57.
Garcia-Retamero, R., & Galesic, M. (2009). Trust in healthcare. In M. W. Kattan (Ed.), *The encyclopedia of medical decision making* (pp. 1153–1155). Thousand Oaks: SAGE.
Garcia-Retamero, R., Galesic, M., & Gigerenzer, G. (2010). Do icon arrays help reduce denominator neglect? *Medical Decision Making, 30*, 672–684.
Garcia-Retamero, R., Galesic, M., & Gigerenzer, G. (2011). Enhancing understanding and recall of quantitative information about medical risks: A cross-cultural comparison between Germany and Spain. *The Spanish Journal of Psychology, 14*, 218–226.
Gigerenzer, G. (2000). *Adaptive thinking: Rationality in the real world*. New York: Oxford University Press.
Gigerenzer, G. (2002). *Calculated risks: How to know when numbers deceive you*. New York: Simon & Schuster.
Gigerenzer, G. (2007). *Gut feelings: The intelligence of the unconscious*. New York: Viking.
Gigerenzer, G. (2008). *Rationality for mortals*. New York: Oxford University Press.
Gigerenzer, G., & Edwards, A. (2003). Simple tools for understanding risks: From innumeracy to insight. *British Medical Journal, 327*, 741–744.
Gigerenzer, G., & Engel, C. (2006). *Heuristics and the law*. Cambridge: MIT Press.
Gigerenzer, G., & Gaissmaier, W. (2011). Heuristic decision making. *Annual Review of Psychology, 62*, 451–482.
Gigerenzer, G., Gaissmaier, W., Kurz-Milcke, E., Schwartz, L. M., & Woloshin, S. (2007). Helping doctors and patients make sense of health statistics. *Psychological Science in the Public Interest, 8*, 53–96.
Gigerenzer, G., & Gray, J. A. M. (2011). *Better doctors, better patients, better decisions: Envisioning Health Care 2020* (Strüngemann Forum Report, Vol. 6). Cambridge: MIT Press.
Gigerenzer, G., Hertwig, R., & Pachur, T. (2011). *Heuristics: The foundations of adaptive behavior*. New York: Oxford University Press.
Gigerenzer, G., Mata, J., & Frank, R. (2009). Public knowledge of benefits of breast and prostate cancer screening in Europe. *Journal of the National Cancer Institute, 101*, 1216–1220.
Gigerenzer, G., Todd, P. M., & the ABC Research Group. (1999). *Simple heuristics that make us smart*. New York: Oxford University Press.
Gigerenzer, G., Wegwarth, O., & Feufel, M. (2010). Misleading communication of risk. *British Medical Journal, 341*, 791–792.
Groman, R., & Ginsburg, J., & The American College of Physicians (2004). Racial and ethnic disparities in health care: A position paper of the American college of physicians. *Annals of Internal Medicine, 141*, 226–232.
Hanson, J. L. (2008). Shared decision making: Have we missed the obvious? *Archives of Internal Medicine, 168*, 1368–1370.
Heesen, C., Kopke, S., Richter, T., & Kasper, J. (2007). Shared decision making and self-management in multiple sclerosis—a consequence of evidence. *Journal of Neurology, 254*, 116–121.
Huerta, E. E., & Macario, E. (1999). Communicating health risk to ethnic groups: Reaching Hispanics as a case study. *Journal of the National Cancer Institute Monographs, 25*, 23–26.
James, X., Hawkins, A., & Rowel, R. (2007). An assessment of the cultural appropriateness of emergency preparedness communication for low income minorities. *Journal of Homeland Security and Emergency Management, 4*, 1–24.
Larkey, L. K., & Gonzalez, J. (2007). Storytelling for promoting colorectal cancer prevention and early detection among Latinos. *Patient Education and Counseling, 67*, 272–278.
Lipkus, I. M. (2007). Numeric, verbal, and visual formats of conveying health risks: Suggested best practices and future recommendations. *Medical Decision Making, 27*, 696–713.
Lipkus, I. M., & Peters, E. (2009). Framework and practical insights understanding the role of numeracy in health: Proposed theoretical insights. *Health Education and Behavior, 36*, 1065–1081.

Lipkus, I. M., Samsa, G., & Rimer, B. K. (2001). General performance on a numeracy scale among highly educated samples. *Medical Decision Making, 21*, 37–44.
Murray, A. S., Stevenson, E., Kerr, F., & Burns, C. (2010). "A heartbeat moment:" Qualitative study of GP views of patients bringing health information from the internet to a consultation. *The British Journal of General Practice, 60*, 88–94.
Okan, Y., Galesic, M., & Garcia-Retamero. (2010). Graph comprehension in medical contexts: An eye-tracking study. 13th Biennial European Conference of the Society for Medical Decision Making. *Hall in Tyrol*, Austria.
Okan, Y., Garcia-Retamero, R., Galesic, M., & Cokely, E. (2012). When higher bars do not represent larger quantities: On individual differences in the use of spatial-to-conceptual mappings in graph comprehension. *Spatial Cognition and Computation, 12*, 195–218.
Paling, J. (2003). Strategies to help patients understand risks. *British Medical Journal, 327*, 745–748.
Peters, E., Hibbard, J. H., Slovic, P., & Dieckmann, N. F. (2007). Numeracy skill and the communication, comprehension, and use of risk and benefit information. *Health Affairs, 26*, 741–748.
Peters, E., Västfjäll, D., Slovic, P., Mertz, C. K., Mazzocco, K., & Dickert, S. (2006). Numeracy and decision making. *Psychological Science, 17*, 407–413.
Renn, O., & Rohrmann, B. (2000). *Cross-cultural risk perception: A survey of empirical studies*. Dordrecht: Kluwer.
Reyna, V. R., Nelson, W. L., Han, P., & Dieckmann, N. F. (2009). How numeracy influences risk comprehension and medical decision making. *Psychological Bulletin, 135*, 943–973.
Schwartz, L. M., Woloshin, S., Black, W. C., & Welch, H. G. (1997). The role of numeracy in understanding the benefit of screening mammography. *Annals of Internal Medicine, 127*, 966–972.
Sudore, R. L., Landefeld, C. S., Pérez-Stable, E. J., Bibbins-Domingo, K., Williams, B. A., & Schillinger, D. (2009). Unraveling the relationship between literacy, language proficiency, and patient–physician communication. *Patient Education and Counseling, 75*, 398–402.
Taylor-Clark, K., Koh, H., & Viswanath, K. (2007). Perceptions of environmental health risks and communication barriers among low-SEP and racial/ethnic minority communities. *Journal of Health Care for the Poor and Underserved, 18*, 165–183.
Vaughn, E. (1995). The significance of socioeconomic and ethnic diversity for the risk communication process. *Risk Analysis, 15*, 169–180.
Ward, B., Bertera, E. M., & Hoge, P. (1997). Developing and evaluating a Spanish TEL-MED message on breast cancer. *Journal of Community Health, 22*, 127–135.
Woller-Carter, M. M., Okan, Y., Cokely, E. T., & Garcia-Retamero, R. (2012). Communicating risks with graphs: An eye-tracking study. *Proceedings of the Human Factors and Ergonomics Society Annual Meeting, 56*, 1723–1727.
Zhu, L., & Gigerenzer, G. (2006). Children can solve Bayesian problems: The role of representation in mental computation. *Cognition, 98*, 287–308.

Chapter 15
Appendix: Numeracy and Graph Literacy Scales

15.1 Introduction

In the Appendix, we present four scales used in many of the studies reported in this book, each in English, German, and Spanish. The scales have promising psychometric properties and are suitable for use in most clinical and research circumstances. They were originally developed in English and translated into German and Spanish by a native speaker with excellent knowledge of English, back-translated into English by another person with equivalent language skills, and compared with the original English version. Any inconsistencies were resolved by a native speaker and an excellent English speaker familiar with the research objectives. Finally, the English, German, and Spanish versions were compared and edited by a bilingual German–English or Spanish–English speaker.

We first present an objective numeracy scale that consists of nine items adapted from Schwartz et al. (1997) and Lipkus et al. (2001; see Galesic and Garcia-Retamero 2010 and Chap. 2). The items of this scale were selected based on their correlation with the total score, other items, and their difficulty, as found in a pilot study conducted on samples drawn from opt-in Web panels in Germany ($n=461$) and the USA These items were used successfuly to differentiate low and high numeracy people in a number of studies in Germany, the USA, and Spain (Galesic and Garcia-Retamero 2011a, b; Garcia-Retamero and Cokely 2012; Garcia-Retamero and Galesic 2009, 2010a, b, 2011).

Second, we present a subjective numeracy scale adapted from Fagerlin et al. (2007) and Zikmund-Fisher et al. (2007) that consists of seven items. Our research showed that measures of numeracy using this scale correspond to objective measures and are not dependent on the context in which they are measured (e.g., before or after answering several difficult numerical questions), which speak to its wide applicability (Galesic and Garcia-Retamero 2010).

Third, we present the Berlin Numeracy Test (Cokely et al. 2012), a psychometrically sound statistical numeracy test that could be used with highly educated,

R. Garcia-Retamero and M. Galesic (eds.), *Transparent Communication of Health Risks: Overcoming Cultural Differences*, DOI 10.1007/978-1-4614-4358-2_15,

high-ability samples. To complete the test, participants are asked 2–3 questions (of four possible questions). Questions are adaptively selected based on participants' past success in answering previous questions using an adaptive scoring algorithm (see Fig. 3.1 for test structure). Cokely and colleagues conducted 21 validation studies showing that the Berlin Numeracy Test provides sound assessment with high discriminability across diverse samples, cultures, education levels, and languages (see Chap. 3).

Finally, we present a graph literacy scale developed by Galesic and Garcia-Retamero (2011c, see also Chap. 4). The scale consists of 13 items and measures three abilities related to graph comprehension (see Friel et al. 2001) (1) the ability to *read the data*, that is, to find specific information in the graph; (2) the ability to *read between the data*, that is, to find relationships in the data as shown on the graph; and (3) the ability to *read beyond the data*, or make inferences and predictions from the data. The graph literacy scale was validated in a survey conducted on probabilistic national samples in Germany and the USA (Galesic and Garcia-Retamero 2011c; Garcia-Retamero and Galesic 2010b). The scale was also successfully used in Spain (Okan et al. 2012).

15.2 Objective Numeracy Scale in English

Q1. Imagine that we flip a fair coin 1,000 times. What is your best guess about how many times the coin would come up heads in 1,000 flips?
_______ times out of 1,000 (*Correct answer: ≥400 and ≤600*)

Q2. In the Bingo Lottery, the chance of winning a $10 prize is 1 %. What is your best guess about how many people would win a $10 prize if 1,000 people each buy a single ticket to Bingo Lottery?
_______ person(s) out of 1,000 (*Correct answer: 10*)

Q3. In Daily Times Sweepstakes, the chance of winning a car is 1 in 1,000. What percent of tickets to Daily Times Sweepstakes win a car?
_______ % of tickets (*Correct answer: 0.1*)

Q4. Imagine that we roll a fair, six-sided die 1,000 times. Out of 1,000 rolls, how many times do you think the die would come up even (2, 4, or 6)?
_______ times out of 1,000 (*Correct answer: ≥400 and ≤600*)

Q5. Which of the following numbers represents the biggest risk of getting a disease? (*order of options randomized*) (*Correct answer: a*)
(a) 1 in 10
(b) 1 in 100
(c) 1 in 1,000

Q6. Which of the following represents the biggest risk of getting a disease? (*order of options randomized*) (*Correct answer: c*)
(a) 1 %
(b) 5 %
(c) 10 %

Q7. If the chance of getting a disease is 10 %, how many people would be expected to get the disease out of 1,000?
_______ people (*Correct answer: 100*)

Q8. If the chance of getting a disease is 20 out of 100, this would be the same as having a _______% chance of getting the disease. (*Correct answer: 20*)

Q9. If Person A's chance of getting a disease is 1 in 100 in 10 years, and Person B's risk is double that of A, what is B's risk?
_______ (*Correct answer: 2 % in 10 years, or 2 in 100 in 10 years, or 1 % in 5 years, or 1 in 100 in 5 years*)

15.3 Objective Numeracy Scale in German

Q1. Stellen Sie sich vor, wir werfen ein normale Münze 1.000 mal. Einmal angenommen, auf einer Seite ist ein Kopf abgebildet: Wie viele Male, denken Sie, wird die Münze mit dem Kopf oben landen?
_______ Mal von 1.000 (*Correct answer: ≥400 and ≤600*)

Q2. Bei einer Bingo-Lotterie liegt die Chance, €10 zu gewinnen, bei 1 %. Was schätzen Sie: Wie viele von 1.000 Leuten werden diese €10 gewinnen, wenn jeder ein Einzel-Ticket für die Bingo-Lotterie kauft?
_______ Person(en) von 1.000 (*Correct answer: 10*)

Q3. Bei einer Verlosung ist die Chance, ein Auto zu gewinnen, 1 zu 1.000. Wieviel Prozent der Lose gewinnen ein Auto?
_______ % der Lose (*Correct answer: 0.1*)

Q4. Stellen Sie sich vor, wir werfen einen normalen, sechsseitigen Würfel 1.000 mal. Was meinen Sie: Bei wie vielen dieser 1.000 Würfe wird er eine gerade Zahl zeigen (also 2, 4 oder 6)?
_______ Mal von 1.000 (*Correct answer: ≥400 and ≤600*)

Q5. Welche der folgenden Angaben repräsentiert das größte Risiko, eine Krankheit zu bekommen? (*order of options randomized*) (*Correct answer: a*)
(a) 1 in 10
(b) 1 in 100
(c) 1 in 1.000

Q6. Welche der folgenden Angaben repräsentiert das größte Risiko, eine Krankheit zu bekommen? (*order of options randomized*) (*Correct answer: c*)
(a) 1 %
(b) 5 %
(c) 10 %

Q7. Wenn die Wahrscheinlichkeit, eine Krankheit zu bekommen, 10 % beträgt, was ist zu erwarten: Wie viele von 1.000 Menschen werden die Krankheit bekommen?
_______ Menschen (*Correct answer: 100*)

Q8. Wenn die Wahrscheinlichkeit, eine Krankheit zu bekommen, bei 20 von 100 liegt, dann entspricht das einer Wahrscheinlichkeit von _______ %, die Krankheit zu bekommen. (*Correct answer: 20*)

Q9. Wenn die Wahrscheinlichkeit für Person A, eine Krankheit zu bekommen, bei 1 von 100 in 10 Jahren liegt und die Wahrscheinlichkeit für Person B doppelt so hoch ist wie für A: Wie hoch ist dann die Wahrscheinlichkeit für B?
_______ (*Correct answer: 2 % in 10 years, or 2 in 100 in 10 years, or 1 % in 5 years, or 1 in 100 in 5 years*)

15.4 Objective Numeracy Scale in Spanish

Q1. Imagine que lanzamos una moneda no trucada en 1.000 ocasiones. Haga una estimación: ¿Cuántas veces saldrá cara en los 1.000 intentos?
_______ veces en los 1.000 intentos (*Correct answer:* $\geq$*400 and* $\leq$*600*)

Q2. La probabilidad de ganar un premio de 10 Euros en la lotería es del 1 %. Haga una estimación: ¿Cuántas personas ganarán el premio de 10 Euros en un grupo de 1.000 personas si cada una compra una participación de lotería?
_______ persona(s) en un grupo de 1.000 (*Correct answer: 10*)

Q3. En un concurso de un periódico local la probabilidad de ganar un coche es de 1 entre 1.000. ¿Qué porcentaje de participaciones en dicho concurso ganaría el coche?
_______ % de las participaciones (*Correct answer: 0.1*)

Q4. Imagine que lanzamos un dado no trucado en 1.000 ocasiones. ¿En cuántas de estas 1.000 ocasiones cree que saldrá un número par (2, 4, 6)?
En _______ ocasiones de 1.000 (*Correct answer:* $\geq$*400 and* $\leq$*600*)

Q5. ¿Cuál de las siguientes cantidades representa un riesgo mayor de contraer una enfermedad? (*order of options randomized*) (*Correct answer: a*)
(a) 1 de 10
(b) 1 de 100
(c) 1 de 1.000

Q6. ¿Cuál de las siguientes cantidades representa un riesgo mayor de contraer una enfermedad? (*order of options randomized*) (*Correct answer: c*)
(a) 1 %
(b) 5 %
(c) 10 %

Q7. Si la probabilidad de contraer una enfermedad es del 10 %, ¿cuántas personas espera que contraigan la enfermedad en un grupo de 1,000?
_______ personas (*Correct answer: 100*)

Q8. Si la probabilidad de contraer una enfermedad es de 20 en 100, esto implicaría que hay una probabilidad del
_______ % de contraer la enfermedad. (*Correct answer: 20*)

Q9. Si el riesgo de que una persona llamada A contraiga una enfermedad es de 1 entre 100 en diez años, y el riesgo de que la contraiga una persona llamada B es el doble que A, ¿cuál es el riesgo de que la contraiga B?
_______ (*Correct answer: 2 % in 10 years, or 2 in 100 in 10 years, or 1 % in 5 years, or 1 in 100 in 5 years*)

15.5 Subjective Numeracy Scale in English

Q1. How good are you at working with fractions?
Not at all good—Extremely good (*six-point scale*)

Q2. How good are you at working with percentages?
Not at all good—Extremely good (*six-point scale*)

Q3. How good are you at figuring out how much a shirt will cost if it is 25 % off?
Not at all good—Extremely good (*six-point scale*)

Q4. When reading the newspaper, how helpful do you find tables and graphs that are parts of a story?
Not at all—Extremely (*six-point scale*)

Q5. When people tell you the chance of something happening, do you prefer that they use words ("it rarely happens") or numbers ("there's a 1 % chance")?
Always prefer words—Always prefer numbers (*six-point scale*)

Q6. When you hear a weather forecast, do you prefer predictions using percentages (e.g., "there will be a 20 % chance of rain today") or predictions using only words (e.g., "there is a small chance of rain today")?
Always prefer words—Always prefer percentages (*six-point scale*)

Q7. How often do you find numerical information to be useful?
Never—Very often (*six-point scale*)

15.6 Subjective Numeracy Scale in German

Q1.Wie gut sind Sie im Bruchrechnen?
sehr gut—überhaupt nicht gut (*six-point scale*)

Q2. Wie gut sind Sie im Umgang mit Prozentwerten?
sehr gut—überhaupt nicht gut (*six-point scale*)

Q3.Wie gut sind Sie darin einzuschätzen, wie viel ein Pullover bei einer 25 %-igen Preisreduzierung kosten wird?
sehr gut—gut überhaupt nicht gut (*six-point scale*)

Q4. Wenn Sie eine Tageszeitung lesen, wie nützlich finden Sie Tabellen und Diagramme als Teil eines Artikels?
überhaupt nicht nützlich—sehr nützlich (*six-point scale*)

Q5. Wenn Ihnen jemand etwas über die Wahrscheinlichkeit erzählt, dass ein bestimmtes Ereignis eintreffen wird, bevorzugen Sie es dann, wenn dazu Worte benutzt werden ("passiert selten") oder wenn Zahlenwerte benutzt werden ("es gibt eine 1 %-ige Wahrscheinlichkeit")?
Bevorzuge immer Worte—bevorzuge immer Zahlenwerte (*six-point scale*)

Q6. Wenn Sie den Wetterbericht hören, bevorzugen Sie es dann, wenn die Vorhersagen in Prozentwerten ausgedrückt werden (z.B. "es gibt heute eine 20%ige Regenwahrscheinlichkeit") oder in Worten (z.B. "heute ist die Regenwahrscheinlichkeit gering")?
Bevorzuge immer Worte—bevorzuge immer Prozentwerte (*six-point scale*)

Q7. Wie oft finden Sie Informationen, die in Zahlen ausgedrückt sind, nützlich?
nie—sehr oft (*six-point scale*)

15.7 Subjective Numeracy Scale in Spanish

Q1. ¿Hasta qué punto es usted bueno(a) haciendo cálculos con fracciones?
No soy bueno(a) en absoluto—Soy excelente (*six-point scale*)

Q2. ¿Hasta qué punto es usted bueno(a) haciendo cálculos con porcentajes?
No soy bueno(a) en absoluto—Soy excelente (*six-point scale*)

Q3. ¿Hasta qué punto es usted bueno(a) deduciendo el precio de una camisa que tiene una rebaja del 25 %?
No soy bueno(a) en absoluto—Soy excelente (*six-point scale*)

Q4. Cuando lee un periódico, ¿hasta qué punto le resultan útiles las tablas y gráficas que ilustran el texto?

No me resultan útiles en absoluto—Me resultan muy útiles (*six-point scale*)

Q5. Cuando alguien le dice la probabilidad de que ocurra algo, ¿prefiere que utilice palabras (por ejemplo, "ocurre raramente") o números (por ejemplo, "hay una probabilidad del 1 % de que ocurra")?
Siempre prefiero palabras—Siempre prefiero números (*six-point scale*)

Q6. Cuando escucha la predicción del tiempo, ¿prefiere que la hagan utilizando porcentajes (por ejemplo, "la probabilidad de que llueva hoy es del 20 %") o sólo palabras (por ejemplo, "la probabilidad de que llueva hoy es pequeña")?
Siempre prefiero palabras—Siempre prefiero porcentajes (*six-point scale*)

Q7. ¿Con qué frecuencia encuentra útil la información numérica?
Nunca—Muy frecuentemente (*six-point scale*)

15.8 Berlin Numeracy Test in English

Q1. Out of 1,000 people in a small town 500 are members of a choir. Out of these 500 members in a choir 100 are men. Out of the 500 inhabitants that are not in a choir 300 are men. What is the probability that a randomly drawn man is a member of the choir? Please indicate the probability in percent.
_______ (*Correct answer: 25 %*)

Q2a. Imagine we are throwing a five-sided die 50 times. On average, out of these 50 throws how many times would this five-sided die show an odd number (1, 3 or 5)?
_______ out of 50 throws (*Correct answer: 30*).

Q2b. Imagine we are throwing a loaded die (six sides). The probability that the die shows a six is twice as high as the probability of each of the other numbers. On average, out of 70 throws how many times would the die show the number 6?
_______ out of 70 throws (*Correct answer: 20*)

Q3. In a forest 20 % of mushrooms are red, 50 % brown, and 30 % white. A red mushroom is poisonous with a probability of 20 %. A mushroom that is not red is poisonous with a probability of 5 %. What is the probability that a poisonous mushroom in the forest is red?
_______ (*Correct answer: 50 %*)

15.9 Berlin Numeracy Test in German

Q1. Von 1.000 Leuten in einer Kleinstadt sind 500 Mitglied im Gesangsverein. Von diesen 500 Mitgliedern im Gesangsverein sind 100 Männer. Von den 500 Einwohnern, die nicht im Gesangsverein sind, sind 300 Männer. Wie groß ist die

Wahrscheinlichkeit, dass ein zufällig ausgewählter Mann ein Mitglied des Gesangsvereins ist?
______ (*Correct answer: 25 %*)

Q2a. Stellen Sie sich vor, wir werfen einen fünfseitigen Würfel 50 mal. Bei wie vielen dieser 50 Würfe würde dieser fünfseitige Würfel erwartungsgemäß eine ungerade Zahl zeigen (1, 3 oder 5)?
______ von 50 Würfen (*Correct answer: 30*)

Q2b. Stellen Sie sich vor, wir werfen einen gezinkten Würfel (6 Seiten). Die Wahrscheinlichkeit, dass der Würfel eine 6 zeigt, ist doppelt so hoch wie die Wahrscheinlichkeit jeder der anderen Zahlen. Von 70 Würfen, bei wie vielen dieser 70 Würfe würde dieser Würfel erwartungsgemäß eine 6 zeigen?
______ von 70 Würfen (*Correct answer: 20*)

Q3. In einem Wald sind 20 % der Pilze rot, 50 % braun und 30 % weiß. Ein roter Pilz ist mit einer Wahrscheinlichkeit von 20 % giftig. Ein Pilz, der nicht rot ist, ist mit einer Wahrscheinlichkeit von 5 % giftig. Wie hoch ist die Wahrscheinlichkeit, dass ein giftiger Pilz im Wald rot ist?
______ (*Correct answer: 50 %*)

15.10 Berlin Numeracy Test in Spanish

Q1. De las 1.000 personas que viven en un pequeño pueblo, 500 son miembros de un coro. De esos 500 miembros del coro, 100 son hombres. De los 500 habitantes que no pertenecen a un coro, 300 son hombres. ¿Cuál es la probabilidad de que un hombre seleccionado al azar sea miembro del coro? Por favor, indique la probabilidad empleando para ello un porcentaje.
______ (*Correct answer: 25 %*)

Q2a. Imagine que tiramos un dado de cinco caras 50 veces. En promedio, de estas 50 tiradas ¿cuántas veces cree que saldría un número impar (1, 3, o 5) en este dado de cinco caras?
______ de 50 tiradas (*Correct answer: 30*)

Q2a. Imagine que tiramos un dado trucado de 6 caras. La probabilidad de que salga un 6 al tirar el dado es el doble que la probabilidad de que salga uno de los demás números. En promedio, en 70 tiradas, ¿cuántas veces cree que saldría el número 6?
______ de 70 tiradas (*Correct answer: 20*)

Q3. En un bosque, el 20 % de las setas son rojas, el 50 % son marrones, y el 30 % son blancas. La probabilidad de que una seta roja sea venenosa es del 20 %. La

probabilidad de que una seta que no sea roja sea venenosa es del 5 %. ¿Cuál es la probabilidad de que en el bosque una seta venenosa sea roja?
______ (*Correct answer: 50 %*)

15.11 Graph Literacy Scale in English

Here is some information about cancer therapies.

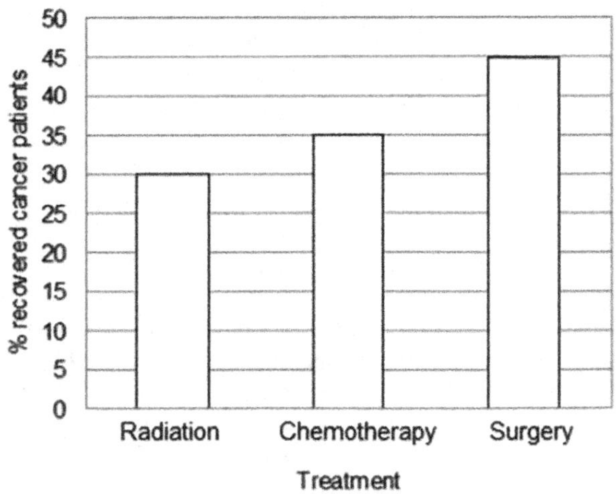

Q1. What percentage of patients recovered after chemotherapy?
______________% (*Correct answer: 35*)

Q2. What is the difference between the percentage of patients who recovered after a surgery and the percentage of patients who recovered after radiation therapy?
______________ (*Correct answer: 15*)

Here is some information about different forms of cancer.

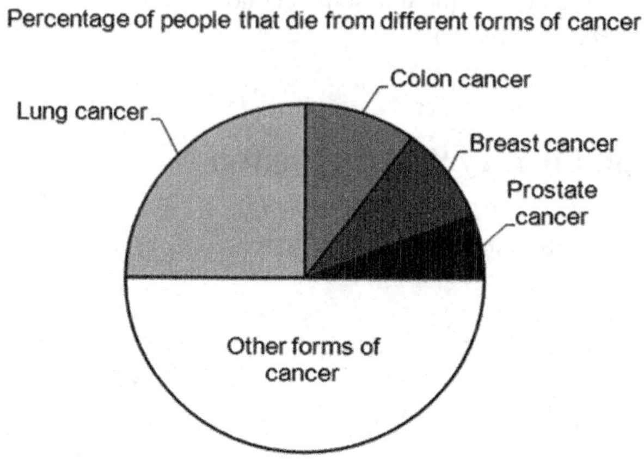

Q3. Of all the people who die from cancer, approximately what percentage dies from lung cancer? ________% (*Correct answer:* ≥*24 and* ≤*26*) Q4. Approximately what percentage of people who die from cancer die from colon cancer, breast cancer, and prostate cancer taken together? ________% (*Correct answer:* ≥*24 and* ≤*26*)

Here is some information about an imaginary disease called Adeolitis.

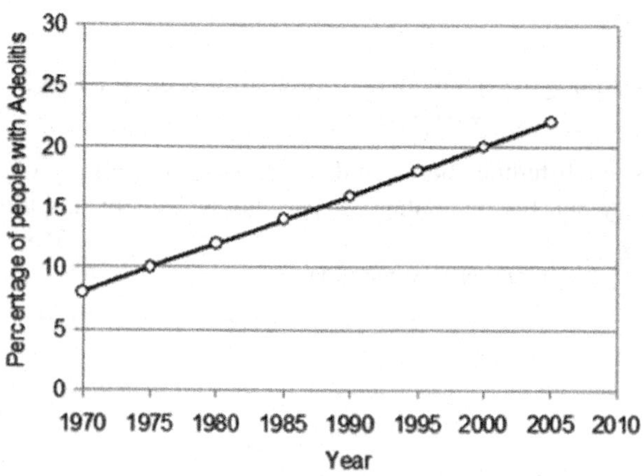

Q5. Approximately what percentage of people had Adeolitis in the year 2000?

_______________% (*Correct answer: 20*)

Q6. When was the increase in the percentage of people with Adeolitis higher? (*Correct answer: 3*)

From 1975 to 1980............................1
From 2000 to 2005............................2
Increase was the same in both intervals....3
Don't know.....................................4

Q7. According to your best guess, what will the percentage of people with Adeolitis be in the year 2010? (*Correct answer: ≥23 and ≤25*)

_______________%

The following figure shows the number of men and women among patients with disease X. The total number of circles is 100.

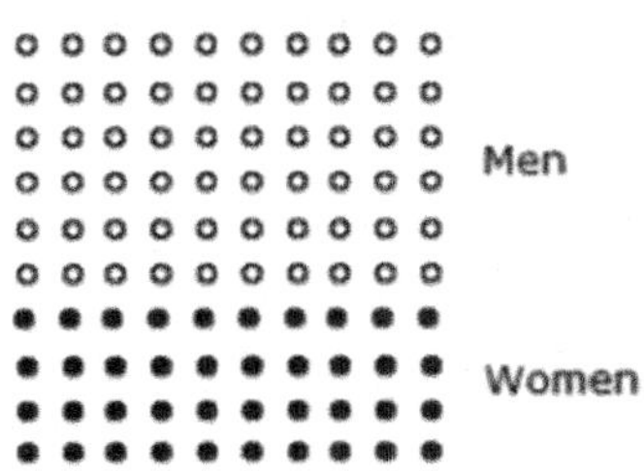

Q8. Of 100 patients with disease X, how many are women? (*Correct answer: 40*)

_______________women

Q9. How many more men than women are there among 100 patients with disease X? (*Correct answer: 20*)

_______________ men

In a magazine you see two advertisements, one on page 5 and another on page 12. Each is for a different drug for treating heart disease, and each includes a graph showing the effectiveness of the drug compared to a placebo (sugar pill).

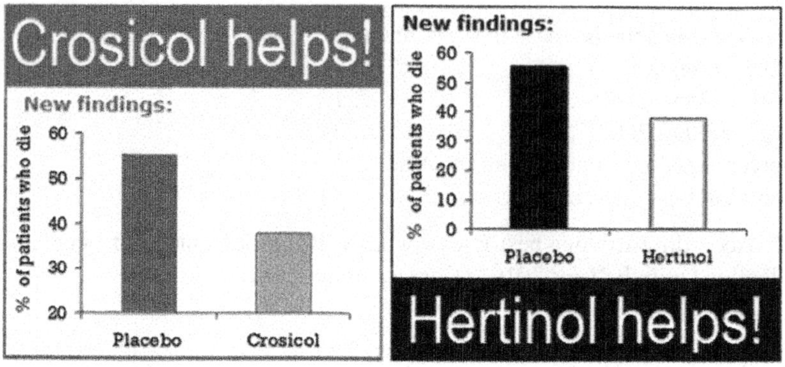

Q10. Compared to the placebo, which treatment leads to a larger decrease in the percentage of patients who die? (*Correct answer: 3*)
Crosicol…....................1
Hertinol…………………2
They are equal…….........3
Can't say……..…………4

In a newspaper you see two advertisements, one on page 15 and another on page 17. Each is for a different treatment of psoriasis, and each includes a graph showing the effectiveness of the treatment over time.

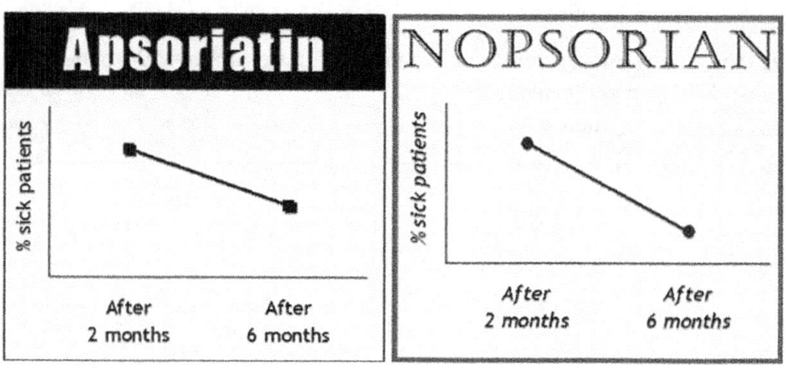

Q11. Which of the treatments contributes to a larger decrease in the percentage of sick patients? (*Correct answer: 4*)
Apsoriatin 1
Nopsorian 2
They are equal..............3
Can't say.....................4

Here is some information about the imaginary diseases Coliosis and Tiosis.

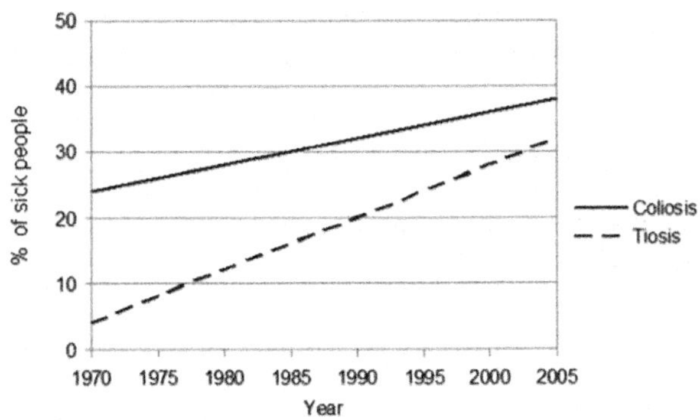

Q12. Between 1980 and 1990, which disease had a higher increase in the percentage of people affected? (*Correct answer: 2*)
Coliosis 1
Tiosis 2
The increase was equal.......3
Can't say.........................4

Here is some information about cancer therapies.

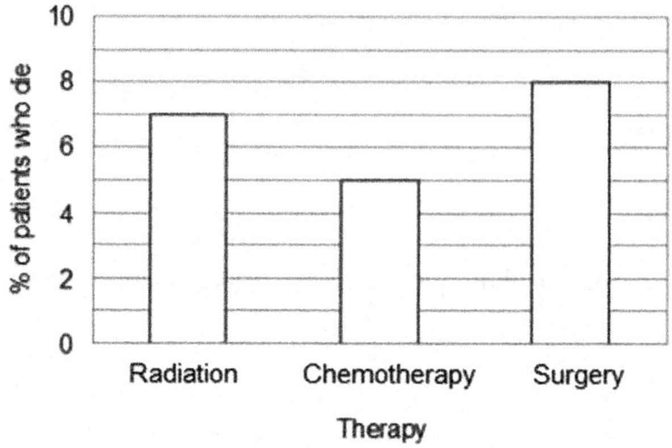

Q13. What is the percentage of cancer patients who die after chemotherapy?
(*Correct answer: 5*)
_______________%

15.12 Graph Literacy Scale in German

Sie erhalten nun einige Informationen über Krebsbehandlungen.

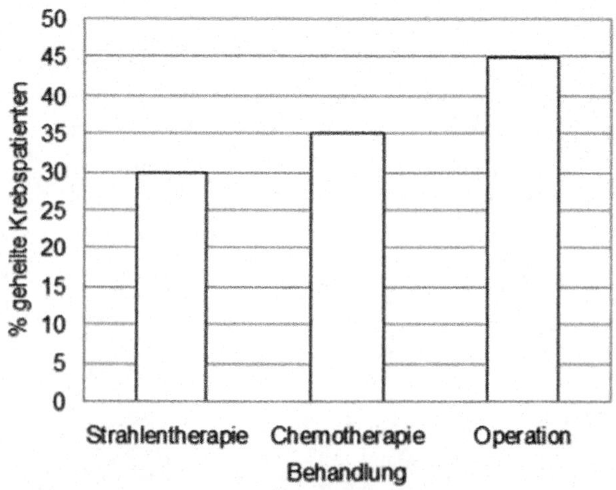

Q1. Wie hoch ist der Prozentanteil der Patienten, die nach einer Chemotherapie geheilt waren?
_______________% (*Correct answer: 35*)

Q2. Wie groß ist der Unterschied zwischen dem Prozentanteil von Patienten, die nach einer Operation geheilt waren und dem Prozentanteil von Patienten, die nach einer Strahlentherapie geheilt waren?
_______________ (*Correct answer: 15*)

Sie erhalten nun einige Informationen über Krebserkrankungen.

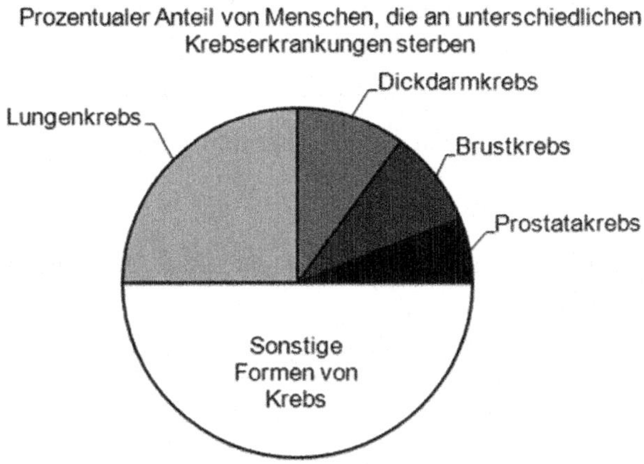

Q3. Von allen Menschen, die an Krebs sterben: Ungefähr welcher Prozentanteil von ihnen stirbt an Lungenkrebs?
________% (*Correct answer:* $\geq$*24 and* $\leq$*26*)

Q4. Von allen Menschen, die an Krebs sterben: Ungefähr welcher Prozentanteil von ihnen stirbt an Dickdarmkrebs, Brustkrebs und Prostatakrebs zusammengenommen?
________% (*Correct answer:* $\geq$*24 and* $\leq$*26*)

Sie erhalten nun einige Informationen zu einer fiktiven Krankheit namens Adeolitis.

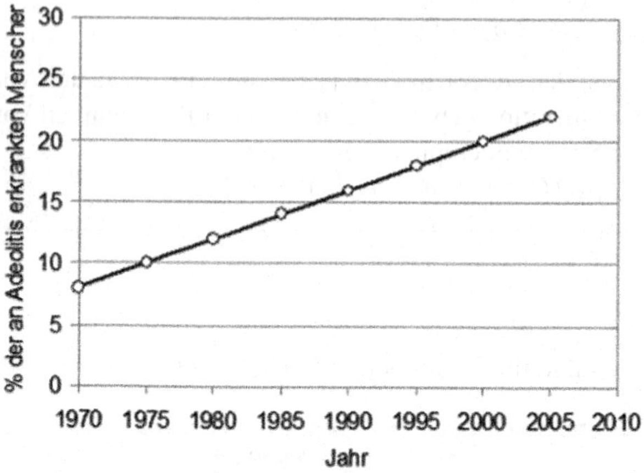

Q5. Ungefähr welcher Prozentanteil der Menschen litt im Jahr 2000 an Adeolitis?

______________% (*Correct answer: 20*)

Q6. In welchem Zeitraum stieg der Prozentanteil von Menschen mit Adeolitis stärker? (*Correct answer: 3*)

von 1975 bis 1980.......................................1
von 2000 bis 2005.......................................2
die Steigerung war in beiden Zeiträumen gleich hoch..3
weiß ich nicht 4

Q7. Was schätzen Sie: Welcher Prozentanteil der Menschen wird im Jahr 2010 an Adeolitis leiden? (*Correct answer: ≥23 and ≤25*)

______________%

Die folgende Abbildung zeigt, wie viele Männer und Frauen es unter den Patienten gibt, die unter der Krankheit X leiden. Die Summe der Kreise ist 100.

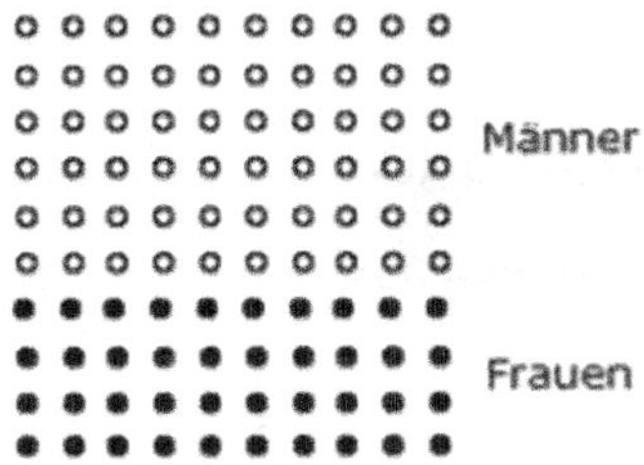

Q8. Wie viele Frauen befinden sich unter 100 Patienten mit der Krankheit X? (*Correct answer: 40*)
______________Frauen

Q9. Wie viel mehr Männer als Frauen sind unter den 100 Patienten mit der Krankheit X? (*Correct answer: 20*)
______________ Männer

In einer Zeitschrift sehen Sie zwei Anzeigen. Jede wirbt für ein anderes Medikament gegen Herzerkrankungen. In jeder wird ein Schaubild gezeigt, das die Wirksamkeit dieses Medikamentes im Vergleich zu einem Placebo, also einer Pille aus Zucker, verdeutlicht.

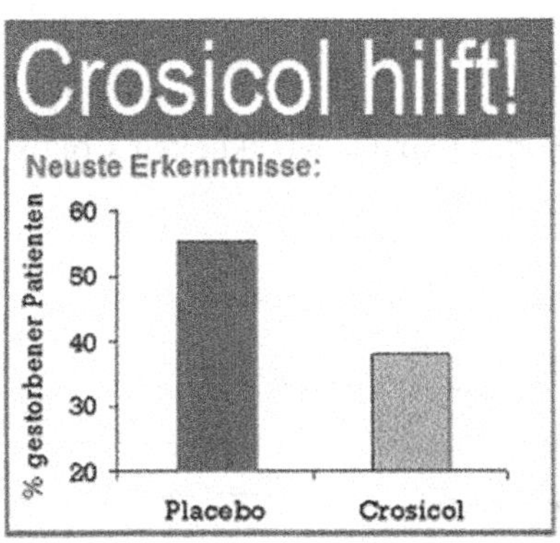

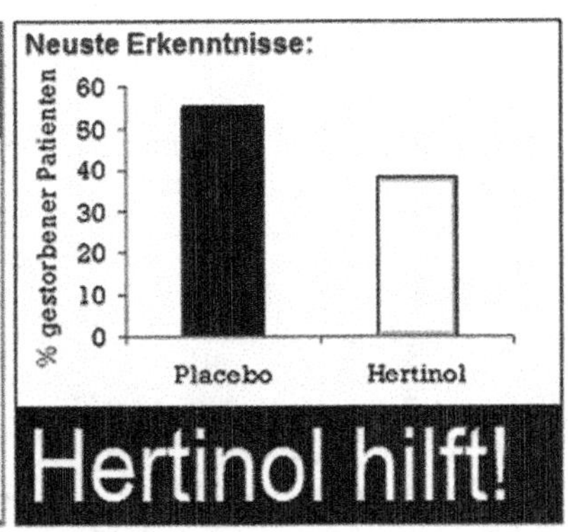

Q10. Im Vergleich zum Placebo: Bei welchem Medikament sinkt der Prozentanteil der Patienten, die sterben, stärker? (*Correct answer: 3*)
Crosicol.......................1
Hertinol.......................2
Bei beiden gleich.............3
Kann man nicht sagen.....4

In einer Tageszeitung sehen Sie zwei Anzeigen. Jede wirbt für ein anderes Medikament gegen die Hautkrankheit Psoriasis. Jede Anzeige beinhaltet ein Schaubild, in dem die Wirkung dieses Medikamentes im Laufe der Behandlung dargestellt wird.

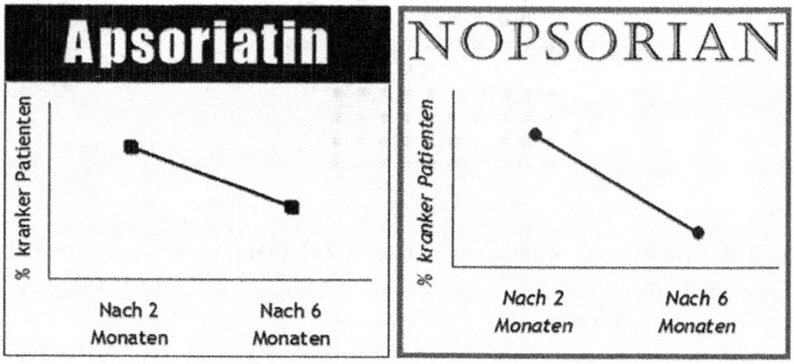

Q11. Bei welcher Behandlungsmethode sinkt der Prozentanteil kranker Patienten stärker? (*Correct answer: 4*)
Apsoriatin....................1
Nopsorian.........................2
Bei beiden gleich 3
Kann man nicht sagen.......4

Sie erhalten nun einige Information über die fiktiven Krankheiten Coliosis und Tiosis.

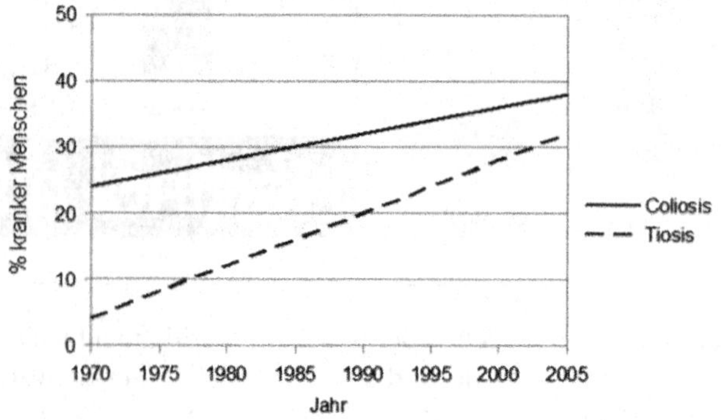

Q12. Bei welcher Krankheit stieg zwischen 1980 und 1990 die Prozentzahl der erkrankten Menschen stärker? (*Correct answer:* 2)
Coliosis..............................1
Tiosis......,..........................2
Bei beiden gleich..................3
Kann man nicht sagen.........4

Sie erhalten nun einige Informationen über Krebsbehandlungen.

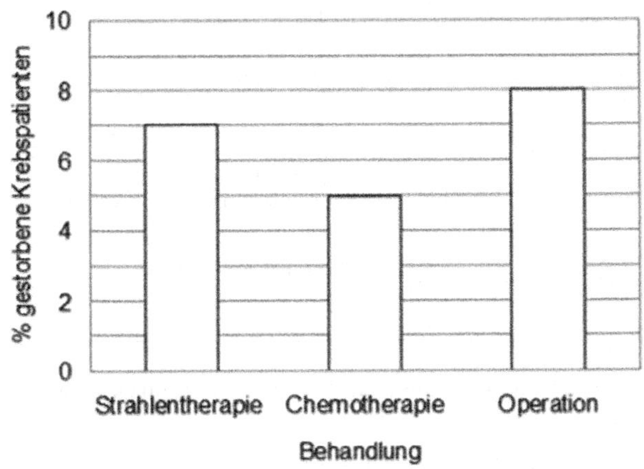

Q13. Welcher Prozentanteil der Krebspatienten stirbt nach einer Chemotherapie? (*Correct answer:* 5)
_______________%

15.13 Graph Literacy Scale in Spanish

A continuación, le presentamos información sobre varios tratamientos para el cáncer.

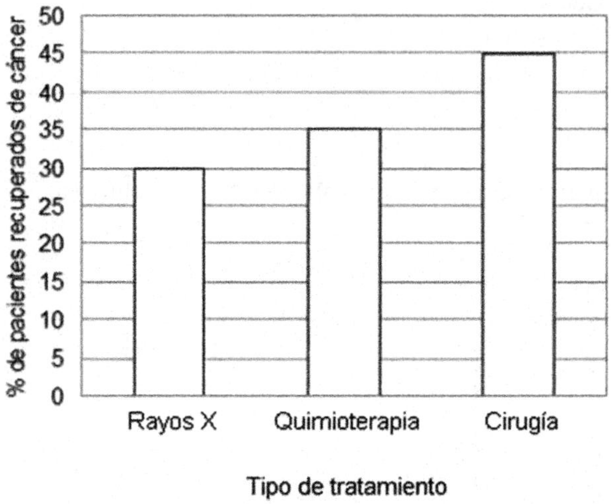

Q1. ¿Qué porcentaje de pacientes se han recuperado tras recibir quimioterapia?
______________% (*Correct answer: 35*)

Q2. ¿Qué diferencia hay entre el porcentaje de pacientes que se ha recuperado tras recibir cirugía y el porcentaje de pacientes que se ha recuperado tras recibir rayos X?
______________ (*Correct answer: 15*)

A continuación, le presentamos información sobre varios tipos de cáncer.

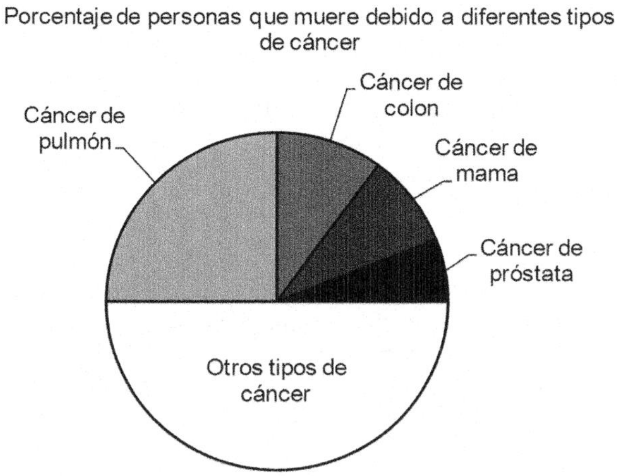

Q3. De entre todas las personas que mueren de cáncer, aproximadamente ¿qué porcentaje muere de cáncer de pulmón?
________% (*Correct answer:* $\geq$*24and* $\leq$*26*)

Q4. Aproximadamente, ¿qué porcentaje de personas que muere por cáncer, fallece por cáncer de colon, cáncer de mama, y cáncer de próstata en conjunto?
________% (*Correct answer:* $\geq$*24and* $\leq$*26*)

A continuación, le presentamos información sobre un trastorno llamado Adeolitis.

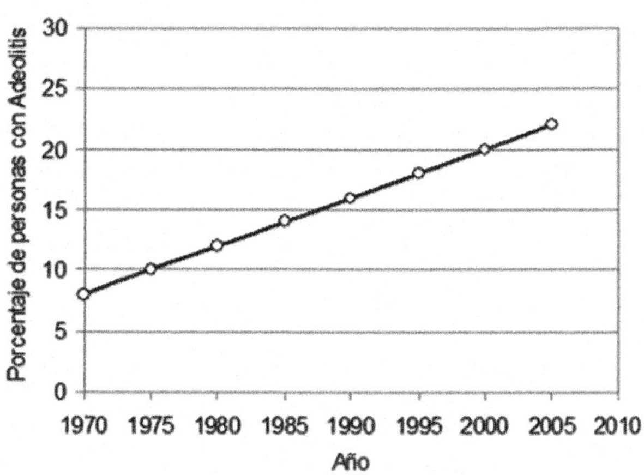

Q5. Aproximadamente, ¿qué porcentaje de personas sufrió Adeolitis en el año 2000?

______________% (*Correct answer: 20*)

Q6. ¿Cuándo se produjo un incremento mayor en el porcentaje de personas que sufre Adeolitis? (*Correct answer: 3*)

Entre 1975 y 1980..1
Entre 2000 y 2005..2
El incremento es igual en ambos intervalos........3
No lo sé..4

Q7. Haga una estimación: ¿qué porcentaje de personas sufrirá Adeolitis en el año 2010? (*Correct answer: ≥23 and ≤25*)

______________%

En la figura que aparece a continuación, se representa mediante círculos el número de hombres y mujeres en un grupo de pacientes que padecen el trastorno X. El número total de círculos es 100.

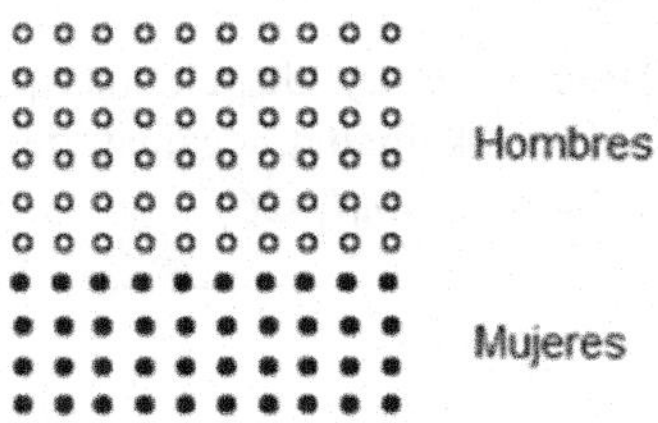

Q8. De entre los 100 pacientes con el trastorno X, ¿cuántos son mujeres? (*Correct answer: 40*)

______________mujeres

Q9. ¿Cuántos más hombres que mujeres hay entre los 100 pacientes que padecen el trastorno X? (*Correct answer: 20*)

______________ hombres

Imagine que ve los siguientes anuncios en las páginas 5 y 12 de una revista, respectivamente. Cada uno de ellos hace referencia a un medicamento diferente para tratar los problemas de corazón, e incluye un gráfico mostrando la efectividad del medicamento comparada con la efectividad de un placebo (una pastilla de sacarina).

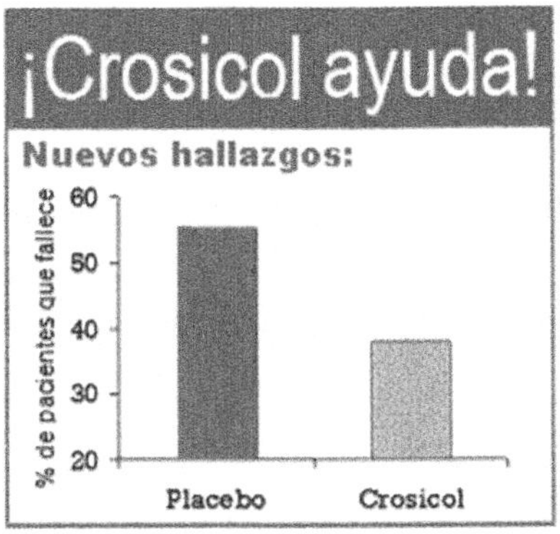

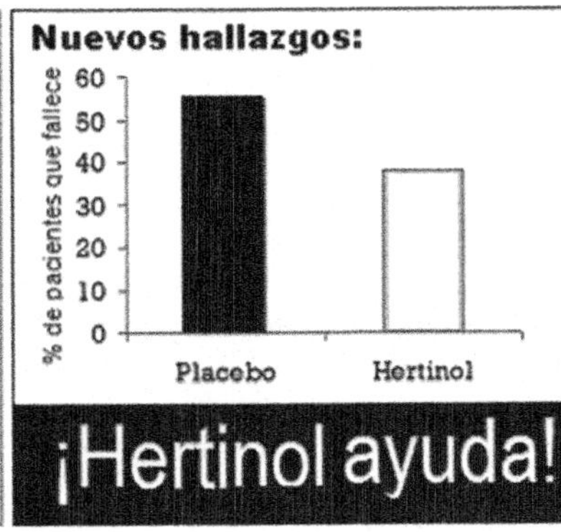

Q10. En comparación con el placebo, ¿qué tratamiento supone un decremento mayor en el porcentaje de pacientes que fallece? (*Correct answer: 3*)
Crosicol..........................1
Hertinol..........................2
Ambos son iguales..........3
No lo sé..........................4

Imagine que lee los siguientes anuncios en el periódico, uno en la página 15 y el otro en la página 17. Cada uno de ellos hace referencia a un tratamiento diferente para la soriasis, e incluye un gráfico mostrando la efectividad del tratamiento en dos momentos temporales.

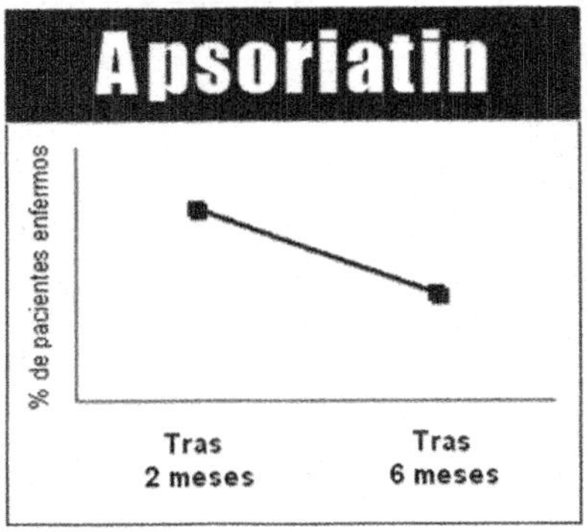

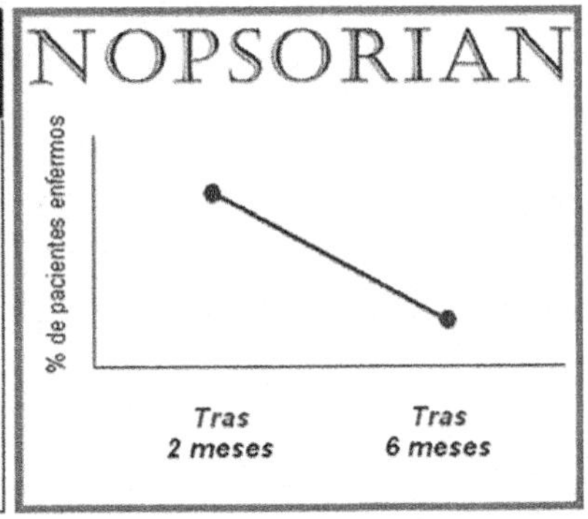

Q11. ¿Qué tratamiento implica un decremento mayor en el porcentaje de pacientes enfermos? (*Correct answer: 4*)
Apsoriatin....................1
Nopsorian.......................2
Ambos son iguales.........3
No lo sé............................4

A continuación, le presentamos información sobre dos enfermedades llamadas Coliosis y Tiosis.

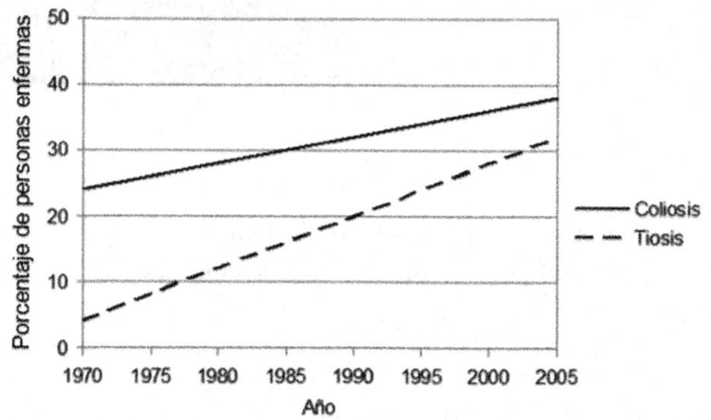

Q12. ¿Qué enfermedad presenta un incremento mayor en el porcentaje de personas afectadas entre 1980 y 1990? (*Correct answer: 2*)
Coliosis...............................1
Tiosis......,.........................2
Ambas son iguales................ 3
No lo sé..........................4

A continuación, le presentamos información sobre las terapias contra el cáncer.

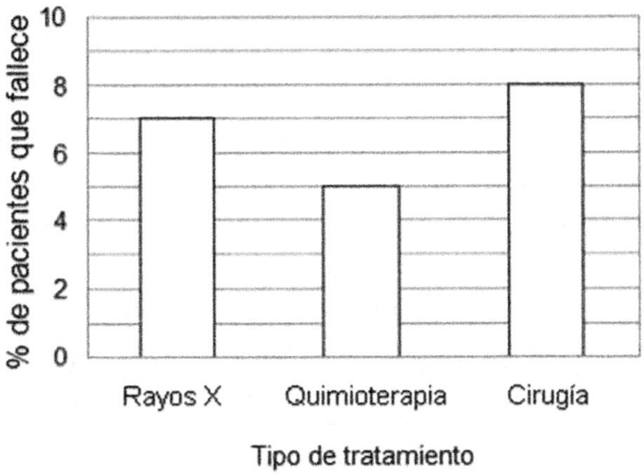

Q13. ¿Qué porcentaje de pacientes con cáncer fallece tras recibir quimioterapia? (*Correct answer: 5*)

_______________%

References

Cokely, E. T., Galesic, M., Schulz, E., Ghazal, S., & Garcia-Retamero, R. (2012). Measuring risk literacy: The Berlin numeracy test. *Judgment and Decision Making, 7*, 25–47.

Fagerlin, A., Zikmund-Fisher, B. J., Ubel, P. A., Jankovic, A., Derry, H. A., & Smith, D. M. (2007). Measuring numeracy without a math test: Development of the Subjective Numeracy Scale. *Medical Decision Making, 27*, 672–680.

Friel, S. N., Curcio, F. R., & Bright, G. W. (2001). Making sense of graphs: Critical factors influencing comprehension and instructional implications. *Journal for Research in Mathematics Education, 32*, 124–158.

Galesic, M., & Garcia-Retamero, R. (2010). Statistical numeracy for health: A cross-cultural comparison with probabilistic national samples. *Archives of Internal Medicine, 170*, 462–468.

Galesic, M., & Garcia-Retamero, R. (2011a). Communicating consequences of risky behaviors: Life expectancy versus risk of disease. *Patient Education and Counseling, 82*, 30–35.

Galesic, M., & Garcia-Retamero, R. (2011b). Do low-numeracy people avoid shared decision making? *Health Psychology, 30*, 336–341.

Galesic, M., & Garcia-Retamero, R. (2011c). Graph literacy: A cross-cultural comparison. *Medical Decision Making, 31*, 444–457.

Garcia-Retamero, R., & Cokely, E. (2012). Communicating risks with visual aids: Mapping the influence of skills, attitudes, and message frames on condom use. Manuscript under review.

Garcia-Retamero, R., & Galesic, M. (2009). Communicating treatment risk reduction to people with low numeracy skills: A cross-cultural comparison. *American Journal of Public Health, 99*, 2196–2202.

Garcia-Retamero, R., & Galesic, M. (2010a). How to reduce the effect of framing on messages about health. *Journal of General Internal Medicine, 25*, 1323–1329.

Garcia-Retamero, R., & Galesic, M. (2010b). Who profits from visual aids: Overcoming challenges in people's understanding of risks. *Social Science and Medicine, 70*, 1019–1025.

Garcia-Retamero, R., & Galesic, M. (2011). Using plausible group sizes to communicate information about medical risks. *Patient Education and Counseling, 84*, 245–250.

Lipkus, I. M., Samsa, G., & Rimer, B. K. (2001). General performance on a numeracy scale among highly educated samples. *Medical Decision Making, 21*, 37–44.

Okan, Y., Garcia-Retamero, R., Cokely, E. T., & Maldonado, A. (2012). Individual differences in graph literacy: Overcoming denominator neglect in risk comprehension. *Journal of Behavioral Decision Making*, doi: 10.1002/bdm.751.

Schwartz, L. M., Woloshin, S., Black, W. C., & Welch, H. G. (1997). The role of numeracy in understanding the benefit of screening mammography. *Annals of Internal Medicine, 127*, 966–972.

Zikmund-Fisher, B. J., Smith, D. M., Ubel, P. A., & Fagerlin, A. (2007). Validation of the subjective numeracy scale: Effects of low numeracy on comprehension of risk communications and utility elicitations. *Medical Decision Making, 27*, 663–671.

Index

R. Garcia-Retamero and M. Galesic (eds.), *Transparent Communication of Health Risks: Overcoming Cultural Differences*, DOI 10.1007/978-1-4614-4358-2,

CPSIA information can be obtained at www.ICGtesting.com
Printed in the USA
LVOW04*1912250215

428343LV00009B/79/P

9 781461 443575